Diagnostic Tests

made

Incredibly Easy!®

Springhouse
Springhouse, Pennsylvania

D1294145

Staff

Publisher
Judith A. Schilling McCann, RN, MSN

Creative Director
Jake Smith

Clinical Director
Joan M. Robinson, RN, MSN, CCRN

Clinical Editors
Collette Bishop Hendler, RN, CCRN (clinical project manager); Pamela Kovach, RN, BSN; Anita Lockhart, RN,C, MSN; Beverly Ann Tscheschlog, RN, BS

Editors
Brenna H. Mayer (senior associate editor), Naina Chohan, Cheryl Duksta, Ty Eggenberger, Stacey Ann Follin, Kirk Robinson

Copy Editors
Jaime L. Stockslager (supervisor), Kimberly Bilotta, Amy Furman, Shana Harrington, Pamela Wingrod

Designers
Arlene Putterman (associate design director), Mary Ludwicki (art director), Lynn Foulk

Illustrators
Scott Thorn Barrows, Barbara Cousins, John Cymerman, Mark Lefkowitz, Judy Newhouse, Bot Roda, Mary Stangl, Nina Wallace, Larry Ward

Electronic Production Services
Diane Paluba (manager), Joyce Rossi Biletz

Manufacturing
Patricia Dorshaw (senior manager), Beth Janae Orr

Associate Editor (Electronic)
Liz Schaeffer

Editorial Assistants
Danielle Jan Barsky, Beverly Lane, Linda Ruhl, Elfriede Young

Indexer
Barbara Hodgson

The clinical treatments described and recommended in this publication are based on research and consultation with nursing, medical, and legal authorities. To the best of our knowledge, these procedures reflect currently accepted practice. Nevertheless, they can't be considered absolute and universal recommendations. For individual applications, all recommendations must be considered in light of the patient's clinical condition and, before administration of new or infrequently used drugs, in light of the latest package-insert information. The authors and publisher disclaim responsibility for any adverse effects resulting from the suggested procedures, from any undetected errors, or from the reader's misunderstanding of the text.

Printed in the United States of America.

IEDXT - D N
03 02 01   10 9 8 7 6 5 4 3 2 1

Library of Congress Cataloging-in-Publication Data

Diagnostic tests made incredibly easy!.
    p. ; cm.
    Includes index.
    1. Diagnosis. 2. Nursing assessment. 3. Nursing.
I. Springhouse Corporation.
    [DNLM: 1. Diagnostic Techniques and Procedures—Nurses' Instruction. 2. Diagnostic Techniques and Procedures—Problems and Exercises. WB 18.2 D536 2002]
RT48.5 .D533 2002
616.07'5—dc21   2001049609
ISBN 1-58255-137-5 (alk. paper)

Contents

Contributors and consultants		*iv*
Foreword		*v*
1	Hematology and coagulation tests	1
2	Blood chemistry tests	23
3	Hormone tests	85
4	Immunologic tests	125
5	Urine tests	177
6	Other specimen tests	211
7	Cultures	239
8	Biopsy	253
9	Endoscopy	273
10	Ultrasonography	291
11	Radiography	305
12	Computed tomography and magnetic resonance imaging	339
13	Nuclear medicine scans	357
14	Monitoring, catheterization, and miscellaneous tests	369
Appendices and index		*399*
	Normal laboratory test values	*400*
	Guide to uncommon diagnostic tests	*401*
	Index	*406*

Contributors and consultants

Margaret E. Barnes, RN, MSN
Staff Development Educator
Sisters of Charity Hospital
Buffalo

Thomas A. Brabson, DO, FACOEP, FACEP
Emergency Physician
Albert Einstein Medical Center
Philadelphia

Barbara S. Buckner, RN, BSN
Staff Nurse
Harton Regional Medical Center
Tullahoma, Tenn.

Christine S. Clayton, RN, MS
Nurse Practitioner and Clinical Nurse
Specialist
Sioux Valley Hospital and University
Medical Center
Sioux Falls, S.Dak.

Ellen P. Digan, MA, MT(ASCP)
Professor of Biology; Coordinator, MLT
Program
Manchester (Conn.) Community College

Diane Dixon, PA-C, MA, MMSC
Assistant Professor, Department of PA
Studies
University of South Alabama
Mobile

Kathleen Ellstrom, RN, CS, PhD, CNS
Pulmonary Clinical Nurse Specialist
University of California at Los Angeles
Medical Enterprise

Peggi Guenter, RN, PhD
Editor-in-Chief, Nutrition in Clinical Practice
American Society for Parenteral and
Enteral Nutrition
Silver Spring, Md.

Victoria Hackett, HT(ASCP)
Histotechnology Specialist
Health Network Labs
Allentown, Pa.

Connie S. Heflin, RN, MSN
Professor
Paducah (Ky.) Community College

Marianne Hoy, RN, MSN
Director of Nursing
Cumberland County College
Vineland, N.J.

Elaine G. Lange, RN, MSN, CCRN, ANP-C
Adult Nurse Practitioner
Deerfield Valley Health Center
Wilmington, Vt.

Hal S. Larsen, PhD, MT, CLS
Associate Dean, School of Allied Health
Texas Tech University Health Sciences
Center
Lubbock

Michel E. Lloyd, MT(ASCP), SBB
Technical Coordinator, Blood Bank
St. Luke's Hospital
Bethlehem, Pa.

Julia A. McAvoy, RN, MSN, CCRN
Clinical Nurse Specialist, Critical Care
The Washington (Pa.) Hospital

Cathy D. McNew, MS, CRNP
Adult Epilepsy Nurse Practitioner
Pennsylvania State Geisinger Health
System
Hershey, Pa.

Teresa A. Richardson, BS, MT
Medical Technologist—Generalist
St. Luke's Quakertown (Pa.) Hospital

Mary Jean Rutherford, MEd, MT(ASCP), SC
Associate Professor and CLS Programs
Director
Arkansas State University
Jonesboro

Bruce Austin Scott, RN,CS, MSN
Nursing Instructor, San Joaquin Delta
College
Staff Nurse, St. Joseph's Behavioral Health
Center
Stockton, Calif.

Sylvia J. Smith, RN, CRNP
OB/GYN Nurse Practitioner
Rosedale Women's Care, P.C.
Pottstown, Pa.

Patricia D. Weiskittel, RN, MSN, CNN, CS
Renal Clinical Nurse Specialist
University Hospital
Cincinnati

Jay W. Wilborn, MEd, MT(ASCP)
Program Director
Garland County Community College
Hot Springs, Ark.

Denise Zacher, RN, MSN, CCRN
Administrative Supervisor
Taylor Hospital
Ridley Park, Pa.

Foreword

When a doctor requests a complete blood count, glucose test, mammogram, or total cholesterol test, you probably have a clear idea of how the test fits into the patient's diagnostic workup. Chances are, you would have no problem explaining to the patient or his family why the test was ordered and what the results might mean. For most health care professionals, these tests are part of the daily routine.

But what if the doctor orders a fibrin split products test? A plasma renin activity test? Transcranial Doppler studies? Thallium imaging? Unless you deal with these tests nearly every day, you may be unfamiliar with their why's and wherefore's. You may not even know exactly what they are.

As a health care professional, your involvement with laboratory tests and other diagnostic procedures may encompass the entire spectrum of events before, during, and after the test. You may be responsible for making sure the test is ordered correctly, preparing the patient for the test, assisting during the test, providing emotional support if the test is difficult or painful, getting the specimen prepared properly and sent to the laboratory promptly in the appropriate container, monitoring for test complications, and providing posttest care.

Even for a common test, some of these responsibilities could pose a challenge if your memory or knowledge base has gaps. If the test is uncommon, new, complex, or high tech, you may lack even basic information. In either situation, you need a handy reference packed with reliable information, such as why the test is ordered, how it's likely to affect the patient, and what the results indicate. In the best of all possible worlds, this reference would be accurate, up-to-date, organized for easy use, written in plain English, and a pleasure to look at and read. It would even contain some light-hearted elements to make learning fun.

Well, congratulations! The book you're holding measures up on all counts. *Diagnostic Tests Made Incredibly Easy* helps the health care professional and student find clear, concise, direct answers to questions about hundreds of diagnostic tests. Using a consistent format throughout, it succinctly describes each test, summarizes normal test results, explains what abnormal results may mean, and discusses what steps to take before, during, and after the test. The test purpose and interfering factors (such as medications) are highlighted separately in the margin for quick access.

The book's 14 chapters are organized by test type. Chapters 1 through 7 cover the most commonly used clinical laboratory tests. You'll find these chapters essential for reviewing basic facts about frequently ordered routine tests — hematology and coagulation tests, blood chemistry tests, hormone and immunologic tests, urine tests, other specimen tests, and cultures.

Most of the remaining chapters focus on a particular diagnostic technique — biopsy, endoscopy, ultrasonography, radiography, computed tomography and magnetic resonance imaging, and nuclear medicine scans. The final chapter discusses tests used for monitoring (such as fetal monitoring tests, electroencephalography, and cardiac monitoring and catheterization) as well as miscellaneous tests (including pulmonary function tests).

Each chapter starts with a summary of key topics and ends with a quick quiz (which includes answers and rationales) to reinforce learning. Charts and tables provide additional information on test procedures and test interpretation, while an appendix on normal laboratory test values makes *Diagnostic Tests Made Incredibly Easy* even more useful.

What's more, playful cartoons make the book *fun* to read. Abundant illustrations highlight important steps of a test or show the anatomic area affected by a test procedure. A special section of full-color photographs depicts patients undergoing echocardiography and endoscopic ultrasonography. It also takes you inside computed tomographs of abnormal brains. Appendices provide information on normal laboratory test values and describe uncommon diagnostic tests.

Throughout the book, special logos highlight essential information:

Warning alerts you to the factors that can interfere with test results.

Memory jogger helps you remember difficult information.

Peak technique tells how to perform or assist with a particular test.

Now I get it explains important aspects of a test in clear, easily understood terms.

Advice from the experts offers expert guidance on interpreting test results.

Listen up discusses patient teaching points.

To sum it all up, *Diagnostic Tests Made Incredibly Easy* is a valuable resource for health care professionals and students who need information about diagnostic tests but don't have the time to develop an expertise or stay current in all test procedures. The book is unique not just for the wealth of information it contains but for the way it presents that information — with a gentle humor that keeps you entertained and engaged. I highly recommend the book.

Hal Larsen, PhD, MT(ASCP), CLS(NCA)
Associate Dean
School of Allied Health
Texas Tech University Health Sciences Center
Lubbock

Hematology and coagulation tests

Just the facts

In this chapter, you'll learn:

♦ about hematology and coagulation tests

♦ what patient care is associated with these tests

♦ what factors can interfere with test results

♦ what hematology and coagulation test results may indicate.

A look at hematology and coagulation tests

Hematology tests determine whether specific blood levels are higher or lower than normal and can be useful in the diagnosis of such diseases as anemia, leukemia, and infection. **Coagulation** tests are performed for patients with bleeding disorders, coagulopathies, vascular injury, or trauma. They're also necessary to guide anticoagulant therapy.

Explain and reassure

The first step in preparing a patient for a hematology test is to explain the test. Your patient should always know what's happening to him and why. Use simple, direct language and avoid jargon. If the patient is a child, is elderly, or is otherwise unable to understand your instructions, you may also need to explain the test to a parent or caregiver.

Get to the point

Hematology and coagulation tests, except for bleeding time, require a blood sample, and some patients may be a little uneasy about needles. Before taking a blood sample,

Some patients are afraid of needles, so take an extra second to put your patient at ease.

explain that some brief discomfort may accompany the needle puncture or the application of a tourniquet.

Handle with care

Try to use a large-gauge needle when drawing the blood specimen, and handle blood samples carefully *to prevent the breakdown of red blood cells* or *hemolysis,* which may interfere with test results. Observe standard precautions. Also, after taking a blood sample, check the venipuncture site for bleeding. If a hematoma develops at the venipuncture site, apply warm soaks.

Hematology tests

White blood cell count

The white blood cell (WBC), or leukocyte, count measures the number of WBCs in a microliter of whole blood. This is done through the use of electronic devices. A WBC count can be useful in diagnosing infection and inflammation as well as in monitoring a patient's response to chemotherapy or radiation therapy. WBC counts can also help determine whether further tests are needed.

Counter culture

WBC counts can vary depending on a number of factors. On any given day, counts may vary by as much as 2,000 cells/µl (SI, 2×10^9/L) because of the effects of stress, strenuous exercise, or other factors. The count also can rise or fall significantly with certain diseases.

What it all means

The WBC count normally ranges from 4,000 to 10,000/µl (SI, 4 to 10×10^9/L). It's useful for diagnosing the severity of a disease process. However, the WBC differential gives more specific information about which type of WBC is being affected and is, therefore, more diagnostically useful.

The lowdown on levels

An elevated WBC count (leukocytosis) commonly signals infection, such as an abscess, meningitis, appendicitis, or tonsillitis. A high count may also indicate leukemia or tissue necrosis caused by burns, myocardial infarction, or gangrene.

A low WBC count (leukopenia) indicates bone marrow depression, which may result from viral infections or from toxic re-

WBC counts help diagnose infection and inflammation as well as determine the need for further tests.

actions, such as those following treatment with antineoplastics, ingestion of mercury or other heavy metals, or exposure to benzene or arsenicals. Leukopenia also accompanies influenza, typhoid fever, measles, infectious hepatitis, mononucleosis, and rubella.

To monitor your progress, you'll need to have multiple WBC tests while you're being treated for an infection.

What needs to be done

• Tell the patient that he should avoid strenuous exercise for 24 hours before the test to avoid altered readings and that he should also avoid ingesting a large meal before the test.
• Perform a venipuncture, and collect the sample in a 7-ml tube containing EDTA.
• Completely fill the sample collection tube, and invert it gently several times to adequately mix the sample and anticoagulant.

White blood cell differential

A white blood cell (WBC) differential can provide more specific information about a patient's immune system. In a WBC differential, the laboratory classifies 100 or more WBCs in a stained film of blood according to five major types of leukocytes — neutrophils, eosinophils, basophils, lymphocytes, and monocytes — and determines the percentage of each type.

Relatively speaking

The differential count is the relative number of each type of WBC in the blood. Multiply the percentage value of each type by the total WBC count to obtain the absolute number of each type of WBC.

A WBC differential helps evaluate the body's ability to fight infection. It also helps detect allergic reactions, parasitic infections, and leukemia.

What it all means

Here are the normal percentages of each WBC type in adults:
• neutrophils — 54% to 75% (SI, 0.54 to 0.75)
• eosinophils — 1% to 4% (SI, 0.01 to 0.04)
• basophils — 0% to 1% (SI, 0 to 0.01)
• monocytes — 2% to 8% (SI, 0.02 to 0.08)
• lymphocytes — 25% to 40% (SI, 0.25 to 0.40).

The lowdown on levels

Abnormally high levels of WBCs are associated with allergic reactions and parasitic infections. Once the normal values for the patient have been determined, an assessment can be made.

How disease affects WBC differential values

White blood cell (WBC) differential aids diagnosis because some disorders affect only one WBC type. Below, each cell type is listed as well as the corresponding effect and its causes.

Cell type	How affected
Neutrophils	**Increases count** • Infections: osteomyelitis, otitis media, septicemia, gonorrhea, endocarditis, chickenpox, herpes • Ischemic necrosis caused by myocardial infarction, burns, cancer • Metabolic disorders: diabetic acidosis, eclampsia, uremia, thyrotoxicosis • Stress response • Inflammatory diseases: rheumatic fever, rheumatoid arthritis, acute gout, vasculitis, myositis **Decreases count** • Bone marrow depression caused by radiation or cytotoxic drugs • Infections: typhoid, hepatitis, influenza, measles, mumps, rubella, infectious mononucleosis • Hypersplenism: hepatic disease and storage diseases • Collagen vascular diseases such as systemic lupus erythematosus • Deficiency of folic acid or vitamin B_{12}
Eosinophils	**Increases count** • Allergic disorders: asthma, hay fever, food or drug sensitivity, serum sickness, angioneurotic edema • Parasitic infections: trichinosis, hookworm, roundworm, amebiasis • Skin diseases: eczema, pemphigus, psoriasis, dermatitis, herpes simplex • Neoplastic diseases: chronic myelocytic leukemia, Hodgkin's disease, metastasis **Decreases count** • Stress response • Cushing's syndrome
Basophils	**Increases count** • Chronic myelocytic leukemia, Hodgkin's disease, ulcerative colitis, chronic hypersensitivity states **Decreases count** • Hyperthyroidism, ovulation, pregnancy, stress
Lymphocytes	**Increases count** • Infections: tuberculosis, hepatitis, infectious mononucleosis, mumps, rubella, cytomegalovirus • Thyrotoxicosis, hypoadrenalism, ulcerative colitis, immune diseases, lymphocytic leukemia **Decreases count** • Severe debilitating illnesses, such as heart failure, renal failure, advanced tuberculosis • Defective lymphatic circulation, high levels of adrenal corticosteroids, immunodeficiency
Monocytes	**Increases count** • Infections: subacute bacterial endocarditis, tuberculosis, hepatitis, malaria • Collagen vascular diseases: systemic lupus erythematosus, rheumatoid arthritis • Carcinomas, monocytic leukemia, lymphomas

Looking at the big picture

Keep in mind that to achieve an accurate diagnosis, differential test results must always be interpreted in relation to the total WBC count. Abnormal differential patterns suggest a range of disease states and other conditions. (See *How disease affects WBC differential values.*)

Danger signs

Some WBC differential findings indicate that immediate action is required. For instance, an absolute neutrophil count of 1,000/µl (SI, 1×10^9/L) or less requires neutropenic precautions, including protective isolation. (See *Drugs that influence the eosinophil count.*)

What needs to be done

• Tell the patient to avoid strenuous exercise before a WBC count to ensure accurate results.
• Perform a venipuncture, and collect the sample in a 7-ml tube containing EDTA.
• Completely fill the collection tube, and invert it gently several times to adequately mix the sample and anticoagulant.

Red blood cell count

Red blood cells (RBCs) are the main component of blood. The RBC count helps assess the blood's oxygen-carrying capacity and can be useful in diagnosing anemia, protein deficiency, and dehydration. An RBC count, also known as an erythrocyte count, is used to find the number of RBCs in a microliter (cubic milliliter) of whole blood. RBCs are commonly counted with electronic devices, which provide fast, accurate results. The RBC count itself provides no information about the size, shape, or concentration of hemoglobin (Hb) within the cells, but it may be used to calculate two erythrocyte indices: mean corpuscular volume and mean corpuscular Hb.

What it all means

Normal RBC values vary depending on a number of factors. In adult males, the RBC count ranges from 4.5 to 5.5 million/µl (SI, 4.5 to 5.5×10^{12}/L) of venous blood; in adult females, the count ranges from 4 to 5 million/µl (SI, 4 to 5×10^{12}/L) of venous blood; and

---

Drugs that influence the eosinophil count

Many drugs can affect the accuracy of the eosinophil count by increasing or decreasing it. Some of these drugs are listed below.

Increases count
• Anticonvulsants
• Gold compounds
• isoniazid
• Penicillins
• Phenothiazines
• rifampin
• streptomycin
• Sulfonamides
• Tetracyclines

Decreases count
• indomethacin
• procainamide

All right now, count off! An RBC count helps gather information about the blood's oxygen-carrying capacity and helps support other hematology tests in the diagnosis of anemia and polycythemia.

in children, from 4.6 to 4.8 million/µl (SI, 4.6 to 4.8 × 10^{12}/L) of venous blood. In full-term neonates, values range from 4.4 to 5.8 million/µl (SI, 4.4 to 5.8 × 10^{12}/L) of capillary blood at birth, fall to 3 to 3.8 million/µl (SI, 3 to 3.8 × 10^{12}/L) at age 2 months, and increase slowly thereafter. Values are also generally higher in people living at high altitudes.

The lowdown on levels

An elevated RBC count may indicate absolute or relative polycythemia. A depressed count may indicate anemia, fluid overload, or hemorrhage lasting more than 24 hours. (See *RBC count interference.*)

What needs to be done

• For adults and older children, draw venous blood into a 7-ml tube containing EDTA. For younger children, collect capillary blood in a microcollection device.
• Completely fill the collection tube, and invert it gently several times to mix the sample and anticoagulant.

Warning!

RBC count interference

The following factors may alter RBC count results:
• high white blood cell count, which falsely elevates the RBC count in semiautomated and automated counters
• diseases that cause RBCs to clump, leading to a falsely decreased RBC count.

Hemoglobin

Hemoglobin (Hb), which transports oxygen, is the main component of a red blood cell (RBC). Each RBC contains about 250 million molecules of Hb. Therefore, Hb concentration correlates closely with the RBC count. Hb level is a good indicator of anemia.

What it all means

Hb concentration varies depending on the patient's age and sex and on the type of blood sample drawn.

Through the ages

The following values reflect normal Hb concentrations (in number of grams per deciliter):
• *neonates:* 17 to 22 (SI, 170 to 220 g/L)
• *1 week:* 15 to 20 (SI, 150 to 200 g/L)
• *1 month:* 11 to 15 (SI, 110 to 150 g/L)
• *children:* 11 to 13 (SI, 110 to 130 g/L)
• *adult males:* 14 to 17.4 (SI, 140 to 174 g/L)
• *males after middle age:* 12.4 to 14.9 (SI, 124 to 149 g/L)
• *females:* 12 to 16 (SI, 120 to 160 g/L)
• *females after middle age:* 11.7 to 13.8 (SI, 117 to 138 g/L).

A hemoglobin test can help diagnose anemia or polycythemia and help monitor therapy.

The lowdown on levels

Low Hb concentration may indicate anemia, recent hemorrhage, or fluid retention, which can cause hemodilution; elevated Hb suggests hemoconcentration from polycythemia or dehydration. (See *Hb test interference.*)

What needs to be done

• For adults and older children, perform a venipuncture and collect the sample in a 7-ml tube containing EDTA. For younger children and infants, collect the sample by fingerstick or heelstick in a microcollection device containing EDTA.
• Completely fill the collection tube, and invert it gently several times to adequately mix the sample and anticoagulant.

Warning!

Hb test interference

Very high white blood cell counts or red blood cells that resist lysis may falsely elevate Hb values.

Hematocrit

Hematocrit (HCT) levels reflect the proportion of blood occupied by red blood cells (RBCs). The HCT test is a common, reliable test that measures the percentage by volume of packed RBCs in a whole-blood sample; for example, an HCT of 40% (SI, 0.40) means that a 100-ml sample contains 40 ml of packed RBCs. The packing of RBCs is achieved by centrifugation of anticoagulated whole blood in a capillary tube, which tightly packs RBCs without causing hemolysis.

What it all means

HCT values vary depending on the patient's sex and age, the type of sample, and the laboratory performing the test.

The following ranges represent normal HCT values for different age-groups:
• *neonates:* 55% to 68% (SI, 0.55 to 0.68)
• *1 week:* 47% to 65% (SI, 0.47 to 0.65)
• *1 month:* 37% to 49% (SI, 0.37 to 0.49)
• *3 months:* 30% to 36% (SI, 0.3 to 0.36)
• *1 year:* 29% to 41% (SI, 0.29 to 0.41)
• *10 years:* 36% to 40% (SI, 0.36 to 0.4)
• *adult males:* 42% to 52% (SI, 0.42 to 0.52)
• *adult females:* 36% to 48% (SI, 0.36 to 0.48).

Hematocrit aids in diagnosing abnormal states of hydration, polycythemia, and anemia and in calculating erythrocyte indices.

The lowdown on levels

Low HCT suggests anemia, hemodilution, or massive blood loss; high HCT indicates indicates polycythemia or hemoconcentration resulting from blood loss and dehydration. (See *HCT test interference*, page 8.)

What needs to be done

• For adults, perform a venipuncture and collect the sample in a 7-ml tube containing EDTA. For younger children and infants, collect the sample by fingerstick or heelstick in a microcollection device containing EDTA.
• Completely fill the collection tube, and invert it gently several times to adequately mix the sample and anticoagulant.
• Send the sample to the laboratory immediately.

Platelet count

Platelets, or thrombocytes, are the smallest formed elements in the blood. Platelets promote coagulation by supplying phospholipids to the intrinsic clotting pathway, helping to form a hemostatic plug for vascular injuries.

The platelet count is one of the most important screening tests of platelet function. Accurate counts are vital for monitoring severe increases or decreases in the number of platelets in the blood. A platelet count that falls below 50,000/µl (SI, 50×10^9/L) can cause spontaneous bleeding; when the count drops below 5,000/µl (SI, 5×10^9/L), fatal central nervous system bleeding or massive GI hemorrhage is possible.

What it all means

A normal platelet count ranges from 140,000 to 400,000/µl (SI, 140 to 400×10^9/L) in adults and from 150,000 to 450,000/µl (SI, 150 to 450×10^9/L) in children.

The lowdown on levels

An increased platelet count (thrombocytosis) can result from hemorrhage, infectious disorders, cancers, iron deficiency anemia, or inflammatory disease as well as from recent surgery, pregnancy, or splenectomy. In such cases, the platelet count returns to normal after the patient recovers from the primary disorder. However, the count remains high in primary thrombocythemia, myelofibrosis with myeloid metaplasia, polycythemia vera, and chronic myelogenous leukemia.

A decreased platelet count (thrombocytopenia) can result from aplastic (undeveloped) or hypoplastic (underdeveloped) bone marrow; infiltrative bone marrow disease, such as leukemia or disseminated infection; ineffective platelet development caused by folic acid or vitamin B_{12} deficiency; pooling of platelets in an enlarged spleen; increased platelet destruction caused by drugs or immune disorders; disseminated intravascular coagulation; or mechanical injury to platelets. (See *Platelet count interference.*)

Warning!

HCT test interference

Hemoconcentration caused by tourniquet constriction for longer than 1 minute typically raises HCT by 2.5% to 5% and may alter HCT test results.

They may sound alike, but they aren't! A platelet count helps measure thrombo**cytopenia** (decreased blood platelet level) and thrombo**cytosis** (elevated blood platelet level).

What needs to be done

• Perform a venipuncture, and collect the sample in a 7-ml tube containing EDTA.
• Completely fill the collection tube, and invert it gently several times to adequately mix the sample and anticoagulant.

Red cell indices

There are three main red cell indices, which are ascertained through the use of other blood tests. Using the results of the red blood cell (RBC) count, hematocrit (HCT), and total hemoglobin (Hb) test, the red cell indices (also known as erythrocyte indices) provide important information about Hb concentration and weight and the size of an average RBC. The red cell indices include:
• mean corpuscular volume (MCV)
• mean corpuscular Hb (MCH)
• mean corpuscular Hb concentration (MCHC).

Eyes on the size

MCV, the ratio of HCT (packed cell volume) to the RBC count, expresses the average size of the erythrocytes and indicates whether they're undersized (microcytic), oversized (macrocytic), or normal (normocytic).

A weighty issue

MCH, the ratio of Hb weight to the RBC count, gives the weight of Hb in an average RBC.

Rating the ratio

MCHC, the ratio of Hb weight to HCT, defines the Hb concentration in 100 ml of packed RBCs. It helps distinguish normally colored (normochromic) RBCs from paler (hypochromic) RBCs.

What it all means

The range of normal red cell indices is as follows:
• *MCV:* 82 to 98 mm^3 (SI, 82 to 98 fl)
• *MCH:* 26 to 34 pg (SI, 26 to 34 pg)
• *MCHC:* 31 to 37 g/dl (SI, 310 to 370 g/L).

The lowdown on levels

The red cell indices help to classify anemias. Low MCV and MCHC indicate microcytic, hypochromic anemias caused by iron deficiency anemia, pyridoxine-responsive anemia, or thalassemia. A high MCV suggests macrocytic anemias caused by megaloblastic anemias that are in turn caused by

Warning!

Platelet count interference

• Acetazolamide, acetohexamide, antineoplastics, brompheniramine maleate, carbamazepine, chloramphenicol, ethacrynic acid, furosemide, gold salt, indomethacin, isoniazid, mephenytoin, oral diazoxide, phenytoin, salicylates, thiazide and thiazide-like diuretics, tricyclic antidepressants, and menstruation decrease platelet count.
• High altitudes, persistent cold temperatures, strenuous exercise, and excitement increase platelet count.

Red cell indices help diagnose and classify anemias.

folic acid or vitamin B_{12} deficiency, inherited disorders of deoxyribonucleic acid synthesis, or reticulocytosis. (See *Red blood cell indices interference*.)

Because MCV reflects the average volume of many cells, a value within the normal range can encompass RBCs of varying size, from microcytic to macrocytic.

What needs to be done

• Perform a venipuncture, and collect the sample in a 7-ml tube containing EDTA.
• Completely fill the collection tube, and invert it gently several times to adequately mix the sample and anticoagulant.

Erythrocyte sedimentation rate

The erythrocyte sedimentation rate (ESR) measures the degree of erythrocyte, or red blood cell (RBC), settling during a specified time period. As the RBCs descend in the tube, they displace an equal volume of plasma upward, which slows the downward progress of other settling blood elements.

Early indicator

The ESR is a sensitive but nonspecific test that's commonly the earliest indicator of disease when other chemical or physical signs are normal. The ESR typically rises significantly in widespread inflammatory disorders caused by infection or autoimmune mechanisms; such elevations may be prolonged in localized inflammation and malignancy.

What it all means

Normal ESR ranges from 0 to 10 mm/hour (SI, 0 to 10 mm/hour) in males and from 0 to 20 mm/hour (SI, 0 to 20 mm/hour) in females; rates gradually increase with age.

The ESR rises in pregnancy, acute or chronic inflammation, tuberculosis, blood cell dyscrasias, rheumatic fever, rheumatoid arthritis, and some cancers. Anemia also tends to raise ESR because less upward displacement of plasma occurs to retard the relatively few sedimenting RBCs.

Polycythemia, sickle cell anemia, hyperviscosity (excessively thick blood), or low plasma fibrinogen or globulin levels tend to depress ESR.

Warning!

Red blood cell indices interference

• Falsely elevated RBC count, caused by a high white blood cell count in semiautomated and automated counters, invalidates MCV and MCH results.
• Falsely elevated Hb values invalidate MCH and MCHC results.
• Diseases that cause RBCs to clump together falsely decrease RBC count.

ESR helps monitor inflammatory or malignant disease and diagnose occult disease, such as tuberculosis, tissue necrosis, or connective tissue disease.

What needs to be done

• Perform a venipuncture, and collect the sample in a 7-ml tube containing EDTA or a 4.5-ml tube with sodium citrate added. (Check with the laboratory to determine preference.)
• Completely fill the collection tube, and invert it gently several times to adequately mix the sample and anticoagulant.
• Send the sample to the laboratory immediately after examining it for clots or clumps. The sample must be tested within 2 to 4 hours.

Methemoglobin levels detect methemoglobinemia, which can be congenital or result from radiation or toxic effects of chemicals or drugs.

Methemoglobin

Methemoglobin (MetHb, Hb M) is a variety of hemoglobin (Hb) formed when the heme portion of deoxygenated Hb is oxidized to a ferric state. When this oxidization occurs, the heme is incapable of combining with oxygen and transporting it to the tissues, and the patient becomes cyanotic. Patients exposed to nitrites have an increased risk of becoming cyanotic.

What it all means

Normal MetHb levels fall between 0% and 1.5% (SI, 0 to 0.015) of total Hb.

The lowdown on levels

Increased MetHb levels may indicate acquired or hereditary methemoglobinemia or carbon monoxide poisoning. These levels can also be caused by certain drugs or substances.

Decreased MetHb levels may occur in pancreatitis. (See *MetHb test interference.*)

What needs to be done

• Obtain a patient history that includes the patient's hematologic status and any Hb disorders, conditions that produce nitrite, and exposure to sources of nitrites in drugs.
• Tell the patient to avoid such medications as benzocaine, nitrates, and sulfonamides.
• Perform a venipuncture, and collect a sample in a 7-ml heparinized tube.
• Completely fill the collection tube, and invert it gently several times.
• Place the collection tube on ice, and send it to the laboratory immediately.

Warning!

MetHb test interference

The following factors can increase MetHb levels:
• inorganic nitrate in the diet
• such drugs as aniline dyes, nitroglycerin, benzocaine, chlorates, lidocaine, nitrates, nitrites, sulfonamides, radiation, and primaquine.

Sickle cell test

Sickle cells (Hb S) are severely deformed erythrocytes. The sickle cell test (also known as the Hb S test) helps identify sickle cell anemia. The disorder is found almost exclusively in blacks. More than 50,000 Americans have sickle cell disease.

The sickle cell test identifies sickle cell disease and sickle cell trait.

Spontaneous sickling

People who are homozygous for Hb S usually show abundant spontaneously sickled red blood cells (RBCs) on a peripheral blood smear. People who are heterozygous for Hb S alone or with another hemoglobin (Hb) deformity may have normal RBCs that can be easily changed to sickled forms by lowering oxygen tension. This sickling tendency can be identified by sealing a drop of blood between a glass slide and coverslip and adding a deoxygenating agent. The RBCs can then be observed under a microscope and compared to a central slide containing blood and saline solution. If the patient's Hb is of the S variation, the cells will assume the crescent (sickle) shape, and the test is positive.

May produce erroneous results

Although the sickle cell test is useful as a rapid screening procedure, it may produce erroneous results; consequently, Hb electrophoresis should be performed if sickle cell trait is strongly suspected.

What it all means

Results of this test are reported as positive or negative. A normal, or negative, test suggests the absence of Hb S. A positive test may indicate the presence of sickle cells, but Hb electrophoresis is needed to distinguish between homozygous and heterozygous forms. (See *Sickle cell test interference.*)

What needs to be done

• Check the patient history for a blood transfusion within the past 3 months.
• Perform a venipuncture, and collect the sample in a 7-ml tube containing EDTA. For younger children, collect capillary blood in a microcollection device.
• Completely fill the collection tube, and invert it gently several times to adequately mix the sample and anticoagulant.

Warning!

Sickle cell test interference

Hb concentration under 10%, elevated sickle cell levels in infants younger than age 6 months, and a blood transfusion within the past 3 months may produce false-negative results.

Iron and total iron-binding capacity

An iron assay is used to measure the amount of iron bound to transferrin in blood plasma. Total iron-binding capacity (TIBC) is a measure of the amount of iron that would appear in plasma if all the transferrin were saturated with iron. The percentage of saturation is obtained by dividing the serum iron result by the TIBC, which reveals the actual amount of saturated transferrin. Normally, transferrin is about 30% saturated.

A serum iron assay helps diagnose hemochromatosis.

What it all means

Reference values are as follows:
- *serum iron:* 60 to 170 µg/dl (SI, 10.7 to 30.4 µmol/L) for men; 50 to 130 µg/dl (SI, 9 to 23.3 µmol/L) for women
- *TIBC:* 300 to 360 µg/dL (SI, 54 to 64 µmol/L) for adults
- *saturation:* 20% to 50% (SI, 0.2 to 0.5) for men and women.

The lowdown on levels

In iron deficiency, serum iron levels drop and TIBC increases to decrease the saturation. In cases of chronic inflammation, such as in rheumatoid arthritis, serum iron may be low in the presence of adequate body stores but TIBC may be unchanged or may drop to preserve normal saturation.

Iron overload may not alter serum levels until relatively late but, in general, serum iron increases and TIBC remains the same to increase the saturation. (See *Iron and TIBC test interference.*)

What needs to be done

- Check the patient history and hold drugs such as chloramphenicol, corticotropin, iron supplements, and oral contraceptives, as ordered. If such medications must be continued, note this on the laboratory request.
- Perform a venipuncture, and collect the sample in a 7-ml clot-activator tube.
- As ordered, resume administration of any medications that were withheld for the test.

Ferritin

Ferritin, a major iron-storage protein found in reticuloendothelial cells (cells lining vascular and lymph vessels), normally appears in small quantities in serum. In healthy adults, serum ferritin levels are directly related to the amount of available iron stored in the body and can be measured accurately by radioimmunoassay. Unlike many other blood studies, the serum ferritin test isn't affected

---

Warning!

Iron and TIBC test interference

- Use of chloramphenicol and oral contraceptives can cause false-positive test results.
- Corticotropin can produce false-negative test results.
- Iron supplements can cause false-positive serum iron values but false-negative TIBC.

by moderate hemolysis of the sample or by the patient's use of drugs.

What it all means

Normal serum ferritin values vary with age and sex as follows:
- *men:* 20 to 300 ng/ml (SI, 20 to 300 µg/L)
- *women:* 20 to 120 ng/ml (SI, 20 to 120 µg/L)
- *6 months to 15 years:* 7 to 140 ng/ml (SI, 7 to 140 µg/L)
- *2 to 5 months:* 50 to 200 ng/ml (SI, 50 to 200 µg/L)
- *1 month:* 200 to 600 ng/ml (SI, 200 to 600 µg/L)
- *neonates:* 25 to 200 ng/ml (SI, 25 to 200 µg/L).

The lowdown on levels

High serum ferritin levels may indicate acute or chronic hepatic disease, iron overload, leukemia, acute or chronic infection or inflammation, Hodgkin's disease, or chronic hemolytic anemias; in these disorders, iron stores in bone marrow may be normal or significantly increased. Serum ferritin levels are characteristically normal or slightly elevated in patients who have chronic renal disease.

Low serum ferritin levels indicate chronic iron deficiency. (See *Ferritin test interference.*)

What needs to be done

- Review the patient history for a recent transfusion.
- Perform a venipuncture, and collect the sample in a 10-ml tube without additives.

Ferritin levels help screen for iron deficiency and iron overload, measure iron storage, and distinguish between iron deficiency and chronic inflammation.

Coagulation tests

Bleeding time

The bleeding time test measures the duration of bleeding after a standardized skin incision. Bleeding time depends on the elasticity of the blood vessel wall and the number and function of platelets.

Not recommended for all

The bleeding time test usually isn't recommended for a patient whose platelet count is less than 75,000/µl (SI, 75×10^9/L). However, some patients with altered platelet morphology may have normal bleeding times despite low platelet counts.

Warning!

Ferritin test interference

A recent transfusion may elevate serum ferritin levels.

What it all means

Normal bleeding time is 3 to 6 minutes (SI, 3 to 60 m).

Bleeding overtime

Prolonged bleeding time may indicate the presence of disorders associated with thrombocytopenia, such as Hodgkin's disease, acute leukemia, disseminated intravascular coagulation, hemolytic disease of the neonate, Schönlein-Henoch purpura, severe hepatic disease, or severe deficiency of factors I, II, V, VII, VIII, IX, or XI. Prolonged bleeding time in a person with a normal platelet count suggests a platelet function disorder and requires further investigation with clot retraction, prothrombin consumption, and platelet aggregation tests. (See *Bleeding time interference.*)

What needs to be done

• Check for a recent history of drugs that prolong bleeding time. If the patient has taken such drugs, check with the laboratory for special instructions. If the test is being used to identify a suspected bleeding disorder, it should be postponed and the drugs discontinued as ordered; if it's being used preoperatively to assess hemostatic function, it should proceed as scheduled.
• Wrap a pressure cuff around the patient's upper arm, and inflate it to 40 mm Hg. Select an area on the forearm that's free from superficial veins, and clean it with antiseptic. Let the skin dry completely before making the incisions. Apply the appropriate template lengthwise to the forearm. Use a lancet to make two incisions, each 1 mm deep and 9 mm long. Start the stopwatch. Without touching the cuts, gently blot the blood drops with filter paper every 30 seconds until bleeding stops in both cuts. Average the time of the two cuts, and record the results.
• If the bleeding doesn't diminish after 15 minutes, discontinue the test.
• For a patient with a bleeding tendency (such as hemophilia), maintain a pressure bandage over the incision for 24 to 48 hours to prevent further bleeding. If the template method was used, keep the edges of the cuts aligned to minimize scarring. Otherwise, a piece of gauze held in place by an adhesive bandage is sufficient. Check the test area frequently.
• As ordered, resume administration of medications discontinued before the test.

The bleeding time test assesses the body's ability to stop bleeding and detects congenital and acquired platelet function disorders.

Warning!

Bleeding time interference

Sulfonamides, thiazide diuretics, antineoplastics, anticoagulants, nonsteroidal anti-inflammatory drugs, aspirin and aspirin compounds, and some nonnarcotic analgesics may prolong bleeding time.

Partial thromboplastin time

The partial thromboplastin time (PTT) test evaluates all the clotting factors of the intrinsic pathway—except platelets—by measuring the time it takes a clot to form after adding calcium and phospholipid emulsion to a plasma sample. The PTT test also helps monitor a patient's response to heparin therapy.

What it all means

Normally, a fibrin clot forms 21 to 35 seconds (SI, 21 to 35 s) after the addition of reagents. For a patient on anticoagulant therapy, check with the attending doctor to find out the desirable values for the therapy being delivered.

May signal deficiency

Prolonged PTT may indicate a deficiency of certain plasma clotting factors, the presence of heparin, or the presence of fibrin split products, fibrinolysins, or circulating anticoagulants that are antibodies to specific clotting factors.

What needs to be done

• Tell the patient receiving heparin therapy that this test may be repeated at regular intervals to assess his response to treatment.
• Perform a venipuncture, and collect the sample in a 7-ml tube with sodium citrate added.
• Completely fill the collection tube, invert it gently several times, and send it to the laboratory on ice.
• For a patient on anticoagulant therapy, additional pressure may be needed at the venipuncture site to control bleeding.

The PTT test screens for deficiencies of the clotting factors and monitors response to heparin therapy.

Prothrombin time

Prothrombin, or factor II, is a plasma protein produced by the liver. The prothrombin time test (commonly known as pro time, or PT) measures the time required for a fibrin clot to form in a citrated plasma sample after the addition of calcium ions and tissue thromboplastin (factor III). It's an excellent screening procedure for overall evaluation of extrinsic coagulation factors V, VII, and X and of prothrombin and fibrinogen. PT is the test of choice for monitoring oral anticoagulant therapy.

What it all means

Normally, PT ranges from 10 to 14 seconds (SI, 10 to 14 s). In a patient receiving warfarin therapy, PT is usually maintained between 1½ and 2 times the normal control value. (See "International Normalized Ratio.")

The PT test evaluates the extrinsic coagulation system and monitors response to oral anticoagulant therapy.

Prolonged PT

Prolonged PT may indicate hepatic disease or deficiencies in fibrinogen, prothrombin, vitamin K, or factors V, VII, or X (specific assays can pinpoint such deficiencies). Or, it may result from ongoing oral anticoagulant therapy. Prolonged PT that exceeds 2½ times the control value is commonly associated with abnormal bleeding. (See *PT test interference*.)

What needs to be done

• Check the patient history for use of medications that may affect test results, such as vitamin K or antibiotics.
• Perform a venipuncture, and collect the sample in a 7-ml siliconized tube.
• Completely fill the collection tube, and invert it gently several times to adequately mix the sample and anticoagulant. If the tube isn't filled to the correct volume, an excess of citrate appears in the sample.

Warning!

PT test interference

• Antihistamines, corticosteroids, digoxin, diuretics, glutethimide, progestin-estrogen combinations, pyrazinamide, vitamin K, and xanthines may shorten PT.
• Alcohol overuse and administration of corticotropin, anabolic steroids, I.V. heparin, indomethacin, methimazole, phenylbutazone, phenytoin, propylthiouracil, quinidine, thyroid hormones, or vitamin A may prolong PT.

International Normalized Ratio

The International Normalized Ratio (INR) system is the best means of standardizing measurement of prothrombin time to monitor oral anticoagulant therapy.

What it all means

Normal INR for those receiving warfarin therapy is 2.0 to 3.0 (SI, 2.0 to 3.0). For those with mechanical prosthetic heart valves, an INR of 2.5 to 3.5 (SI, 2.5 to 3.5) is suggested.

Increased INR values may indicate disseminated intravascular coagulation, cirrhosis, hepatitis, vitamin K deficiency, salicylate intoxication, uncontrolled oral anticoagulation, or massive blood transfusion.

What needs to be done

• Perform a venipuncture, and collect the sample in a 7-ml tube with sodium citrate added.
• Completely fill the collection tube; otherwise, excess citrate will appear in the sample.
• Gently invert the tube several times to thoroughly mix the sample and anticoagulant.
• Put the sample on ice, and send it to the laboratory promptly.

The INR system evaluates the effectiveness of oral anticoagulant therapy.

Activated clotting time

Activated clotting time, or automated coagulation time, measures the time it takes whole blood to clot. This test is commonly performed during procedures that require extracorporeal (occurring outside the body) circulation, such as cardiopulmonary bypass, ultrafiltration, hemodialysis, and extracorporeal membrane oxygenation (ECMO).

> Activated clotting time monitors the effects of heparin and protamine sulfate in heparin neutralization. It also detects severe deficiencies in clotting factors — except factor VII.

What it all means

In a patient who isn't receiving anticoagulants, normal activated clotting time is 107 ±13 seconds (SI, 107 ±13 s). During cardiopulmonary bypass, heparin is titrated to maintain an activated clotting time between 400 and 600 seconds (SI, 400 to 600 s). During ECMO, heparin is titrated to maintain activated clotting time between 220 and 260 seconds (SI, 220 to 260 s).

What needs to be done

• Explain to the patient that the test requires a blood sample, which is usually drawn from an existing vascular access site; therefore, no venipuncture is necessary.
• Explain that two samples will be drawn. The first one will be discarded so that any heparin in the tubing doesn't interfere with the results.
• If the sample is drawn from a line with a continuous infusion, stop the infusion before drawing the sample.
• Withdraw 5 to 10 ml of blood from the line and discard it.
• Withdraw a clean sample of blood into the special tube containing celite provided with the activated clotting time unit.
• Activate the activated clotting time unit, and wait for the signal to insert the tube.
• Flush the vascular access site according to your facility's protocol.

> Plasma thrombin time detects a fibrinogen deficiency or defect, helps diagnose DIC and hepatic disease, and monitors treatment with heparin or thrombolytic agents.

Plasma thrombin time

The plasma thrombin time test measures how quickly a clot forms when a standard amount of bovine thrombin is added to a platelet-poor plasma sample from the patient and to a normal plasma control sample. After thrombin is added, the clotting time for each sample is compared with the other and recorded. Because thrombin rapidly converts fibrinogen to a fibrin clot, this test (also known as the thrombin clotting time test) allows a quick but imprecise estimation of plasma fibrinogen levels, which are a function of clotting time.

What it all means

Normal thrombin times range from 10 to 15 seconds (SI, 10 to 15 s) and should be within 2 seconds of the control. Test results are usually reported with a normal control value.

Prolonged thrombin time

A prolonged thrombin time may indicate heparin therapy, hepatic disease, disseminated intravascular coagulation (DIC), or fibrinogen defect or deficiency. Patients with prolonged thrombin times may require quantitation of fibrinogen levels; in suspected DIC, the test for fibrin split products is also necessary. (See *Plasma thrombin time test interference*.)

Warning!

Plasma thrombin time test interference

Heparin, fibrinogen, or fibrin degradation products may prolong clotting time.

What needs to be done

- If possible, withhold heparin therapy before the test as ordered. If heparin must be continued, note this on the laboratory request.
- Perform a venipuncture, and collect the sample in a 7-ml siliconized tube.
- Completely fill the collection tube, and invert it gently several times to adequately mix the sample and anticoagulant. If the tube isn't filled to the correct volume, excess citrate appears in the sample.
- Send the sample to the laboratory immediately.

Plasma fibrinogen

The plasma fibrinogen test measures the plasma concentration of fibrinogen available for coagulation. Fibrinogen (factor I) isn't normally present in serum; it's converted to fibrin by thrombin during clotting. Because fibrin is a necessary part of a blood clot, fibrinogen deficiency can produce mild to severe bleeding disorders. When fibrinogen levels drop below 100 mg/dl (SI, 1 g/L), accurate interpretation of all coagulation tests that have a fibrin clot as an end point becomes difficult.

The plasma fibrinogen test helps diagnose suspected clotting or bleeding disorders caused by fibrinogen abnormalities.

What it all means

Fibrinogen levels normally range from 200 to 400 mg/dl (SI, 2 to 4 g/L).

The lowdown on levels

Depressed fibrinogen levels may indicate congenital afibrinogenemia (absence of fibrinogen), hypofibrinogenemia (deficiency of fibrinogen), dysfibrinogenemia (abnormal fibrinogen), disseminated intravascular coagulation, fibrinolysis, severe hepatic disease, bone marrow lesions, or cancer of the prostate, pancreas, or lung. Obstetric complications or trauma may also cause low levels.

Elevated levels may indicate cancer of the stomach, breast, or kidney or an inflammatory disorder, such as pneumonia or glomerulonephritis. (See *Plasma fibrinogen test interference.*)

What needs to be done

• Assess the patient for contraindications to this test, such as active bleeding or acute infection or illness. This test is also contraindicated in patients who have received a blood transfusion within the past 4 weeks.
• Check the patient history for use of anticoagulants or oral contraceptives. Note such drugs on the laboratory request.
• If the patient is receiving heparin therapy, notify the laboratory; such therapy requires the use of a different reagent.
• Perform a venipuncture, and collect the sample in a 7-ml tube with sodium citrate added.
• Completely fill the collection tube, invert it gently several times, and send it to the laboratory immediately.

Warning!

Plasma fibrinogen test interference

The following factors may alter plasma fibrinogen test results:
• fibrinogen levels that are elevated during the third trimester of pregnancy and in postoperative patients
• transfusion of blood products within 4 weeks of the test.

Fibrin split products

After a fibrin clot forms in response to vascular injury, the fibrinolytic system acts to break down the clot by converting plasminogen into the fibrin-dissolving enzyme plasmin. Plasmin breaks down fibrin and fibrinogen into fragments known as fibrin split products (FSP) or fibrin degradation products. An excess of these products in the circulation causes anticoagulant activity. This excess may lead to coagulation disorders, which may be due to fibrinogenolysis or such clotting excesses as disseminated intravascular coagulation (DIC).

A test for FSP detects FSP in the circulation and helps determine the presence and approximate severity of a hyperfibrinolytic state such as in as DIC.

Reaction detected

FSP are detected by a reaction, in which diluted serum left in a blood sample after clotting is mixed on a slide with latex particles that carry antibodies to some of the split products. Clumping of the latex particles occurs if FSP are present in the serum dilution.

What it all means

Serum normally contains less than 10 µg/ml (SI, less than 10 mg/L) of FSP. A quantitative assay shows levels of less than 3 µg/ml (SI, less than 3 mg/L).

Reasons for rising

FSP levels rise in primary fibrinolytic states because of increased levels of circulating profibrinolysin; they rise; in secondary states, because of DIC and subsequent fibrinolysis. Levels also increase in alcoholic cirrhosis, preeclampsia, abruptio placentae, heart disease, sunstroke, burns, intrauterine death, pulmonary embolus, deep vein thrombosis (transient increase), and myocardial infarction (after 1 or 2 days). FSP levels usually exceed 100 µg/ml (SI, 100 mg/L) in active renal disease or kidney transplant rejection. (See *FSP test interference*.)

What needs to be done

• Check the patient history for use of medications (especially heparin) that may affect the accuracy of test results.
• Draw the sample before administering heparin to help avoid false-positive test results.
• Perform a venipuncture and draw 2 ml of blood into a plastic syringe. Transfer the sample to the tube provided by the laboratory. The tube contains a soybean trypsin inhibitor and bovine thrombin. Evacuated tubes are available in kits designed to provide a rapid semiquantitative analysis of FSP. Follow the manufacturer's directions for specimen collection and handling.
• Gently invert the collection tube several times to adequately mix the contents. The blood clots within 2 seconds and must then be sent to the laboratory immediately to be incubated at 98.6° F (37° C) for 30 minutes before testing proceeds.

Warning!

FSP test interference

• Pretest administration of heparin causes false-positive results.
• Fibrinolytic drugs, such as streptokinase, tissue plasminogen activator, and large doses of barbiturates increase FSP levels.

Quick quiz

1.   The erythrocyte sedimentation rate (ESR) measures the degree of erythrocyte settling in a blood sample during a specified period. What's the significance of an elevated ESR?
    A.   An inflammatory disorder may be present.
    B.   It distinguishes between hypoproliferative and hyperproliferative anemias.
    C.   An infection is present.
Answer: A. An elevation in the patient's ESR may indicate presence of an inflammatory disorder.

2. Which test provides information about the size and hemoglobin (Hb) weight of an average red blood cell (RBC)?

    A.   Hematocrit
    B.   Red cell indices
    C.   RBC count

Answer: B. Red cell indices provide information about the size, Hb concentration, and Hb weight of an average RBC.

3. Which test provides the best means of standardizing measurement of prothrombin time (PT) to monitor oral anticoagulant therapy?

    A.   Plasma thrombin time
    B.   International Normalized Ratio (INR)
    C.   Partial thromboplastin time

Answer: B. The INR is the best means of standardizing measurement of PT to monitor anticoagulant therapy.

4. Which of the following actions may interfere with results of fibrin split products (FSP) testing?

    A.   Pretest heparin administration
    B.   Filling the collection tube completely with blood
    C.   Failure to administer a fibrinolytic drug before testing

Answer: A. Pretest heparin administration can result in falsely elevated FSP levels.

5. A patient's platelet count may decrease normally in what circumstance?

    A.   During strenuous exercise
    B.   During persistent cold temperatures
    C.   Just before menstruation

Answer: C. The patient's platelet count may decrease normally just before menstruation.

Scoring

☆☆☆   If you answered all five questions correctly, super! Your knowledge is coagulating nicely.

☆☆   If you answered three or four questions correctly, great! You have a high "level" of understanding.

☆   If you answered fewer than three correctly, our diagnosis is test stress. Relax, you'll ace the next test on tests.

Blood chemistry tests

Just the facts

In this chapter, you'll learn:

♦ about blood chemistry tests
♦ what patient care is associated with these tests
♦ what factors can interfere with test results
♦ what blood chemistry test results may indicate.

A look at blood chemistry tests

Laboratory analysis of blood chemistry tests helps evaluate the body's respiratory and metabolic status. Arterial blood gas values provide important information about the adequacy of gas exchange in the lungs, ventilatory function, blood pH, and acid-base balance. Electrolyte levels provide valuable data about the body's acid-base balance and fluid balance.

Takin' care of business

Before obtaining a sample for a blood chemistry test, make sure the patient understands the procedure. Explain the procedure's purpose, and tell the patient that he'll feel some pressure from the tourniquet (if one is used) and may feel brief discomfort from the needle puncture.

If possible, use a large-gauge needle when drawing the sample, and handle the sample carefully to prevent hemolysis, which may interfere with test results. Observe standard precautions. Also, after taking a blood sample, check the venipuncture site for bleeding. If a hematoma develops at the site, apply warm soaks.

Running interference

A number of drugs can interfere with blood chemistry tests. Be sure to check the patient history and make notations as necessary.

Blood gases

Arterial blood gas analysis

Arterial blood gas (ABG) analysis evaluates gas exchange in the lungs by measuring the partial pressures of oxygen (Pao_2) and carbon dioxide ($Paco_2$) as well as the pH of an arterial sample. Pao_2 measures the pressure exerted by the oxygen dissolved in the blood and evaluates the lungs' ability to oxygenate the blood. $Paco_2$ measures the pressure exerted by carbon dioxide dissolved in the blood and reflects the adequacy of ventilation by the lungs. The pH measures the blood's hydrogen ion concentration and is the best way to tell whether blood is too acidic or too alkaline. Bicarbonate (HCO_3^-) is a measure of the bicarbonate ion concentration in the blood, which is regulated by the kidneys. Oxygen saturation (Sao_2) is the oxygen content of the blood expressed as a percentage of the oxygen capacity (the amount of oxygen the blood is capable of carrying if all of the hemoglobin [Hb] were fully saturated). Oxygen content (O_2CT) measures the actual amount of oxygen in the blood and isn't commonly used in blood gas evaluation.

What it all means

Normal ABG values fall within the following ranges:
- *pH:* 7.35 to 7.45 (SI, 7.35 to 7.45)
- *$Paco_2$:* 35 to 45 mm Hg (SI, 4.7 to 5.3 kPa)
- *Pao_2:* 80 to 100 mm Hg (SI, 10.6 to 13.3 kPa)
- *HCO_3^-:* 22 to 26 mEq/L (SI, 22 to 26 mmol/L)
- *Sao_2:* 94% to 100% (SI, 0.94 to 1)
- *O_2CT:* 15% to 23% (SI, 0.15 to 0.23).

The lowdown on levels

Low Pao_2, O_2CT, and Sao_2 levels in combination with a high $Paco_2$ may occur with:
- respiratory muscle weakness or paralysis (as in Guillain-Barré syndrome or myasthenia gravis)
- respiratory center inhibition (from head injury, brain tumor, or drug abuse) or airway obstruction (possibly from a mucus plug or tumor)
- bronchiole obstruction associated with asthma or emphysema
- abnormal ventilation-perfusion ratio.

ABG analysis evaluates pulmonary gas exchange, assesses the ventilatory control system, determines the blood's acid-base balance, and monitors respiratory therapy.

When inspired air contains insufficient oxygen, PaO_2, O_2CT, and SaO_2 also decrease, but $PaCO_2$ may be normal. Such findings are common in:
- pneumothorax
- impaired diffusion between alveoli and blood (such as that caused by interstitial fibrosis)
- arteriovenous shunt that permits blood to bypass the lungs.

Low O_2CT with normal PaO_2, SaO_2, and possibly $PaCO_2$ may result from severe anemia, decreased blood volume, and reduced oxygen-carrying capacity of Hb. (See *ABG analysis interference.*) In addition to clarifying blood oxygen disorders, ABG values can provide considerable information about acid-base disorders.

What needs to be done

- Wait at least 20 minutes before drawing ABG in the following situations:
  – after initiating, changing, or discontinuing oxygen therapy
  – after initiating or changing settings of mechanical ventilation
  – after extubation.
- Tell the patient which site — radial, brachial, or femoral artery — has been selected for the puncture.
- Instruct the patient to breathe normally during the test, and warn him that he may feel brief cramping or throbbing pain at the puncture site. (See *Obtaining an ABG sample.*)
- Include the following information on the laboratory request:
  – room air or amount of oxygen and method of delivery (for example, 40% aerosol face mask)

Warning!

ABG analysis interference

- Bicarbonate, ethacrynic acid, hydrocortisone, metolazone, prednisone, and thiazides may elevate $PaCO_2$.
- Acetazolamide, methicillin, nitrofurantoin, and tetracycline may decrease $PaCO_2$.
- Hypothermia may cause false-low PaO_2 and $PaCO_2$ levels.
- Fever may cause false-high PaO_2 and $PaCO_2$ levels.

Peak technique

Obtaining an ABG sample

Follow the steps below to obtain a sample for an arterial blood gas (ABG) analysis:
- After Allen's test, perform a cutaneous arterial puncture (or if an arterial line is in place, draw blood from the arterial line).
- Use a heparinized blood gas syringe to draw the sample.
- Eliminate all air from the sample, place it on ice immediately, and transport it for analysis.
- Apply pressure to the puncture site for 3 to 5 minutes. If the patient is receiving anticoagulants or has a coagulopathy, hold the puncture site longer than 5 minutes, if necessary.
- Tape a gauze pad firmly over the puncture site. If the puncture site is on the arm, don't tape the entire circumference, because this may restrict circulation.

– ventilator settings if on mechanical ventilation (fraction of inspired oxygen, tidal volume, mode, respiratory rate, positive-end respiratory pressure)
– patient's temperature.
• Monitor vital signs and observe for signs of circulatory impairment, such as swelling, discoloration, pain, numbness, or tingling in the bandaged arm or leg.

> The total CO_2 test helps evaluate acid-base balance.

Total carbon dioxide

Carbon dioxide (CO_2) is present in the body as an end product of metabolic processes as well as being present in small amounts in the air. When the pressure of CO_2 in the red cells exceeds 40 mm Hg (SI, 5.3 kPa), CO_2 flows out of the cells and dissolves in plasma. At this point, it combines with water to form carbonic acid, which in turn dissociates into hydrogen and bicarbonate ions.

The total CO_2 test measures the total concentration of all such forms of CO_2 in serum, plasma, or whole blood samples. Because about 90% of CO_2 in serum is in the form of bicarbonate, this test is a close approximation of bicarbonate levels. Total CO_2 content reflects the efficiency of the carbonic acid–bicarbonate buffer system, which maintains acid-base balance and normal pH.

What it all means

Normal CO_2 levels range from 22 to 26 mEq/L (SI, 22 to 26 mmol/L).

Too much

High CO_2 levels may occur in metabolic alkalosis (caused by excessive ingestion or retention of base bicarbonate), respiratory acidosis (from hypoventilation, for example, as in emphysema or pneumonia), primary aldosteronism, and Cushing's syndrome. CO_2 levels may also be elevated after excessive loss of acids, such as in severe vomiting and continuous gastric drainage.

Too little

Decreased CO_2 levels are common in metabolic acidosis (such as diabetic acidosis or renal tube acidosis caused by renal failure). Decreased total CO_2 levels in metabolic acidosis also result from loss of bicarbonate (such as in severe diarrhea or intestinal drainage). Levels also may fall below normal in respiratory alkalosis (for example, from hyperventilation after trauma). (See *Total CO_2 test interference*.)

Uh oh!   *Warning!*

Total CO_2 test interference

• Excessive use of corticotropin, cortisone, or thiazide diuretics or excessive ingestion of alkalis or licorice causes CO_2 levels to rise.
• Salicylates, paraldehyde, methicillin, dimercaprol, ammonium chloride, acetazolamide, or ingestion of ethylene glycol or methyl alcohol causes CO_2 levels to decrease.

What needs to be done

• Perform a venipuncture. Because CO_2 content is usually measured along with electrolytes, a 7-ml clot-activator tube may be used. When this test is performed alone, a heparinized tube is appropriate.
• Fill the tube completely to prevent diffusion of CO_2 into the vacuum.

Electrolytes

Sodium

The serum sodium test measures serum levels of sodium, the major extracellular cation. Sodium affects body water distribution, maintains osmotic pressure of extracellular fluid, and helps promote neuromuscular function; it also helps maintain acid-base balance and influences chloride and potassium levels. Sodium is absorbed by the kidneys; a small amount is lost through the skin.

Relationship with water

Serum sodium levels are evaluated in relation to the amount of water in the body, which is affected by the cellular mechanics of sodium (decreased sodium levels promote water excretion, and increased levels promote retention). For example, a sodium deficit (hyponatremia) refers to a decreased level of sodium in relation to the body's water level.

What it all means

Normally, serum sodium levels range from 135 to 145 mEq/L (SI, 135 to 145 mmol/L)

Sodium imbalance can result from a loss or gain of sodium or from a change in water volume. Remember, serum sodium results must be interpreted in light of the patient's state of hydration.

When it's high

Elevated serum sodium levels (hypernatremia) may be caused by inadequate water intake, water loss that exceeds sodium loss (such as in diabetes insipidus, impaired renal function, prolonged hyperventilation and, occasionally, severe vomiting or diarrhea), and sodium retention (such as in aldosteronism). Hypernatremia can also result from excessive sodium intake.

The serum sodium test evaluates fluid-electrolyte and acid-base balance as well as related neuromuscular, renal, and adrenal functions.

When it's low

Abnormally low serum sodium levels (hyponatremia) may result from inadequate sodium intake or excessive sodium loss caused by profuse sweating, GI suctioning, diuretic therapy, diarrhea, vomiting, adrenal insufficiency, burns, or chronic renal insufficiency with acidosis. Urine sodium determinations are frequently more sensitive to early changes in sodium balance and should always be evaluated simultaneously with serum sodium findings. (See *Sodium test interference.*)

What needs to be done

Perform a venipuncture, and collect the sample in a 7-ml clot-activator tube.

Sodium test interference

• Most diuretics, lithium, chlorpropamide, and vasopressin suppress serum sodium levels.
• Corticosteroids and antihypertensives (such as methyldopa, hydralazine, and reserpine) elevate serum sodium levels.

Potassium

Potassium is the major intracellular cation. The intracellular concentration of potassium is 150 to 160 mEq/L (SI, 150 to 160 mmol/L), and the extracellular concentration is 3.5 to 5 mEq/L (SI, 3.5 to 5 mmol/L). Evaluation of serum potassium measures the extracellular levels of this electrolyte.

Keeps cells neutral

Potassium is important in maintaining cellular electrical neutrality. The sodium-potassium active transport pump maintains the ratio of intracellular potassium to extracellular potassium that determines the resting membrane potential necessary for nerve impulse transmission. Disturbances in this ratio alter cardiac rhythms, transmission and conduction of nerve impulses, and muscle contraction.

What it all means

Normally, serum potassium levels range from 3.5 to 5 mEq/L (SI, 3.5 to 5 mmol/L).

A mess of potassium...

Hyperkalemia (elevated potassium level) occurs with:
• increased potassium intake
• shift in the concentration from intracellular to extracellular fluid
• decreased renal excretion
• infusion of stored whole blood
• penicillin G
• replacement potassium

Potassium is measured to determine potassium excess or depletion and to detect the origin of arrhythmias.

- acidosis
- insulin deficiency
- burns
- crushing injuries
- diabetic ketoacidosis
- extensive surgery
- myocardial infarction
- renal failure.

...or less of potassium?

Hypokalemia (decreased potassium level) occurs with depletion of total body potassium caused by shifts from extracellular fluid to intracellular fluid.

Depletion of total body potassium occurs with:
- diabetic ketoacidosis and insulin administration without potassium supplements
- GI and renal disorders
- vomiting
- diarrhea
- gastric suctioning
- diuretics
- excessive aldosterone secretion
- excessive licorice ingestion. (See *Potassium test interference.*)

What needs to be done

- Perform a venipuncture, and collect the sample in a 7-ml clot-activator tube.
- Draw the sample immediately after applying the tourniquet, because a delay may elevate the potassium level by allowing intracellular potassium to leak into the serum.
- Educate patients at risk for hypokalemia about increasing dietary intake of potassium-rich foods.

Magnesium

Magnesium is a commonly overlooked electrolyte vital to neuromuscular function. Magnesium activates many essential enzymes and affects the metabolism of nucleic acids and proteins. It also helps transport sodium and potassium across cell membranes and, through its effect on the secretion of parathyroid hormone, influences intracellular calcium levels.

Magnesium is measured to evaluate electrolyte status and assess neuromuscular or renal function. The serum magnesium test, a quantitative analysis, measures serum levels of magnesium, which is (after potassium) the most abundant intracellular cation.

> **Warning!**
>
> ## Potassium test interference
>
> The following factors may cause elevated potassium levels:
> - repeated fist clenching before venipuncture
> - excessive or rapid potassium infusion, spironolactone or penicillin G potassium therapy, or renal toxicity from administration of amphotericin B, methicillin, or tetracycline.

> Magnesium is measured to evaluate electrolyte status and assess neuromuscular and renal function.

An absorbing topic

Most magnesium is found in bone and in intracellular fluid; a small amount is found in extracellular fluid. Magnesium is absorbed by the small intestine and is excreted in the urine and feces.

What it all means

Normally, serum magnesium levels range from 1.3 to 2.1 mg/dl (SI, 0.65 to 1.05 mmol/L).

Renal failure

Elevated serum magnesium levels (hypermagnesemia) that aren't caused by magnesium administration or ingestion most commonly occur in renal failure, when the kidneys excrete inadequate amounts of magnesium. Adrenal insufficiency (Addison's disease) can also elevate serum magnesium levels.

Chronic alcoholism

Decreased serum magnesium levels (hypomagnesemia) most commonly result from chronic alcoholism. Other causes include malabsorption syndrome, diarrhea, faulty absorption after bowel resection, prolonged bowel or gastric aspiration, acute pancreatitis, primary aldosteronism, severe burns, hypercalcemic conditions (including hyperparathyroidism), and use of certain diuretics. (See *Magnesium test interference.*)

What needs to be done

• Tell the patient he shouldn't use magnesium salts, such as milk of magnesia or Epsom salts, for at least 3 days before the test.
• Perform a venipuncture, without a tourniquet if possible, and collect the sample in a 7-ml clot-activator tube.
• Educate patients at risk for hypermagnesemia about antacids, laxatives, and mineral supplements that contain magnesium.

Phosphates

Phosphates are essential in the storage and utilization of energy, calcium regulation, red blood cell function, acid-base balance, bone formation, and metabolism of carbohydrates, protein, and fat. Tests for phosphates measure serum levels of phosphates, the dominant cellular anions.

Warning!

Magnesium test interference

• Excessive use of antacids or cathartics or excessive infusion of magnesium sulfate raises magnesium levels.
• Prolonged I.V. infusions without magnesium suppress levels (excessive use of diuretics decreases magnesium levels).
• I.V. administration of calcium gluconate may falsely decrease serum magnesium levels.

Phosphate levels help diagnose acid-base imbalance and endocrine, renal, skeletal, and calcium disorders.

Linked to calcium

The intestine absorbs a considerable amount of phosphates from dietary sources, but adequate levels of vitamin D are necessary for their absorption. The kidneys regulate phosphate excretion and retention. Because calcium and phosphates interact in a reciprocal relationship, urinary excretion of phosphates increases or decreases in inverse proportion to serum calcium levels.

Abnormal phosphate levels result more commonly from improper excretion than from abnormal ingestion or absorption from dietary sources.

What it all means

Normally, serum phosphate levels in adults range from 2.7 to 4.5 mg/dl (SI, 0.87 to 1.45 mmol/L). In children, the normal range is 4.5 to 6.7 mg/dl (SI, 1.45 to 1.78 mmol/L).

The lowdown on levels

Decreased phosphate levels (hypophosphatemia) may result from malnutrition, malabsorption syndromes, hyperparathyroidism, renal tubular acidosis, or treatment of diabetic acidosis. In children, low phosphate levels can suppress normal growth.

Elevated phosphate levels (hyperphosphatemia) may result from skeletal disease, healing fractures, hypoparathyroidism, acromegaly, diabetic acidosis, high intestinal obstruction, and renal failure. Elevated phosphate levels are rarely clinically significant; however, if prolonged, they can alter bone metabolism by causing abnormal calcium phosphate deposits. (See *Phosphate test interference.*)

What needs to be done

• Perform a venipuncture (without using a tourniquet, if possible), and collect the sample in a 7-ml clot-activator tube.

Warning!

Phosphate test interference

The following factors may alter phosphate test results:

• extended I.V. infusion of dextrose 5% in water, the use of phosphate-binding antacids, and the use of acetazolamide, insulin, and epinephrine

• excessive vitamin D intake and use of anabolic corticosteroids or androgens, which may elevate serum phosphate levels.

Calcium

Total calcium measurement is the most commonly performed test for evaluation of serum calcium levels. Approximately 1% of the total calcium in the body circulates in the blood. Of this, about 50% is bound to plasma proteins and 40% is ionized, or free.

Calcium gets around

Evaluation of serum calcium levels measures the total amount of calcium circulating in the blood. Evaluation of ionized calcium levels measures the fraction of serum calcium that's in the ionized form, which is the most physiologically active form of serum calcium. The other 99% of the calcium in the body is stored in the bones and teeth.

Many laboratories don't have the equipment to measure ionized calcium levels. Because of this, serum albumin should be measured at the same time serum calcium is measured because the serum calcium level decreases 0.8 mg/dl for every 1-g decrease in the serum albumin level. The measured serum calcium is then adjusted upward by the amount of decrease in serum albumin. Ionized calcium is estimated to be approximately half of the adjusted calcium value.

What it all means

Normal calcium values are as follows:
- *total calcium:* 8.2 to 10.2 mg/dl (SI, 2.05 to 2.54 mmol/L) in adults; 8.6 to 11.2 mg/dl (SI, 2.15 to 2.79 mmol/L) in children
- *ionized calcium:* 4.65 to 5.28 mg/dl (SI, 1.1 to 61.32 mmol/L).

Going overboard with calcium...

Hypercalcemia, may occur in patients with hyperparathyroidism and parathyroid tumors (because of oversecretion of parathyroid hormone), Paget's disease of the bone, multiple myeloma, metastatic carcinoma, multiple fractures, or prolonged immobilization. Elevated serum calcium levels may also result from inadequate excretion of calcium, such as in adrenal insufficiency and renal disease; from excessive calcium ingestion; or from overuse of antacids such as calcium carbonate.

The total calcium level helps evaluate endocrine function, calcium metabolism, and acid-base balance. It also guides therapy for renal failure, renal transplant, endocrine disorders, malignancies, cardiac disease, and skeletal disorders.

Warning!

Calcium test interference

The following factors may alter calcium test results:
- excessive ingestion of vitamin D or its derivatives (dihydrotachysterol, calcitriol)
- use of androgens, calciferol-activated calcium salts, progestins-estrogens, or thiazide diuretics, which may elevate levels
- chronic laxative use
- excessive transfusions of citrated blood
- administration of acetazolamide, corticosteroids, or mithramycin.

...or missing the calcium boat

Hypocalcemia may result from hypoparathyroidism, total parathyroidectomy, or malabsorption. Decreased serum levels of calcium may follow calcium loss in patients with Cushing's syndrome, renal failure, acute pancreatitis, or peritonitis. (See *Calcium test interference.*)

What needs to be done

Perform a venipuncture (without using a tourniquet, if possible), and collect the sample in a 7-ml clot-activator tube.

The serum chloride test detects acid-base imbalance and helps evaluate fluid status.

Chloride

Interacting with sodium, chloride helps maintain the osmotic pressure of blood and therefore helps regulate blood volume and arterial pressure. Chloride levels also affect acid-base balance. Serum concentrations of this electrolyte are regulated by aldosterone secondarily to regulation of sodium. Chloride is absorbed from the intestines and is excreted primarily by the kidneys.

The serum chloride test, a quantitative analysis, measures serum levels of chloride, the major extracellular fluid anion.

What it all means

Normal serum chloride levels range from 100 to 108 mEq/L (SI, 100 to 108 mmol/L).

Chloride levels relate inversely to those of bicarbonate and thus reflect acid-base balance. Excessive loss of gastric juices or of other secretions containing chloride may cause hypochloremic metabolic alkalosis; excessive chloride retention or ingestion may lead to hyperchloremic metabolic acidosis.

The lowdown on levels

Elevated serum chloride levels (hyperchloremia) may result from bicarbonate loss caused by diarrhea, severe dehydration, complete renal shutdown, head injury (producing neurogenic hyperventilation), or primary aldosteronism.

Low chloride levels (hypochloremia) are usually associated with low sodium and potassium levels. Possible underlying causes include prolonged vomiting, gastric suctioning, intestinal fistula, chronic renal failure, and Addison's disease. Heart failure or edema resulting in excess extracellular fluid can cause dilutional hypochloremia. (See *Chloride test interference.*)

UH OH **Warning!**

Chloride test interference

• Ammonium chloride, cholestyramine, or excessive I.V. infusion of sodium chloride may elevate serum chloride levels.

• Thiazide diuretics, ethacrynic acid, furosemide, or bicarbonates, or prolonged I.V. infusion of dextrose 5% in water may decrease serum chloride levels.

What needs to be done

Perform a venipuncture, and collect the sample in a 7-ml clot-activator tube.

Anion gap

The anion gap reflects anion-cation balance in the serum and helps distinguish types of metabolic acidosis without expensive, time-consuming measurement of all serum electrolytes. The anion gap test uses serum levels of routinely measured electrolytes—sodium, chloride, and bicarbonate—for a quick calculation based on a simple physical principle: Total concentrations of cations and anions are normally equal, thereby maintaining electrical neutrality in serum.

Because sodium accounts for more than 90% of circulating cations, whereas chloride and bicarbonate together account for 85% of the counterbalancing anions, the gap between measured cation and anion levels represents those anions not routinely measured, including sulfate, phosphates, proteins, and organic acids, such as ketone bodies and lactic acid.

> The anion gap helps distinguish types of metabolic acidosis and monitors renal function and total parenteral nutrition.

What it all means

Normally, the anion gap ranges from 8 to 14 mEq/L (SI, 8 to 14 mmol/L). A normal anion gap doesn't rule out metabolic acidosis.

Normal anion gap acidosis

When acidosis results from loss of bicarbonate in the urine or other body fluids, renal reabsorption of sodium promotes retention of chloride, and the anion gap remains unchanged. Thus, metabolic acidosis associated with excessive chloride levels is known as normal anion gap acidosis.

High anion gap acidosis

When acidosis results from accumulation of metabolic acids, as with lactic acidosis, the anion gap increases above 14 mEq/L (14 mmol/L) with the increase being in unmeasured anions. Metabolic acidosis caused by such accumulation is known as high anion gap acidosis. (See *Understanding anion gap and metabolic acidosis.*)

Because the anion gap determines only total anion-cation balance, it doesn't necessarily reflect abnormal values for individual electrolytes. Further investigation and diagnostic tests are usually necessary to determine the specific cause of metabolic acidosis.

Advice from the experts

Understanding anion gap and metabolic acidosis

Metabolic acidosis with a normal anion gap (8 to 14 mEq/L [SI, 8 to 14 µmol/L]) occurs with bicarbonate loss, such as from:
• hypokalemic acidosis associated with renal tubular acidosis, diarrhea, or ureteral diversions
• hyperkalemic acidosis caused by acidifying agents (for example, ammonium chloride or hydrochloric acid), hydronephrosis, or sickle cell nephropathy.
  Metabolic acidosis with an increased anion gap (above 14 mEq/L [SI, greater than 14 mmol/L]) occurs with accumulation of organic acids, sulfates, or phosphates, such as from:
• renal failure
• ketoacidosis associated with starvation, diabetes mellitus, or alcohol abuse
• lactic acidosis
• ingestion of toxins, such as salicylates, methanol, ethylene glycol (antifreeze), and paraldehyde.

Warning!

Anion gap test interference

A range of medications and other substances can alter the anion gap.

Increases the gap
• Ammonium chloride
• Antihypertensives
• Bicarbonates
• Corticosteroids
• Ethacrynic acid
• furosemide
• Prolonged infusion of dextrose 5% in water
• Salicylates
• Thiazide diuretics

Decreases the gap
• Chlorothiazide diuretics
• chlorpropamide
• cortisone
• Diuretics
• Excessive ingestion of alkalis or licorice
• lithium
• vasopressin

A decreased anion gap (less than 8 mEq/L) is rare but may occur in hypermagnesemia and in paraproteinemic states, such as multiple myeloma and Waldenström's macroglobulinemia. (See *Anion gap test interference.*)

What needs to be done

• Perform a venipuncture, and collect the sample in a 7-ml clot-activator tube.
• As ordered, instruct the patient to resume use of any drugs discontinued for the test.

Proteins and protein metabolites

Blood urea nitrogen

Urea is the chief end product of protein metabolism. Formed in the liver from ammonia and excreted by the kidneys, urea constitutes 40% to 50% of the blood's nonprotein nitrogen. Because the level of reabsorption of urea in the renal tubules is directly related to the rate of urine flow through the kidneys, the blood urea nitrogen (BUN) level is a less reliable indicator of uremia than is the

Warning!

BUN test interference

- Chloramphenicol can depress BUN levels.
- Nephrotoxic drugs, such as aminoglycosides, amphotericin B, and methicillin, can elevate BUN levels.

The BUN test evaluates renal function and helps diagnose renal disease and hydration level.

serum creatine level. The BUN test measures the nitrogen fraction of urea.

What it all means

BUN values normally range from 8 to 20 mg/dl (SI, 2.9 to 7.5 mmol/L, with slightly higher values in elderly patients. Elevated BUN levels occur in renal disease, reduced renal blood flow (such as with dehydration), urinary tract obstruction, and increased protein catabolism (such as occurs in burns).

Depressed BUN levels occur in severe hepatic damage, malnutrition, and overhydration. (See *BUN test interference*.)

What needs to be done

- Tell the patient to avoid a diet high in meat.
- Perform a venipuncture, and collect the sample in a 7-ml clot-activator tube.

Creatinine

A quantitative analysis of serum creatinine levels, the serum creatinine test provides a more sensitive measure of renal damage than do blood urea nitrogen levels because renal impairment is virtually the only cause of creatinine elevation.

Because creatinine levels normally remain constant, elevated levels usually indicate diminished renal function.

Because creatinine levels normally stay constant, elevated levels usually indicate diminished kidney function.

What it all means

Serum creatinine levels in males normally range from 0.8 to 1.2 mg/dl (SI, 62 to 115 µmol/L); in females, they range from 0.6 to 0.9 mg/dl (SI, 53 to 97 µmol/L). Elevated serum creatinine levels generally indicate renal disease that has seriously damaged 50% or more of the nephrons. They may also be associated with gigantism and acromegaly. (See *Creatinine test interference*.)

Warning!

Creatinine test interference

• Ascorbic acid, barbiturates, and diuretics may raise serum creatinine levels.

• Sulfobromophthalein or phenolsulfonphthalein given within the previous 24 hours, can elevate creatinine levels.

• Exceptionally large muscle mass, such as in athletes, may cause above-average creatinine levels, even with normal renal function.

What needs to be done

Perform a venipuncture, and collect the sample in a 7-ml clot-activator tube.

Uric acid

Used primarily to detect gout, the uric acid test measures serum levels of uric acid—the major end metabolite of purine. Purine is a nitrogen-containing compound produced in the digestion of certain dietary proteins.

What it all means

Uric acid concentrations in men normally range from 3.4 to 7 mg/dl (SI, 202 to 416 µmol/L); in women, from 2.3 to 6 mg/dl (SI, 143 to 357 µmol/L).

Serum uric acid testing confirms gout and helps detect kidney dysfunction.

Warning!

Uric acid test interference

• Starvation, a high-purine diet, stress, alcohol abuse, loop diuretics, ethambutol, vincristine, pyrazinamide, thiazides, and low aspirin doses may raise levels.

• Acetaminophen, ascorbic acid, and levodopa may cause false elevations.

• High aspirin doses may decrease levels.

The lowdown on levels

Increased serum uric acid levels may indicate gout or impaired renal function (levels don't correlate with the severity of disease, however). Levels may also rise in heart failure, glycogen storage disease (type I, von Gierke's disease), infections, hemolytic or sickle cell anemia, polycythemia, neoplasms, and psoriasis.

Depressed uric acid levels may indicate defective tubular absorption (such as in Fanconi's syndrome and Wilson's disease) or acute hepatic atrophy. (See *Uric acid test interference*, page 37.)

What needs to be done

• Tell the patient that he must fast for 8 hours before the test.
• Perform a venipuncture, and collect the sample in a 7-ml clot-activator tube.

The protein electrophoresis test helps diagnose protein deficiency and renal disorders as well as GI and neoplastic diseases.

Protein electrophoresis

Protein electrophoresis measures serum albumin and globulins, the major blood proteins, by separating the proteins into five distinct fractions: albumin, alpha$_1$, alpha$_2$, beta, and gamma proteins.

What it all means

Normal protein values are:
• *total serum protein:* 6.4 to 8.3 g/dl (SI, 64 to 83 g/L)
• *albumin:* 3.5 to 5 g/dl (SI, 35 to 50 g/L)
• *alpha$_1$-globulin:* 0.1 to 0.3 g/dl (SI, 1 to 3 g/L)
• *alpha$_2$-globulin:* 0.6 to 1 g/dl (SI, 6 to 10 g/L)
• *beta globulin:* 0.7 to 1.1 g/dl (SI, 7 to 11 g/L)
• *gamma globulin:* 0.8 to 1.6 g/dl (SI, 8 to 16 g/L). (See *Clinical implications of abnormal protein levels* and *Protein electrophoresis interference*, page 40.)

What needs to be done

• This test must be performed on a serum sample to avoid measuring the fibrinogen fraction. (The fibrinogen fraction, if present, would be indistinguishable from certain monoclonal gammopathies.)
• Perform a venipuncture, and collect the sample in a 7-ml clot-activator tube.

Advice from the experts

Clinical implications of abnormal protein levels

Abnormal levels of albumin or globulins occur in many pathologic states, including those listed here.

Increased levels

Total proteins
- Dehydration
- Vomiting, diarrhea
- Diabetic acidosis
- Fulminating and chronic infections
- Multiple myeloma
- Monocytic leukemia
- Chronic inflammatory disease (such as rheumatoid arthritis or early-stage Laënnec's cirrhosis)

Albumin
- Multiple myeloma

Globulins
- Multiple myeloma
- Chronic syphilis
- Tuberculosis
- Subacute bacterial endocarditis
- Collagen diseases
- Systemic lupus erythematosus
- Rheumatoid arthritis
- Diabetes mellitus
- Hodgkin's disease

Decreased levels

Total proteins
- Malnutrition
- GI disease
- Blood dyscrasias
- Essential hypertension
- Hodgkin's disease
- Uncontrolled diabetes mellitus
- Malabsorption
- Hepatic dysfunction
- Toxemia of pregnancy
- Nephrosis
- Surgical and traumatic shock
- Severe burns
- Hemorrhage
- Hyperthyroidism
- Benzene and carbon tetrachloride poisoning
- Heart failure

Albumin
- Malnutrition
- Nephritis, nephrosis
- Diarrhea
- Plasma loss from burns
- Hepatic disease
- Hodgkin's disease
- Hypogammaglobulinemia
- Peptic ulcer
- Acute cholecystitis
- Sarcoidosis
- Collagen diseases
- Systemic lupus erythematosus
- Rheumatoid arthritis
- Essential hypertension
- Metastatic cancer
- Hyperthyroidism

Globulins
- Variable levels in neoplastic and renal diseases, hepatic dysfunction, and blood dyscrasias

Warning!

Protein electrophoresis interference

- Pretest administration of a contrast agent falsely elevates protein test results.
- Cytotoxic drug use may lower serum albumin levels.
- Pregnancy may lower serum albumin levels.

Haptoglobin

The haptoglobin test measures serum levels of haptoglobin, a glycoprotein produced in the liver. Haptoglobin binds with free hemoglobin (Hb) and prevents its accumulation in plasma, permitting clearance by reticuloendothelial cells and conserving body iron.

Hb circulates inside erythrocytes (red blood cells [RBCs]); when aged erythrocytes die, they release free Hb into plasma. Certain anemias, bacterial toxins, mechanical disruption (from a prosthetic heart valve, for example), or antibodies can increase intravascular hemolysis (the breakdown of RBCs and the release of Hb). In acute intravascular hemolysis, haptoglobin levels fall rapidly; low levels may last for 5 to 7 days, until the liver synthesizes more glycoprotein.

What it all means

Serum haptoglobin concentrations, measured in terms of the protein's Hb-binding capacity, normally range from 40 to 180 mg/dl (SI, 0.4 to 1.8 g/L). Nephelometric procedures yield lower results.

Markedly depressed serum haptoglobin levels are characteristic in acute and chronic hemolysis, severe hepatocellular disease, infectious mononucleosis, and transfusion reactions. Hepatocellular disease inhibits the synthesis of haptoglobin. In hemolytic transfusion reactions, haptoglobin levels begin falling after 6 to 8 hours and drop to 40% of pretransfusion levels after 24 hours.

The lowdown on levels

Although haptoglobin is absent in 90% of neonates, levels usually rise to normal by age 4 months. However, in about 1% of the population — including 4% of blacks — haptoglobin is permanently absent; this disorder is known as congenital ahaptoglobinemia.

The haptoglobin test evaluates hemolysis, differentiates hemoglobin from myoglobin in plasma, and assesses hemolytic transfusion reactions.

Warning!

Haptoglobin test interference

Corticosteroids and androgens can elevate haptoglobin levels.

Markedly elevated serum haptoglobin levels occur in diseases marked by chronic inflammatory reactions or tissue destruction, such as rheumatoid arthritis and malignant neoplasms. (See *Haptoglobin test interference.*)

What needs to be done

Perform a venipuncture, and collect the blood sample in a 7-ml clot-activator tube.

Transferrin

Transferrin (also known as siderophilin), a glycoprotein formed in the liver, transports circulating iron obtained from dietary sources and from the breakdown of red blood cells by reticuloendothelial cells.

The transferrin test measures serum transferrin levels to evaluate iron metabolism.

> The transferrin test determines the blood's iron-transporting capacity and evaluates iron metabolism in iron deficiency anemia.

Taking it to the bone

Most of this iron is transported to bone marrow for use in hemoglobin (Hb) synthesis; some is converted to hemosiderin and ferritin and stored in the liver, spleen, and bone marrow. Inadequate transferrin levels may lead to impaired Hb synthesis and, possibly, anemia. Transferrin is normally about 30% saturated with iron. Serum iron levels are usually obtained simultaneously.

What it all means

Normal serum transferrin values range from 200 to 400 mg/dl (SI, 2 to 4 g/L), of which 65 to 170 mg/dl (SI, 0.65 to 1.7 g/L) are usually bound to iron. Depressed serum transferrin levels may indicate inadequate production caused by hepatic damage or excessive protein loss from renal disease. They may also result from acute or chronic infection or from cancer. Elevated serum transferrin levels may indicate severe iron deficiency. (See *Transferrin test interference.*)

What needs to be done

Perform a venipuncture, and collect the sample in a 7-ml clot-activator tube.

Warning!

Transferrin test interference

Late pregnancy or oral contraceptives may raise transferrin levels.

Phenylalanine

The phenylalanine test (also known as the Guthrie test) is a screening method that detects elevated levels of serum phenylalanine, which is a naturally occurring amino acid essential to growth and nitrogen balance.

The phenylalanine test screens infants for PKU.

Metabolic upset

Elevated levels of phenylalanine may indicate phenylketonuria (PKU), a metabolic disorder inherited as an autosomal recessive trait. An infant with PKU usually has normal phenylalanine levels at birth but, after he begins feeding with breast milk or formula (both contain phenylalanine), levels gradually rise because of a deficiency of the liver enzyme that converts phenylalanine to tyrosine. The resulting accumulation of phenylalanine, phenylpyruvic acid, and other metabolites hinders normal development of central nervous system cells, causing mental retardation.

Day three for accuracy

To ensure accurate results, the test must be performed after 3 full days (preferably 4 days) of breast milk or formula feeding. (In some states, a preliminary test is done 25 hours after birth.)

What it all means

In the laboratory, the sample is added to a culture medium containing a phenylalanine-dependent strain of *B. subtilis* and an antagonist to phenylalanine. A negative test, in which the presence of the phenylalanine antagonist inhibits growth of *B. subtilis* around the blood on the filter paper, indicates normal phenylalanine levels (less than 2 mg/dl [SI, less than 121 µmol/L]) and no appreciable danger of PKU.

Danger ahead

Growth of *B. subtilis* on the filter paper indicates that serum phenylalanine levels are high enough to overcome the antagonist. Such a positive test suggests the possibility of PKU. Diagnosis requires exact serum phenylalanine measurement and urine testing. (See *Confirming PKU.*) A positive test may also result from hepatic disease, galactosemia (an inherited autosomal-recessive disorder of galactose metabolism), or delayed development of certain enzyme systems.

What needs to be done

• Perform a heelstick, and collect three drops of blood — one in each circle — on the filter paper.

Confirming PKU

After the Guthrie test detects the possible presence of phenylketonuria (PKU), serum phenylalanine and tyrosine levels are measured to confirm the diagnosis. Phenylalanine hydroxylase is the enzyme that converts phenylalanine to tyrosine. If this enzyme is absent, increasing phenylalanine levels with concomitant decreasing tyrosine levels indicate PKU.

Samples are obtained by venipuncture (femoral or external jugular). Serum phenylalanine levels greater than 4 mg/dl (SI, greater than 242 μmol/L) and low tyrosine levels—with urinary excretion of phenylpyruvic acid—confirm PKU.

• Note the infant's name and birth date and the date of the first breast milk or formula feeding on the laboratory request, and send the sample to the laboratory immediately.
• Reassure the parents of a child who may have PKU that early detection and continuous treatment with a low-phenylalanine diet can prevent permanent mental retardation.

Plasma ammonia

The plasma ammonia test measures plasma levels of ammonia, a nonprotein nitrogen compound that helps maintain acid-base balance. Most ammonia is absorbed from the intestinal tract, where it's produced by bacterial action on protein; a smaller amount of ammonia is produced in the kidneys from hydrolysis of glutamine. Normally, the body uses the nitrogen fraction of ammonia to rebuild amino acids and then converts the ammonia to urea in the liver for excretion by the kidneys. In diseases such as cirrhosis of the liver, ammonia can bypass the liver and accumulate in the blood. Therefore, measurement of plasma ammonia levels may help indicate the severity of hepatocellular damage.

What it all means

Normally, plasma ammonia levels are 15 to 45 μg/dl (SI, 11 to 32 μmol/L) Elevated plasma ammonia levels are common in patients with severe hepatic disease, such as cirrhosis and acute hepatic necrosis, and may lead to hepatic coma. Elevated levels are also possible in patients with Reye's syndrome, severe heart failure, GI hemorrhage, and erythroblastosis fetalis (a type of hemo-

The plasma ammonia test helps monitor severe hepatic disease and the effectiveness of therapy.

lytic anemia in neonates). (See *Plasma ammonia test interference*.)

What needs to be done
• Tell the patient that an overnight fast before the test is required because plasma ammonia levels may vary with protein intake.
• Notify the laboratory before performing the venipuncture so that preliminary preparations can begin.
• Perform a venipuncture, and collect the sample in a 10-ml heparinized tube.
• Make sure bleeding has stopped before removing pressure from the venipuncture site.
• Handle the sample gently, pack it in ice, and send it to the laboratory immediately. *Don't* use a chilled container.
• Watch for signs of impending or established hepatic coma, if plasma ammonia levels are high.

Warning!

Plasma ammonia test interference
• Acetazolamide, thiazides, ammonium salts, and furosemide as well as total parenteral nutrition or a portacaval shunt raise ammonia levels.
• Lactulose, neomycin, and kanamycin depress ammonia levels.

Cardiac enzymes and proteins

Creatine kinase

Creatine kinase (CK) is an enzyme that catalyzes the creatine-creatinine metabolic pathway in muscle cells and brain tissue. Because of its important role in energy production, CK levels reflect normal tissue catabolism; above-normal serum levels indicate trauma to cells with high CK content.

A triad of isoenzymes

CK may be separated into three isoenzymes with distinct molecular structures: CK-BB (CK_1), found primarily in brain tissue; CK-MB (CK_2), found primarily in cardiac muscle (a small amount also appears in skeletal muscle); and CK-MM (CK_3), found mainly in skeletal muscle.

Getting specific

Total serum CK levels were once widely used to detect acute myocardial infarction (MI), but elevated levels caused by skeletal muscle damage reduce the test's specificity for this disorder. Fractionation and measurement of CK isoenzymes has replaced total CK assay to accurately localize the site of increased tissue destruction. In addition, subunits of CK-MM and CK-MB, called isoforms, can be assayed to increase the sensitivity of the test.

CK levels are measured to diagnose acute MI and to monitor the severity of myocardial ischemia after cardiac surgery or catheterization.

What it all means

Total CK values normally range from 55 to 170 U/L (SI, 0.94 to 2.89 µkat/L) for men and from 30 to 135 U/L (SI, 0.51 to 2.3 µkat/L) for women. CK levels may be significantly higher in very muscular people. Infants up to age 1 year have levels two to four times higher than adults, possibly reflecting birth trauma and striated muscle development. The normal ranges for isoenzyme levels are as follows: CK-BB, undetectable; CK-MB, less than 6% (SI, less than 0.06); CK-MM, 90% to 100% (SI, 0.9 to 1).

Detectable CK-BB

CK-MM constitutes over 99% (SI, over 0.99) of total CK normally present in serum. Detectable CK-BB levels may indicate brain tissue injury, certain widespread malignant tumors, severe shock, or renal failure. However, such elevations don't confirm a specific diagnosis.

High CK-MB

CK-MB levels greater than 5% of total CK indicate MI, especially if the lactate dehydrogenase 1 and 2 (LD_1-LD_2) isoenzyme ratio is greater than 1 (flipped LD). In acute MI and after cardiac surgery, CK-MB levels begin to rise in 2 to 4 hours, peak in 12 to 24 hours, and usually return to normal in 24 to 48 hours; persistent elevations or increasing levels indicate ongoing myocardial damage.

Total CK follows roughly the same pattern but rises slightly later. CK-MB levels don't rise in heart failure or during angina pectoris not accompanied by myocardial cell necrosis, although not all researchers agree about this.

Serious skeletal muscle injury that occurs in certain muscular dystrophies, polymyositis, and severe myoglobinuria may produce mildly elevated CK-MB levels because a small amount of this isoenzyme is present in some skeletal muscles.

Rising CK-MM

Rising CK-MM values follow skeletal muscle damage from trauma, such as surgery and I.M. injections, or from diseases, such as dermatomyositis and muscular dystrophy (values may be 50 to 100 times normal). A moderate rise in CK-MM levels develops in patients with hypothyroidism; sharp elevations occur with muscular activity caused by agitation such as an acute psychotic episode.

Total CK

Total CK levels may be elevated in patients with severe hypokalemia, carbon monoxide poisoning, malignant hyperthermia, or alcoholic cardiomyopathy; in those who have recently had a

Warning!

CK test interference

The following factors may raise total CK values:

• halothane and succinylcholine, alcohol, lithium, and large doses of aminocaproic acid

• I.M. injections, cardioversion, invasive diagnostic procedures, recent vigorous exercise or muscle massage, and severe coughing and trauma

• surgery through skeletal muscle.

seizure; and occasionally in those who have suffered pulmonary or cerebral infarctions. (See *CK test interference*, page 45.)

What needs to be done

• If the patient is being evaluated for skeletal muscle disorders, advise him to avoid exercising for 24 hours before the test.
• Advise the patient that he must not take the following before the test: alcohol, aminocaproic acid, lithium, clofibrate, codeine, dexamethasone, digoxin, lithium, morphine, succinylcholine, furosemide, glutethimide, halothane, heroin, imipramine, meperidine, and phenobarbital. If these substances must be continued, note this on the laboratory request.
• Obtain the sample as scheduled. Because timing is important to the diagnosis, be sure to record the date and time the sample was drawn and the number of hours that elapsed since the onset of chest pain.
• Draw the sample before giving an I.M. injection, or wait at least 1 hour after the injection, because muscle trauma raises total CK levels.
• Perform a venipuncture, and collect the sample in a 7-ml tube without additives.
• Send the sample to the laboratory immediately because CK activity diminishes significantly after 2 hours at room temperature.
• Resume medications discontinued before the test, as ordered.

Lactate dehydrogenase

Lactate dehydrogenase (LD) catalyzes (speeds up the chemical reaction) the reversible conversion of muscle lactic acid into pyruvic acid, which ultimately produces cellular energy.

Gimme five

Because LD is present in almost all body tissues, cellular damage causes an elevation of total serum LD, thus limiting its diagnostic usefulness. However, five tissue-specific isoenzymes can be identified and measured. Two of these isoenzymes, LD_1 and LD_2, appear primarily in the heart, red blood cells (RBCs), and kidneys; LD_3, primarily in the lungs; and LD_4 and LD_5, in the liver and the skeletal muscles. Also, the midzone fractions (LD_2, LD_3, LD_4) can be elevated in granulocytic leukemia, lymphomas, and platelet disorders.

Ups and downs

The specificity of LD isoenzymes and their distribution pattern are useful in diagnosing hepatic, pulmonary, and erythrocytic damage. However, their widest use is in aiding diagnosis of acute

LD testing aids in the diagnosis of MI, pulmonary infarction, anemias, and hepatic disease.

myocardial infarction (MI). An LD isoenzyme assay is helpful when creatine kinase (CK) hasn't been measured within 24 hours of an acute MI. The myocardial LD level rises later than CK (12 to 48 hours after infarction begins), peaks in 2 to 5 days, and drops to normal in 7 to 10 days if tissue necrosis doesn't persist.

What it all means

Total LD levels normally range from 71 to 207 U/L (SI, 1.2 to 3.52 µkat/L), depending on the method used. Normal isoenzyme distribution is as follows:

- LD_1: 14% to 26% (SI, 0.14 to 0.26) of total
- LD_2: 29% to 39% (SI, 0.29 to 0.39) of total
- LD_3: 20% to 26% (SI, 0.2 to 0.26) of total
- LD_4: 8% to 16% (SI, 0.08 to 0.16) of total
- LD_5: 6% to 16% (SI, 0.06 to 0.16) of total.

Upside, downside, and flipside

Because many common diseases cause elevations in total LD levels, isoenzyme electrophoresis is usually necessary for diagnosis. In some disorders, total LD may be within normal limits, but abnormal proportions of each isoenzyme indicate specific organ tissue damage. For instance, in acute MI, the concentration of LD_1 is greater than LD_2 within 12 to 48 hours after onset of symptoms. (That is, the LD_1-LD_2 ratio is greater than 1.) This reversal of normal isoenzyme patterns is typical of myocardial damage and is referred to as "flipped LD." (See *LD test interference*.)

What needs to be done

- Tell the patient that if an MI is suspected, the test is likely to be repeated for the next few mornings to monitor progressive changes.
- Draw the samples on schedule to avoid missing peak levels, and mark the collection time on the laboratory request.
- Perform a venipuncture, and collect the sample in a 7-ml clot-activator tube.
- Send the sample to the laboratory immediately or, if transport is delayed, keep the sample at room temperature. Changes in temperature reportedly inactivate LD_5, thus altering isoenzyme patterns.

Troponin I and cardiac troponin T

Troponin I and cardiac troponin T are proteins in the striated cells, part of the calcium-binding complex of the thin myofilaments of myocardial tissue.

Warning!

LD test interference

- Recent surgery or pregnancy can cause elevated LD levels.
- Prosthetic heart valves may also increase LD levels because of chronic hemolysis.

The cardiac troponin test detects and diagnoses acute MI and reinfarction and evaluates possible causes of chest pain.

Troponins mark the spot

Troponins are extremely specific markers of cardiac damage. When injury occurs to the myocardial tissue, these proteins are released into the bloodstream, increasing from normally undetectable blood levels to levels of more than 50 µg/L (SI, 50 µg/L). Elevations in troponin levels can be seen within 1 hour of myocardial infarction and will persist for a week or longer, making this a useful diagnostic tool.

What it all means

Laboratories may give varying results, with some calling a cardiac troponin test positive if it shows any detectable levels and others giving a range for abnormal results.

A gray zone

Normally, troponin I levels are less than 0.35 µg/L (SI, less than 0.35 µg/L). Cardiac troponin T levels are less than 0.1 µg/L (SI, less than 0.1 µg/L). Troponin I levels between 0 and 0.4 µg/L (SI, between 0 and 0.4 µg/L) aren't suggestive of cardiac injury, and levels from 0.5 to 1.9 µg/L (SI, from 0.5 to 1.9 µg/L) are indeterminate for cardiac injury.

A hurtin' heart

Troponin I levels greater than 2 µg/L (SI, greater than 2 µg/L) are suggestive of cardiac injury. Results of a qualitative cardiac troponin T rapid immunoassay that are greater than 0.2 µg/L (SI, greater than 0.2 µg/L) are considered positive for cardiac injury. When quantitative serum assays for cardiac troponin T are done, the upper limit for normal is 0.1 µg/L (SI, 0.1 µg/L). As long as tissue injury continues, the troponin levels will remain high. Troponin levels rise rapidly and are detectable within 1 hour of myocardial cell injury. Troponin I levels aren't detectable in people without cardiac injury. (See *Cardiac troponin test interference.*)

What needs to be done

- Tell the patient that this test helps assess myocardial injury, and multiple samples may be drawn to detect fluctuations in serum levels.
- Obtain each specimen on schedule, and note the date and collection time on each.
- Perform a venipuncture, and collect the specimen in a 7-ml clot-activator tube.

Warning!

Cardiac troponin test interference

The following factors may increase cardiac troponin levels:

- sustained vigorous exercise, which may increase troponin T levels in the absence of significant cardiac damage associated with noncardiac specific troponin T found in these skeletal muscles
- cardiotoxic drugs such as doxorubicin.

Myoglobin

Myoglobin, which is normally found in skeletal and cardiac muscle, functions as an oxygen-binding muscle protein. It's released into the bloodstream in ischemia, trauma, and inflammation of the muscle.

What it all means

Normal myoglobin values are 0 to 0.09 µg/ml (SI, 5 to 70 µ/L). In addition to occurring in myocardial infarction (MI), increased myoglobin levels may occur in acute alcohol intoxication, dermatomyositis, hypothermia (with prolonged shivering), muscular dystrophy, polymyositis, severe burn injuries, trauma, severe renal failure, and systemic lupus erythematosus. (See *Myoglobin test interference.*)

What needs to be done

• Expect to collect blood samples 4 to 8 hours after the onset of an acute MI.
• Tell the patient that the results of this test need to be correlated with other tests for a definitive diagnosis.
• Perform a venipuncture, and collect the sample in a 5-ml tube with no additives.
• Send the sample to the laboratory immediately.

The myoglobin test can detect MI, estimate damage to skeletal or cardiac muscle, and predict flare-ups of polymyositis.

Warning!

Myoglobin test interference

The following factors may alter myoglobin test results:
• radioactive scans performed within 1 week of the test
• recent angina, cardioversion, or improper timing of the test, which may increase levels
• I.M. injection, which may cause a false-positive result.

Carbohydrates

Fasting plasma glucose

Commonly used to screen for diabetes mellitus, the fasting plasma glucose test (also known as the fasting blood sugar test) measures plasma glucose levels following a 12- to 14-hour fast.

What it all means

The normal range for fasting plasma glucose varies according to the laboratory procedure. Generally, normal values after at least an 8-hour fast are 70 to 110 mg (SI, 3.9 to 6.1 mmol/L) of true glucose per deciliter of blood.

Confirming diabetes

A fasting plasma glucose level of 126 mg/dl (SI, 7 mmol/L) or higher obtained on two or more occasions confirms provisional diabetes mellitus. An impaired blood glucose level is 125 mg/dl (SI, 6.9 mmol/L. A borderline or transiently elevated level requires the 2-hour postprandial plasma glucose test or the oral glucose tolerance test to confirm the diagnosis.

Boosting levels

Increased fasting plasma glucose levels can also result from pancreatitis, recent acute illness (such as myocardial infarction), Cushing's syndrome, acromegaly (a metabolic condition characterized by enlargement and elongation of facial bones and extremities), and pheochromocytoma (a tumor of the adrenal medulla). Hyperglycemia may also stem from hyperlipoproteinemia (especially type III, IV, or V), chronic hepatic disease, nephrotic syndrome, brain tumor, sepsis, or gastrectomy with dumping syndrome and is typical in eclampsia, anoxia, and seizure disorders.

Depressed levels

Depressed plasma glucose levels can result from hyperinsulinism, insulinoma, von Gierke's disease (glycogen storage disease), functional or reactive hypoglycemia, myxedema, adrenal insufficiency, congenital adrenal hyperplasia, hypopituitarism, malabsorption syndrome and some cases of hepatic insufficiency.

Fast action needed

When using fasting plasma glucose tests to monitor drug or diet therapy in patients with diabetes mellitus, results can be obtained

The fasting plasma glucose test screens for diabetes mellitus and monitors drug or dietary therapy in patients with

Warning!

Fasting plasma glucose test interference

The following factors may increase plasma glucose levels:
- acetaminophen, which may cause false-positive findings
- recent illness, infection, or pregnancy
- chlorthalidone, thiazide diuretics, furosemide, triamterene, oral contraceptives (estrogen-progestogen combination), benzodiazepines, phenytoin, phenothiazines, lithium, epinephrine, arginine, phenolphthalein, dextrothyroxine, dizoxide, large doses of nicotinic acid, corticosteroids, and recent I.V. glucose infusions as well as ethacrynic acid (which may also cause hyperglycemia or, in large doses, hypoglycemia in patients with uremia).

The following factors may decrease plasma glucose levels:
- beta-adrenergic blockers, ethanol, clofibrate, insulin, oral antidiabetic agents, and monoamine oxidase inhibitors
- strenuous exercise.

that require immediate action. Most patients develop symptoms when blood glucose is between 50 to 60 mg/dl (SI, 2.8 to 3 mmol/L). Symptoms include fatigue, malaise, nervousness, mood changes, irritability, trembling, tension, headache, hunger, cold sweats, rapid heart rate, and palpitations. Without immediate reversal of the hypoglycemia with parenteral or I.V. glucose, the blood glucose level will continue to fall. Evidence of progressive central nervous system disturbance includes blurry or double vision, inability to concentrate, confusion, motor weakness, hemiplegia, seizures, loss of consciousness, irreversible brain damage, and death.

Plasma glucose levels higher than 300 mg/dl (15 mmol/L) can also be an urgent situation. Treatment with appropriate insulin dosages can correct the hyperglycemia. (See *Fasting plasma glucose test interference*.)

What needs to be done

- Tell the patient he must fast for 12 to 14 hours before the test.

> Sweating can signify hypoglycemia.

- Advise the patient to avoid drugs that affect test results, as ordered. Advise the patient with diabetes that he'll receive his medication after the test.
- Instruct the patient to report the symptoms of hypoglycemia (weakness, restlessness, nervousness, hunger, and sweating).
- Perform a venipuncture, and collect the sample in a 5-ml clot-activator tube.
- Specify on the laboratory request the time the patient last ate, the sample collection time, and the time he received the last pretest dose of insulin or oral antidiabetic drug (if applicable).
- Send the sample to the laboratory immediately because blood glucose levels decrease when the sample is left at room temperature. If transport is delayed, refrigerate the sample.
- Provide a balanced meal or a snack. As ordered, resume administration of medications withheld before the test.

Two-hour postprandial plasma glucose

The 2-hour postprandial test is a valuable screening tool for detecting diabetes mellitus. This procedure is performed on patients who have symptoms of diabetes (polydipsia, polyuria, and polyphagia) or on patients whose fasting plasma glucose test results suggest diabetes.

What it all means

In a person without diabetes, postprandial glucose values are less than 145 mg/dl (SI, less than 8 mmol/L); levels are slightly elevated in people over age 50. (See *Postprandial glucose levels by age.*)

The lowdown on levels

Two-hour postprandial plasma glucose values of 150 mg/dl (SI, 8.3 mmol/L) or more indicate possible diabetes mellitus. Values greater than 200 mg/dl (SI, 11.1 mmol/L) confirm the diagnosis. High levels may also result from pancreatitis, Cushing's syndrome, acromegaly, or pheochromocytoma. Hyperglycemia may also be caused by hyperlipoproteinemia (especially type III, IV, or V), chronic hepatic disease, nephrotic syndrome, brain tumor, sepsis, gastrectomy with dumping syndrome, eclampsia, anoxia, or convulsive disorders.

Depressed glucose levels can result from hyperinsulinism, insulinoma, von Gierke's disease, functional or reactive hypoglycemia, myxedema, adrenal insufficiency, congenital adrenal hyperplasia, hypopituitarism, malabsorption syndrome, and

> The 2-hour postprandial test helps diagnose diabetes mellitus and monitors drug or diet therapy in patients with diabetes.

some cases of hepatic insufficiency. (See *Two-hour postprandial plasma glucose test interference.*)

What needs to be done

• Advise the patient to eat a balanced meal containing 100 g of carbohydrate (recommended by the American Diabetes Association) before the test and then fast for 2 hours. The patient should avoid smoking and strenuous exercise after the meal.
• Perform a venipuncture, and collect the sample in a 5-ml clot-activator tube.

Advice from the experts

Postprandial glucose levels by age

The greatest difference in normal and diabetic insulin responses — and thus in the plasma glucose level — occurs about 2 hours after a glucose challenge. Normal glucose values can fluctuate according to the patient's age (as shown below). After age 50, for example, normal levels rise markedly and steadily, sometimes reaching 160 mg/dl or higher. In younger patients, glucose levels over 145 mg/dl suggest incipient diabetes and require further evaluation.

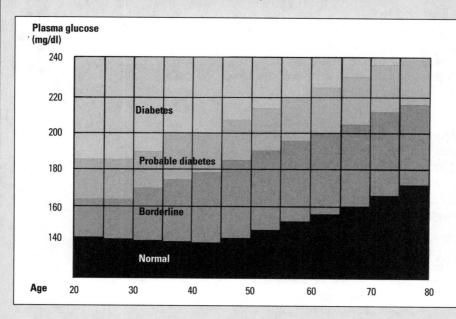

Warning!

Two-hour postprandial plasma glucose test interference

The following factors may raise plasma glucose levels:
• chlorthalidone, thiazide diuretics, furosemide, oral contraceptives, benzodiazepines, phenytoin, phenothiazines, lithium, epinephrine, large doses of nicotinic acid, corticosteroids, and recent I.V. glucose infusions
• recent illness, infection, or pregnancy
• acetaminophen (may cause false-positive findings).
    The following factors may depress plasma glucose levels:
• beta-adrenergic blockers, amphetamines, ethanol, clofibrate, insulin, oral antidiabetic agents, and monoamine oxidase inhibitors
• strenuous exercise.

• Specify on the laboratory request the time the patient last ate, the sample collection time, and the time he received the last pretest dose of insulin or oral antidiabetic drug (if applicable). If the sample is to be drawn by a technician, tell the technician the exact time the venipuncture must be performed.
• Send the sample to the laboratory immediately, or refrigerate it.
• As ordered, resume diet, normal activity, and administration of medications that were discontinued before the test.

Oral glucose tolerance

The oral glucose tolerance test (OGTT) is the most sensitive method of evaluating borderline cases of diabetes mellitus in selected patients. Plasma and urine glucose levels are monitored for 3 hours after a challenge dose of glucose to assess insulin secretion and the body's ability to metabolize glucose. (See *Administering oral glucose solutions.*)

> The OGTT confirms diabetes mellitus and helps diagnose hypoglycemia and malabsorption syndrome.

What it all means

Normal plasma glucose levels peak at 160 to 180 mg/dl (SI, 8.8 to 9.9 mmol/L) within 30 minutes to 1 hour after administration of an oral glucose test dose, and return to fasting levels or lower in 2 to 3 hours. Urine glucose tests remain negative throughout.

Intolerant...

Depressed glucose tolerance, in which levels peak sharply before falling slowly to fasting levels, may confirm diabetes or may result from Cushing's disease, hemochromatosis (a rare disease of iron metabolism), pheochromocytomas, or central nervous system lesions.

...or too tolerant

Increased glucose tolerance, in which levels may peak at less than normal, may indicate insulinoma, malabsorption syndrome, adrenocortical insufficiency (Addison's disease), hypothyroidism, or hypopituitarism. (See *OGTT interference.*)

What needs to be done

• Tell the patient that he must maintain a high-carbohydrate diet for 3 days and then fast for 10 to 16 hours before the test.
• Advise the patient not to smoke, drink coffee or alcohol, or exercise strenuously for 8 hours before or during the test.
• Tell the patient that the test usually requires five blood samples and five urine specimens. Have him bring a book or other quiet di-

Administering oral glucose solutions

The oral glucose load in a glucose tolerance test usually varies from 50 to 100 g. The American Diabetes Association recommends a glucose dose of 40 g/m^2 of body surface area (as calculated by a nomogram based on height and weight).

Many patients become nauseated after drinking the overly sweet glucose solution. To make the solution more palatable, dissolve it in water, flavor it with lemon juice, and chill it. Alternatively, substitute Glucola, a carbonated drink, for the appropriate amount of glucose.

 Warning!

OGTT interference

The following factors may alter OGTT results:
• Carbohydrate deprivation before the test can produce an abnormal increase followed by a delayed decrease.
• Chlorthalidone, thiazide diuretics, furosemide, triamterene, oral contraceptives, benzodiazepines, phenytoin, phenothiazines, lithium, epinephrine, caffeine, large doses of nicotinic acid, corticosteroids, and recent I.V. glucose infusions may increase levels.
• Beta-adrenergic blockers, amphetamines, ethanol, insulin, oral antidiabetic drugs, and monoamine oxidase inhibitors may decrease levels.
• Recent infection, fever, pregnancy, or acute illness, such as myocardial infarction, may elevate levels.

version; the procedure usually takes 3 hours but can last as long as 6 hours.
• Remind the patient that the symptoms of hypoglycemia (weakness, restlessness, nervousness, hunger, and sweating) should be reported immediately.
• Between 7 a.m. and 9 a.m., draw a fasting blood sample in a 7-ml clot-activator tube. Collect a urine specimen at the same time, if your facility includes this as part of the test. After collecting these samples, administer the test load of oral glucose, and record the time of ingestion. Encourage the patient to drink the entire glucose solution within 5 minutes.
• Draw blood samples 30 minutes, 1 hour, 2 hours, and 3 hours after giving the loading dose, using 7-ml clot-activator tubes. Collect urine specimens at the same intervals. Tell the patient to lie down if he feels faint from the numerous venipunctures. Encourage him to drink water throughout the test to promote adequate urine excretion.
• Send blood and urine samples to the laboratory immediately, or refrigerate them. Specify when the patient last ate and the blood and urine collection times. As appropriate, record the time the patient received his last pretest dose of insulin or oral antidiabetic drug.
• If the patient develops severe hypoglycemia, notify the doctor. Draw a blood sample, record the time on the laboratory request, and discontinue the test. Have the patient drink a glass of orange juice or administer glucose I.V. to reverse the reaction.
• Provide a balanced meal or a snack, but observe for a hypoglycemic reaction.
• As ordered, resume administration of medications withheld for the test.

Glycosylated hemoglobin

The glycosylated hemoglobin (Hb) test (also known as the total fasting Hb or glycohemoglobin test) helps monitor the effectiveness of diabetes therapy. Glycosylated Hb levels reflect the average blood glucose level during the preceding 2 to 3 months. This test requires only one venipuncture every 6 to 8 weeks and can therefore be used for evaluating long-term effectiveness of diabetes therapy.

The glycosylated Hb test assesses control of diabetes mellitus.

What it all means

Glycosylated Hb values are reported as a percentage of the total Hb within a red blood cell. Because Hb A_{1c} is present in a larger quantity than the other minor Hbs, it's commonly measured and reported separately. Hb A_{1a} and Hb A_{1b} account for about 1.6% and 0.8%, respectively; Hb A_{1c} accounts for approximately 5%; and total glycosylated hemoglobin accounts for 4% to 7%.

Under control

Good diabetic control is indicated when the glycosylated Hb value is less than 8%.

Out of control

A value greater than 10% indicates poor control. Glycosylated Hb levels approach normal range as therapy begins to control diabetes. (See *Glycosylated Hb test interference*.)

What needs to be done

• Perform a venipuncture, and collect the sample in a 5-ml tube containing EDTA.
• Fill the collection tube completely, and invert it gently several times to adequately mix the sample and anticoagulant.
• Schedule the patient for an appointment in 6 to 8 weeks for appropriate follow-up testing.

Oral lactose tolerance test

The oral lactose tolerance test measures plasma glucose levels after ingestion of a challenge dose of lactose. It's used to screen for lactose intolerance caused by lactase deficiency. Absence of deficiency of lactase causes undigested lactose to remain in the intestinal tract, producing abdominal cramps and watery diarrhea.

Warning!

Glycosylated Hb test interference

• Hemolytic anemia, chronic blood loss, or abnormal hemoglobins (S, C, or D) may lower results.
• Hyperglycemia, thalassemia, or chronic renal failure; dialysis; a recent splenectomy; or elevated triglyceride or Hb F levels may elevate results.

Congenital or secondary?

Congenital lactase deficiency is rare; lactose intolerance is usually acquired as lactase levels decline with age.

What it all means

Normally, plasma glucose levels rise more than 20 mg/dl (SI, more than 1.1 mmol/L) over fasting levels within 15 to 60 minutes after ingestion of the lactose loading dose. A rise in plasma glucose of less than 20 mg/dl (SI, less than 1.1 mmol/L) indicates lactose intolerance. Accompanying signs and symptoms provoked by the test also suggest but don't confirm the diagnosis because such symptoms may develop in patients with normal lactase activity after a loading dose of lactose. Small-bowel biopsy with lactase assay may be done to confirm the diagnosis. (See *Oral lactose tolerance test interference.*)

What needs to be done

• Tell the patient to fast and avoid strenuous activity for 8 hours before the test.
• After the patient has fasted for 8 hours, perform a venipuncture and collect a blood sample in a 7-ml tube with sodium fluoride and potassium oxalate added.
• Administer the test load of lactose—for an adult, 50 g of lactose dissolved in 400 ml of water; for a child, 50 g/m^2 of body surface area. Record the time of ingestion.
• Watch for symptoms of lactose intolerance—abdominal cramps, nausea, bloating, flatulence, and watery diarrhea—caused by the loading dose.
• Draw blood samples at 30, 60, and 120 minutes after giving the loading dose, using 7-ml tubes with sodium fluoride and potassium oxalate added.
• Send blood samples to the laboratory immediately, or refrigerate them if transport is delayed. Note the collection time on the laboratory request.
• As ordered, instruct the patient to resume diet, activity, and medications withheld before the test.

Lactic acid and pyruvic acid

Lactic acid is an intermediate product of carbohydrate metabolism and is normally metabolized by the liver. Lactic acid is present in blood as lactate ion and is derived primarily from muscle cells and red blood cells. Blood lactate concentration depends on

The oral lactose tolerance test detects lactose intolerance.

Warning!

Oral lactose tolerance test interference

The following factors may alter oral lactose tolerance test results:
• delayed emptying of stomach contents, which may depress glucose levels
• thiazide diuretics, oral contraceptives, benzodiazepines, propranolol, and insulin
• glycolysis, which may cause false-negative results.

the production rate and the metabolism rate; lactate levels may rise significantly during exercise.

Deficient or adequate oxygen?

Together, lactate and pyruvate form a reversible reaction that's regulated by oxygen supply. When oxygen levels are deficient, pyruvate converts to lactate; when they're adequate, lactate converts to pyruvate.

Lactic acidosis?

When the hepatic system fails to metabolize lactate sufficiently, or when excess pyruvate converts to lactate because of tissue hypoxia and circulatory collapse, lactic acidosis may result. Measurement of blood lactate levels is recommended for all patients with symptoms of lactic acidosis such as Kussmaul's respirations.

Lactate measurement assesses tissue oxidation and helps determine the cause of lactic acidosis.

What it all means

Blood lactate values range from 0.93 to 1.65 mEq/L (SI, 0.93 to 1.6 mmol/L); pyruvate levels range from 0.08 to 0.16 mEq/L (SI, 0.08 to 0.16 mmol/L). Normally, the lactate-pyruvate ratio is less than 10:1.

When lactate levels are high

Elevated blood lactate levels associated with hypoxia may result from strenuous muscle exercise, shock, hemorrhage, septicemia, myocardial infarction, pulmonary embolism, or cardiac arrest. When no reason for diminished tissue perfusion is apparent, increased lactate levels may result from systemic disorders (such as diabetes mellitus, leukemias, lymphomas, hepatic disease, and renal failure) or from enzymatic defects (such as in von Gierke's disease and fructose 1,6-diphosphatase deficiency).

Lactic acidosis

Lactic acidosis can follow ingestion of large doses of acetaminophen or ethanol, as well as I.V. infusion of epinephrine, glucagon, fructose, or sorbitol.

What needs to be done

• Tell the patient that he must abstain from food overnight and rest for at least 1 hour before the test.
• Because venostasis may raise blood lactate levels, it's best to avoid using a tourniquet; if you do use one, release it at least 2 minutes before collecting the sample, so the blood can circulate.

Tell the patient he must not clench his fist during the venipuncture.
• Perform a venipuncture, and collect the sample in a 5-ml tube with sodium fluoride and potassium oxalate added.
• Because lactate and pyruvate are extremely unstable, place the sample container in an ice-filled cup and send it to the laboratory immediately.
• As ordered, instruct the patient to resume his normal diet.

Pancreatic enzymes

Amylase

Amylase (alpha-amylase or AML) is an enzyme that helps the body digest starch and glycogen in the mouth, stomach, and intestine. In cases of suspected acute pancreatic disease, measurement of serum or urine amylase is the most important laboratory test. Alpha-amylase is synthesized primarily in the pancreas and the salivary glands and secreted into the GI tract.

Serum amylase measurement helps distinguish between acute pancreatitis and other causes of abdominal pain and helps evaluate possible pancreatic injury.

What it all means

Serum amylase levels for adults age 18 and older normally range from 25 to 85 U/L (SI, 0.39 to 1.45 µkat/L). After the onset of acute pancreatitis, serum amylase levels begin to rise in 2 hours, peak at 12 to 48 hours, and return to normal in 3 to 4 days. Determination of urine levels should follow normal serum amylase results to rule out pancreatitis.

Elevations and depressions

Moderate serum elevations may accompany pancreatic injury from perforated peptic ulcer, pancreatic cancer, acute salivary gland disease, impaired renal function, or obstruction of the common bile duct, the pancreatic duct, or the ampulla of Vater. Levels may be slightly elevated in a patient who is asymptomatic or who has an unusual response to therapy.

Depressed amylase levels can occur in patients with chronic pancreatitis, pancreatic cancer, cirrhosis, hepatitis, and toxemia of pregnancy. (See *Amylase test interference*, page 60.)

What needs to be done

• Tell the patient that he must abstain from alcohol for 24 hours before the test.

Warning!

Amylase test interference

Elevate levels
- Aminosalicylic acid, azathioprine, bethanechol, chloride salts, cholinergics, corticoteroids, ethacrynic acid, ethyl alcohol, fluoride salts, furosemide, indomethacin, mercaptopurine, narcotics, pancreozymin, rifampin, oral contraceptives, sulfasalazine, and thiazide diuretics
- Recent pancreatic surgery, perforated ulcer or intestine, abscess, and spasm of the sphincter of Oddi

Decrease levels
- Citrates
- Oxalates

- If the patient has severe abdominal pain, draw the sample before diagnostic or therapeutic intervention. For accurate results, obtaining an early sample is important.
- Perform a venipuncture, and collect the sample in a 7-ml clot-activator tube.
- Handle the sample gently to prevent hemolysis.
- As ordered, resume administration of drugs discontinued before the test.

Lipase

Lipase is produced in the pancreas and secreted into the duodenum, where it converts triglycerides and other fats into fatty acids and glycerol. Destruction of pancreatic cells, which occurs in acute pancreatitis, releases large amounts of lipase into the blood. Also, obstruction of the pancreatic duct prevents the enzymes from reaching their destination, and large amounts of lipase are diverted to the bloodstream.

The lipase test measures serum lipase levels; it's most useful when performed with a serum or urine amylase test.

The lipase test helps diagnose acute pancreatitis.

What it all means

Serum lipase levels normally are less than 160 U/L (SI, less than 2.72 µkat/L).

Obstruction ahead

High lipase levels lasting up to 14 days suggest acute pancreatitis or pancreatic duct obstruction. Lipase levels may also increase in other pancreatic injuries, such as perforated peptic ulcer with chemical pancreatitis caused by gastric juices, and in patients with a high intestinal obstruction, pancreatic cancer, or renal disease with impaired excretion. (See *Lipase test interference*.)

What needs to be done

- Tell the patient that he must fast overnight before the test.
- Instruct the patient to avoid taking cholinergics, codeine, meperidine, and morphine before the test as ordered. If any of these drugs must be continued, note this on the laboratory request.
- Perform a venipuncture, and collect the sample in a 7-ml clot-activator tube.
- As ordered, resume administration of drugs discontinued before the test.

Warning!

Lipase test interference

Cholinergics, codeine, meperidine, and morphine can cause spasm of the sphincter of Oddi, producing false-positive results.

Hepatic enzymes

Aspartate aminotransferase

Aspartate aminotransferase (AST) is one of two enzymes that catalyze the conversion of the nitrogenous portion of an amino acid to an amino acid residue. This enzyme is essential to energy production in the Krebs cycle (tricarboxylic acid or citric acid cycle). AST is found in the cytoplasm and mitochondria of many cells, primarily in the liver, heart, skeletal muscles, kidneys, and pancreas and, to a lesser extent, in red blood cells. It's released into serum in proportion to cellular damage. The change in AST values over time is a reliable monitoring mechanism.

The AST test helps diagnose acute hepatic disease and MI and helps monitor patients with cardiac and hepatic diseases.

What it all means

AST levels range from 8 to 46 U/L (SI, 0.14 to 0.78 µkat/L) in males and from 7 to 34 U/L (SI, 0.12 to 0.58 µkat/L) in females. Values for children are typically higher. AST levels fluctuate in response to the extent of cellular necrosis and therefore may be temporarily and slightly elevated early in the disease process and extremely elevated during the most acute phase. Depending on when during the course of the disease the initial sample was drawn, AST levels can rise, indicating increasing disease severity and tissue damage, or fall, indicating disease resolution and tissue repair. Thus, the relative change in AST values serves as a reliable monitoring mechanism.

The lowdown on levels

Very high AST levels (more than 20 times normal) may indicate acute viral hepatitis, severe skeletal muscle trauma, extensive surgery, drug-induced hepatic injury, or severe passive liver congestion.

High levels (ranging from 10 to 20 times normal) may indicate severe MI, severe infectious mononucleosis, or alcoholic cirrhosis. They also occur during the initial or resolving stages of conditions listed above that cause very high elevations.

Moderate to high levels (ranging from 5 to 10 times normal) may indicate Duchenne's muscular dystrophy, dermatomyositis, or chronic hepatitis. They also occur during initial and resolving stages of diseases that cause high elevations.

Low to moderate levels (ranging from 2 to 5 times normal) may indicate hemolytic anemia, metastatic hepatic tumors, acute pancreatitis, pulmonary emboli, alcohol withdrawal syndrome, or fatty liver. AST levels also rise slightly after the first few days of biliary duct obstruction. (See *AST test interference*.)

What needs to be done

• Tell the patient that the test usually requires three venipunctures—one at admission and one each day for the next 2 days.
• Tell the patient that he must refrain from taking morphine, codeine, meperidine, chlorpropamide, methyldopa, phenazopyridine, and antituberculosis drugs (such as isoniazid and pyrazinamide) as ordered. If any of these medications must be continued, note this on the laboratory request.
• To avoid missing peak AST levels, draw serum samples at the same time each day.
• Perform a venipuncture, and collect the sample in a 7-ml clot-activator tube.
• As ordered, resume medications discontinued before the test.

Warning!

AST test interference

• Chlorpropamide, opiates, methyldopa, erythromycin, sulfonamides, pyridoxine, dicumarol, and antituberculosis agents as well as large doses of acetaminophen, salicylates, or vitamin A may elevate AST levels.
• Strenuous exercise and muscle trauma associated with I.M. injections raise AST levels.

Alanine aminotransferase

Alanine aminotransferase (ALT) is one of two enzymes that catalyze a reversible amino group transfer reaction in the Krebs cycle. This enzyme is necessary for tissue energy production. ALT is found primarily in the liver — with lesser amounts in the kidneys, heart, and skeletal muscles — and is a relatively specific indicator of acute hepatocellular damage.

What it all means

Normally, serum ALT levels range from 8 to 50 IU/L (SI, 0.14 to 0.85 µkat/L).

Highs and lows

Very high ALT levels (up to 50 times normal) suggest viral or severe drug-induced hepatitis or another hepatic disease with extensive necrosis. In these cases, AST levels are also elevated but usually to a lesser degree. Moderate to high levels may indicate infectious mononucleosis, chronic hepatitis, intrahepatic cholestasis (arrest of bile secretion) or cholecystitis, early or improving acute viral hepatitis, or severe hepatic congestion associated with heart failure.

Slight to moderate ALT elevations, usually with higher increases in AST levels, may appear in any condition that produces acute hepatocellular injury, such as active cirrhosis and drug-induced or alcoholic hepatitis. Marginal elevations occasionally occur in association with acute myocardial infarction, reflecting secondary hepatic congestion or the release of small amounts of ALT from myocardial tissue. (See *ALT test interference*.)

What needs to be done

• Tell the patient that he should avoid hepatotoxic or cholestatic drugs, such as methotrexate, chlorpromazine, salicylates, and nar-

The ALT test helps detect and evaluate treatment of acute hepatic disease. It also helps distinguish between myocardial and hepatic tissue damage and assesses the hepatotoxicity of some drugs.

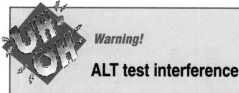

Warning!

ALT test interference

Falsely elevated ALT levels can result from barbiturates, griseofulvin, isoniazid, nitrofurantoin, methyldopa, phenothiazines, phenytoin, salicylates, tetracycline, chlorpromazine, narcotic analgesics, ingestion of lead, or exposure to carbon tetrachloride.

cotics, before the test. If they must be continued, note this on the
laboratory request.
• Perform a venipuncture, and collect the sample in a 7-ml tube
without additives.
• Be aware that ALT activity is stable in serum for up to 3 days at
room temperature.
• As ordered, resume administration of drugs that were withheld
before the test.

The ALP test detects and identifies skeletal diseases. It also detects hepatic lesions.

Alkaline phosphatase

An enzyme most active at a pH of about 10, alkaline phosphatase
(ALP) influences bone calcification and lipid and metabolite transport. Total serum levels reflect the combined activity of several
ALP isoenzymes found in the liver, bones, kidneys, intestinal lining, and placenta.

Bone and liver ALP are always present in adult serum, with liver ALP making up the largest amount—except during the third
trimester of pregnancy, when about half of all ALP originates from
the placenta. The intestinal variant of this enzyme can be a normal component or it can be an abnormal finding associated with
hepatic disease.

What it all means

Total ALP levels normally range from 30 to 85 IU/ml (SI, 42 to
128 U/L).

Although significant ALP elevations are possible with diseases
that affect many organs, they usually indicate skeletal disease or
extrahepatic or intrahepatic biliary obstruction causing cholestasis. Many acute hepatic diseases cause ALP elevations before they
result in any change in serum bilirubin levels. A moderate rise in
ALP levels may reflect acute biliary obstruction from hepatocellular inflammation, inactive cirrhosis, mononucleosis, or viral hepatitis. Moderate increases are also seen in osteomalacia (increased softness of bones) and deficiency-induced rickets.

Climbing the ALPs

Sharp ALP level elevations may result from complete biliary obstruction by malignant or infectious infiltrations or fibrosis. Such
markedly high levels are most common in Paget's disease and, occasionally, in biliary obstruction, extensive bone metastasis, or hyperparathyroidism. Metastatic bone tumors resulting from pancreatic cancer raise ALP levels without a concomitant rise in serum
alanine aminotransferase levels.

Warning!

ALP test interference

The following factors may alter ALP levels:
• recent vitamin D ingestion, which increases levels (from an effect on osteoblastic activity)
• recent infusion of albumin prepared from placental venous blood, which causes a marked increase
• drugs that influence liver function or cause cholestasis, such as barbiturates, chlorpropamide, oral contraceptives, isoniazid, methyldopa, phenothiazines, phenytoin, and rifampin, which can cause a mild increase
• healing long-bone fractures and third-trimester pregnancy, which raise ALP levels
• halothane sensitivity, which may increase ALP levels sharply
• clofibrate, which decreases ALP levels
• patient age (levels typically are elevated in infants, children, adolescents and people over age 45).

A rare low

In rare cases, low ALP levels are associated with hypophosphatasia or with protein or magnesium deficiency. (See *ALP test interference.*)

What needs to be done

• Tell the patient that he must fast for at least 8 hours before the test because fat intake stimulates intestinal ALP secretion.
• Perform a venipuncture, and collect the sample in a 7-ml clot-activator tube.
• Send the sample to the laboratory immediately because ALP activity increases at room temperature in association with a pH rise.
• Tell the patient he may resume a normal diet after the test.

Gamma glutamyl transferase

Gamma glutamyl transferase (GGT), also known as gamma glutamyl transpeptidase, participates in the transfer of amino acids across cellular membranes and, possibly, in glutathione metabolism.

> The GGT test evaluates hepatobiliary disease, assesses liver function, and detects alcohol ingestion. It also distinguishes between skeletal and hepatic disease when serum ALP levels are elevated.

A well-traveled enzyme

Highest concentrations of GGT exist in the renal tubules, where amino acids are reabsorbed from glomerular filtrate, but this enzyme also appears in the liver, biliary tract epithelium, pancreas, lymphocytes, brain, and testes.

What it all means

Normal serum GTT levels range as follows:
- *males:* age 16 and older, 6 to 38 U/L (SI, 0.10 to 0.63 µkat/L)
- *females:* between ages 16 and 45, 4 to 27 U/L (SI, 0.08 to 0.46 µkat/L); age 45 and older, 6 to 37 U/L (SI, 0.10 to 0.63 µkat/L)
- *children:* 3 to 30 U/L (SI, 0.05 to 0.51 µkat/L).

Liver levels

Serum GGT levels rise in any acute hepatic disease as enzyme production increases in response to hepatocellular injury. Moderate increases occur in acute pancreatitis, renal disease, prostatic metastasis, in some patients with epilepsy or brain tumors, and postoperatively. Levels also increase after alcohol ingestion. The sharpest elevations occur in patients with obstructive jaundice or metastatic liver disease. GGT may increase 5 to 10 days after acute myocardial infarction, either as a result of tissue granulation and healing or as an indication of the effects of cardiac insufficiency on the liver. (See *GGT test interference.*)

What needs to be done

- Perform a venipuncture, and collect the sample in a 7-ml tube without additives.
- Know that GGT activity is stable in serum at room temperature for 2 days.

Special enzymes

Acid phosphatase

Acid phosphatases are a group of phosphatase enzymes most active at a pH of about 5. These enzymes appear in the prostate gland and semen and, to a lesser extent, in the liver, spleen, red blood cells, bone marrow, and platelets. Prostatic and erythrocytic enzymes are the major isoenzymes in this group and can

Warning!

GGT test interference

The following factors may alter GGT test results:
- clofibrate and oral contraceptives, which decrease serum GGT levels; aminoglycosides, barbiturates, phenytoin, and glutethimide, which increase serum GGT levels
- moderate intake of alcohol, which causes increased serum GGT levels that may persist for at least 60 hours.

The acid phosphatase test detects prostate cancer and helps monitor prostate cancer therapy.

be isolated in the laboratory; the prostatic isoenzyme is more specific for prostate cancer.

What it all means

Total serum acid phosphatase levels depend on the assay method; they generally range from 0 to 3.7 U/L (SI, 0 to 3.7 U/L).

Moderate and misleading levels

Misleading results may occur if alkaline phosphatase (ALP) levels are high, because acid phosphatase and ALP enzymes are very similar and differ mainly in the optimum pH ranges. Some ALP isoenzymes may react at a lower pH and thus be detected as acid phosphatase.

Acid phosphatase levels rise moderately in patients with prostatic infarction or Gaucher's disease (congenital disease of lipid metabolism), in some patients with Paget's disease, and occasionally in association with other conditions such as multiple myeloma.

Dangerously high levels

High levels of acid phosphatase in the prostate usually indicate a tumor that has spread beyond the prostatic capsule. If the tumor has metastasized to bone, high acid phosphatase levels are accompanied by high ALP levels, reflecting increased osteoblastic activity. (See *Acid phosphatase test interference*.)

What needs to be done

• Don't draw the sample within 48 hours of prostate manipulation (rectal examination).
• Withhold fluorides, phosphates, and clofibrate before the test as ordered. If any of these drugs must be continued, be sure to note this on the laboratory request.
• Perform a venipuncture, and collect the sample in a 7-ml tube without additives. The sample should be iced for delivery to the laboratory. Some laboratories ask for a heparinized tube so they won't have to wait for the sample to clot. If the sample can't be analyzed in less than 30 minutes, it should be frozen.
• Send the sample to the laboratory immediately. Acid phosphatase levels drop by 50% within 1 hour if the sample remains at room temperature without a preservative or if it isn't packed in ice.

Prostate-specific antigen

Until recently, digital rectal examination and measurement of prostatic acid phosphatase were the primary methods of monitoring

Acid phosphatase test interference

The following factors may alter acid phosphatase test results:
• fluorides, phosphates, and oxalates, which can cause false-negative test results; clofibrate, which can cause false-positive results
• prostate massage, catheterization, or rectal examination within 48 hours of the test.

The PSA test screens men older than age 50 for prostate cancer, monitors the course of prostate cancer, and helps evaluate therapy.

the progression of prostate cancer. Now, measurement of prostate-specific antigen (PSA) helps track the course of this disease and evaluates response to treatment.

What it all means

Normal PSA values are as follows:
- *ages 40 to 50:* 2 to 2.8 ng/ml (SI, 2 to 2.8 µg/L)
- *ages 51 to 60:* 2.9 to 3.8 ng/ml (SI, 2.9 to 3.8 µg/L)
- *ages 61 to 70:* 4 to 5.3 ng/ml (SI, 4 to 5.3 µg/L)
- *age 71 and older:* 5.6 to 7.2 ng/ml (SI, 5.6 to 7.2 µg/L).

About 80% of patients with prostate cancer have pretreatment PSA values greater than 4 ng/ml (SI, 4 µg/L). This percentage is higher in advanced stages and lower in early stages.

Not a solo act

However, PSA results alone shouldn't be considered diagnostic for prostate cancer because approximately 20% of patients with benign prostatic hyperplasia also have levels over 4 ng/ml. Further testing, including tissue biopsy and digital rectal examination, is needed to confirm a diagnosis of cancer. (See *PSA test interference.*)

What needs to be done

- Collect the sample either before a digital rectal examination or at least 48 hours after one to avoid falsely elevated PSA levels.
- Perform a venipuncture, and collect the sample in a 7-ml clot-activator tube.
- Send the sample, on ice, to the laboratory immediately.

Warning!

PSA test interference

Excessive doses of chemotherapeutic drugs, such as cyclophosphamide, diethylstilbestrol, and methotrexate may alter PSA test results.

Plasma renin activity

Renin is released into the renal veins in response to sodium depletion and blood loss. Renin secretion from the kidneys is the first stage of the renin-angiotensin-aldosterone cycle, which controls the body's sodium-potassium balance, fluid volume, and blood pressure. The plasma renin activity test is a screening procedure for renovascular hypertension but doesn't confirm it.

What it all means

Levels of plasma renin activity and aldosterone vary with dietary sodium intake, as follows:
- *normal sodium diet:* 1.1 to 4.1 ng/ml/hour (SI, 0.30 to 1.14 ngLs)
- *restricted sodium diet:* 6.2 to 12.4 ng/ml/hour (SI, 1.72 to 3.44 ngLs).

The plasma renin activity test screens for renal origin of hypertension, helps plan treatment of essential hypertension, and helps identify primary aldosteronism.

When renin is up...

Elevated renin levels may occur in essential hypertension (uncommon), malignant and renovascular hypertension, cirrhosis, hypokalemia, hypovolemia caused by hemorrhage, renin-producing renal tumors (Bartter's syndrome), and adrenal hypofunction (Addison's disease). High renin levels may also be found in chronic renal failure with parenchymal disease, end-stage renal disease, and transplant rejection.

...and when it's down

Decreased renin levels may indicate hypervolemia associated with a high-sodium diet, salt-retaining steroids, primary aldosteronism, Cushing's syndrome, licorice ingestion syndrome, or essential hypertension with low renin levels.

High aldosterone

High serum and urine aldosterone levels with low plasma renin activity help identify primary aldosteronism. In the sodium-depleted renin test, low plasma renin confirms this diagnosis and differentiates it from secondary aldosteronism (characterized by increased renin). (See *Plasma renin activity test interference*.)

What needs to be done

- Collect the sample in the morning if possible.
- Instruct the patient to discontinue use of diuretics, antihypertensives, vasodilators, oral contraceptives, and licorice as ordered by the doctor and maintain a normal sodium diet (3 g/day) during this period.
- Explain to the patient that, for the sodium-depleted plasma renin test, he'll receive furosemide (or, if he has angina or cerebrovascular insufficiency, chlorothiazide) and will follow a specific low-sodium diet for 3 days.
- Make sure the patient avoids radioactive treatments for several days before the test.
- If a recumbent sample is ordered, tell the patient to remain in bed at least 2 hours before the sample is obtained because posture influences renin secretion.
- If an upright sample is ordered, have the patient stand or sit upright for 2 hours before the test is performed.
- If renal vein catheterization is ordered, have the patient sign an informed consent form, and explain that the procedure will be done in the radiography department under local anesthetic.

Warning!

Plasma renin activity test interference

The following factors may alter plasma renin activity test results:
- salt-retaining corticosteroid therapy and antidiuretic therapy, which may decrease the level
- oral contraceptives and therapy with diuretics, antihypertensives, or vasodilators, which may increase the level
- radioisotope use within several days before the test
- salt intake, severe blood loss, ingestion of licorice, and pregnancy, which may increase the level.

For a peripheral vein sample

- Perform a venipuncture, and collect the sample in a 7-ml tube that contains EDTA.
- Note on the laboratory slip whether the patient was fasting and whether he was in an upright or supine position during sample collection.

For a renal vein catheterization

- A catheter is advanced to the kidneys through the femoral vein under fluoroscopic control, and samples are obtained from both renal veins and the vena cava.
- After renal vein catheterization, apply pressure to the catheterization site for 10 to 20 minutes to prevent extravasation.
- Monitor vital signs, and check the catheterization site every 30 minutes for 2 hours and then every hour for 4 hours to ensure that the bleeding has stopped. Check distal pulse for signs of thrombus formation and arterial occlusion (cyanosis, loss of pulse, and coolness of skin).

For both methods

- Because renin is unstable, draw the sample into a chilled syringe and collection tube, place it on ice, and send it to the laboratory immediately.
- Completely fill the collection tube, and invert it gently several times to mix the sample and the anticoagulant adequately.

Cholinesterase

The cholinesterase test measures the amounts of two similar enzymes that hydrolyze acetylcholine: acetylcholinesterase (or true cholinesterase) and pseudocholinesterase (also known as serum cholinesterase).

Acetylcholinesterase is present in nerve tissue, the spleen, red blood cells, and the gray matter of the brain. It inactivates acetylcholine at nerve junctions and helps transmit impulses across nerve endings to muscle fibers.

Is something bugging you?

The cholinesterase test has a number of purposes, one of which is to assess for overexposure to insecticides that contain organophosphates.

What it all means

Pseudocholinesterase levels range from 204 to 532 IU/dl (SI, 2.04 to 5.32 kU/L).

> The cholinesterase test evaluates a patient's response to succinylcholine. It also helps identify patients who may have adverse reactions to muscle relaxants.

How low can you go?

Pseudocholinesterase levels are usually normal in early extrahepatic obstruction and decreased in hepatocellular damage, such as hepatitis or cirrhosis. Levels also decline in acute infections, chronic malnutrition, anemia, myocardial infarction, obstructive jaundice, and metastasis.

Very low pseudocholinesterase levels suggest a congenital deficiency or organophosphate insecticide poisoning; levels near zero necessitate emergency treatment. (See *Cholinesterase test interference*.)

What needs to be done

• Perform a venipuncture, and collect the sample in a 7-ml red-top tube.
• If the sample can't be sent to the laboratory within 6 hours after being drawn, refrigerate it.
• As ordered, resume administration of medications discontinued before the test.

Warning!

Cholinesterase test interference

• Cyclophosphamide, monoamine oxidase inhibitors, succinylcholine, neostigmine, quinidine, chloroquine, caffeine, theophylline, epinephrine, ether, barbiturates, atropine, morphine, codeine, phenothiazines, vitamin K, and folic acid can falsely depress levels.
• Pregnancy or recent surgery may alter test results.

Glucose-6-phosphate dehydrogenase

Glucose-6-phosphate dehydrogenase (G6PD), an enzyme found in most body cells, is part of a pathway that metabolizes glucose. The G6PD test, which measures serum G6PD levels, tests for deficiency of this enzyme. G6PD deficiency is a hereditary, sex-linked condition carried on the female X chromosome (with clinical disease found mostly in males) that impairs the stability of the red blood cell (RBC) membrane and makes RBCs susceptible to destruction by strong oxidizing agents.

What it all means

Serum G6PD values vary with the measurement method used but usually range from 4.3 to 11.8 U/g (SI, 0.28 to 0.76 mU/mol) of hemoglobin). They may also be reported simply as normal or abnormal.

Fluorescent spot testing or staining for Heinz bodies or erythrocytes can test for G6PD deficiency. If results are positive, the kinetic quantitative assay for G6PD may be performed. Electrophoretic techniques assess genetic variants of deficiencies (which may cause lifelong, mild, or asymptomatic anemia). Some variants are symptomatic only when the patient experiences stress or illness or is exposed

The G6PD test detects hemolytic anemia caused by G6PD deficiency.

to drugs or agents that elicit hemolytic episodes. (See *G6PD test interference.*)

What needs to be done

• Perform a venipuncture, and collect the sample in a 7-ml tube containing EDTA.
• Completely fill the collection tube, and invert it gently several times to mix the sample and anticoagulant.
• If the sample can't be sent to the laboratory immediately, refrigerate it.

Pyruvate kinase

The erythrocyte enzyme pyruvate kinase (PK) takes part in the anaerobic metabolism of glucose. Abnormally low PK levels are inherited as an autosomal recessive trait and may result in an erythrocyte membrane defect associated with congenital hemolytic anemia.

Although PK deficiency is fairly uncommon, it's the most prevalent congenital hemolytic anemia after glucose-6-phosphate dehydrogenase deficiency. PK assay confirms PK deficiency when red blood cell enzyme deficiency is the suspected cause of anemia.

What it all means

In a routine assay, serum PK levels range from 9 to 22 U/g of hemoglobin (Hb); in the low substrate assay, they range from 1.7 to 6.8 U/g of Hb.

Low serum PK levels confirm a diagnosis of PK deficiency and allow differentiation between PK-deficient hemolytic anemia and other inherited disorders. (See *PK test interference.*)

Warning!

G6PD test interference

• Aspirin, sulfonamides, nitrofurantoin, vitamin K derivatives, primaquine, and fava beans decrease G6PD enzyme activity and precipitate hemolytic episodes.
• Performing the test after a hemolytic episode or a blood transfusion can cause false-negative results.

> The PK assay differentiates PK-deficient hemolytic anemia from other hemolytic anemias. It also detects PK deficiency in asymptomatic, heterozygous inheritance.

Warning!

PK test interference

The following factors may alter PK test results:
• failure to notify the laboratory of a recent blood transfusion
• removal of white blood cells from the sample by the laboratory to prevent false results (PK levels in white blood cells remain normal in hemolytic anemia).

What needs to be done

• Perform a venipuncture, and collect the sample in a 7-ml tube containing EDTA.
• Completely fill the collection tube, and invert it gently several times to mix the sample and anticoagulant.
• Refrigerate the sample if it can't be sent to the laboratory immediately.

Angiotensin-converting enzyme

The angiotensin-converting enzyme (ACE) test measures serum levels of ACE, an enzyme found in high concentrations in lung capillaries and in lesser concentrations in blood vessels and kidney tissue. Its primary function is to help regulate arterial pressure by converting angiotensin I to angiotensin II, a powerful vasoconstrictor.

> The ACE test aids diagnosis of sarcoidosis, monitors response to sarcoidosis therapy, and helps confirm Gaucher's disease or Hansen's disease.

What it all means

Normal serum ACE values for patients age 20 and older range from 8 to 52 U/L (SI, 0.14 to 0.88 µkat/L).

The lowdown on levels

Elevated serum ACE levels may indicate sarcoidosis (a disease characterized by granular tumors that affect any organ or tissue), Gaucher's disease, or Hansen's disease (leprosy), but results must be correlated with the patient's clinical condition. In some patients, elevated ACE levels may result from hyperthyroidism, diabetic retinopathy, or liver disease.

Serum ACE levels decline as the patient responds to steroid or prednisone therapy for sarcoidosis.

What needs to be done

• If the patient is younger than age 20, ask the doctor about postponing the test because ACE levels vary in patients younger than age 20.
• Instruct the patient to fast for 12 hours before the test.
• Avoid using a collection tube with EDTA because this can decrease ACE levels, altering test results.
• Perform a venipuncture, and collect the sample in a 7-ml clot-activator tube.
• Note the patient's age on the laboratory request and send the sample to the laboratory immediately, or freeze it and place it on dry ice until the test can be done.

Lipids and lipoproteins

Triglycerides

Serum triglyceride testing provides quantitative analysis of triglycerides, the main storage form of lipids, which constitute about 95% of fatty tissue. Although not in itself diagnostic, serum triglyceride analysis permits early identification of hyperlipidemia (characteristic in nephrotic syndrome and other conditions) and determination of the risk of coronary artery disease (CAD).

What it all means

Triglyceride values are age- and sex-related. Some controversy exists over the most appropriate normal ranges. Nonetheless, serum values of 40 to 180 mg/dl (SI, 0.11 to 2.01 mmol/L) for adult men and 10 to 190 mg/dl (SI, 0.11 to 2.21 mmol/L) for adult women are widely accepted.

Increased or decreased serum triglyceride levels merely suggest a clinical abnormality; additional tests are required for a definitive diagnosis. For example, measurement of cholesterol may also be necessary, because cholesterol and triglyceride levels vary independently. High levels of triglyceride and cholesterol reflect an increased risk of CAD.

Triglyceride levels help screen for hyperlipidemias, help identify nephrotic syndrome, indicate poorly controlled diabetes mellitus, and help assess the risk of CAD.

Increased levels: Mild, moderate, and severe

A mild to moderate increase in serum triglyceride levels may indicate biliary obstruction, diabetes, nephrotic syndrome, endocrine disorders, or overconsumption of alcohol. Diet and possibly drug therapy are recommended for patients whose fasting triglyceride level exceeds 500 mg/dl (SI, 5.46 mmol/L). The patient should start on a cardiac step 1 diet. Fish oils may also be used to lower triglyceride levels. Markedly increased levels without an identifiable cause reflect congenital hyperlipoproteinemia and necessitate lipoprotein phenotyping to confirm the diagnosis. Severe elevations (greater than 1,000 mg/dl [SI, greater than 11.29 mmol/L]) have a significant association with abdominal pain and pancreatitis. In familial hypertriglyceridemia, patients may exhibit signs, such as eruptive xanthomas (slightly elevated, soft, rounded plaque, usually on the eyelid), corneal arcus (opaque, white ring about the periphery of the cornea), xanthelasma (yellowish tumor found on the eyelids), and lipemia retinalis (a condition in which retinal vessels appear reddish white or white).

Decreased levels

Decreased serum levels are rare, occurring mainly in malnutrition or abetalipoproteinemia (a rare inherited disease characterized by defective apoprotein B synthesis). In the latter, serum is virtually devoid of beta-lipoproteins and triglycerides because the body lacks the capacity to transport preformed triglycerides from the epithelial cells of the intestinal mucosa or from the liver. (See *Triglyceride test interference.*)

What needs to be done

• Be sure to inform the doctor if the patient has an acute illness, infection, fever, or other acute problem that might interfere with the laboratory result.
• Because triglycerides are highly affected by a fat-containing meal, with levels rising and peaking 4 hours after ingesting a meal, tell the patient that he should abstain from food for 10 to 14 hours before the test and from alcohol for 24 hours, but that he may drink water.
• Have the patient sit down for 5 minutes before drawing the blood.
• Perform a venipuncture, collect a sample in a 7-ml tube containing EDTA, and send the sample to the laboratory immediately.
• Avoid prolonged venous occlusion. Remove the tourniquet within 1 minute of application.

Warning!

Triglyceride test interference

• Alcohol ingestion within 24 hours of the test may cause elevated triglyceride levels.
• Long-term use of corticosteroids increases triglyceride levels, as do oral contraceptives, estrogen, ethyl alcohol, furosemide, and miconazole. (Cholestyramine and colestipol hydrochloride either raise or have no effect on triglycerides.)
• Clofibrate, dextrothyroxine, gemfibrozil, and niacin lower triglyceride levels.

Total cholesterol

The total serum cholesterol test measures the circulating levels of free cholesterol and cholesterol esters; it reflects the level of the two forms in which this biochemical compound appears in the body.

What it all means

Total cholesterol levels vary with age and sex. Total cholesterol values for adults and children are as follows:
• *adults:* desirable: less than 205 mg/dl (SI, less than 5.30 mmol/L) for women and less than 190 mg/dl (SI, less than 4.90 mmol/L) for men; borderline-high: up to 240 mg/dl (SI, up to 6.2 mmol/L), depending on sex; high: greater than 240 mg/dl (SI, greater than 6.2 mmol/L).
• *children ages 12 to 18:* desirable: less than 170 mg/dl (SI, less than 4.4 mmol/L); high: greater than 200 mg/dl (SI, greater than 5.15 mmol/L).

Keep the risk in context

The cholesterol level needs to be evaluated in the context of the entire risk factor analysis for each patient. If the level is abnormal, a second cholesterol test should be completed 1 week later to verify the results. Marked fluctuations can occur from day to day. A decision to begin treatment will be based on the number of risk factors and a patient's prior cardiovascular history.

Danger signs

An elevated serum cholesterol level (hypercholesterolemia) may indicate an increased risk of coronary artery disease as well as impending hepatitis, lipid disorders, bile duct blockage, nephrotic syndrome, obstructive jaundice, pancreatitis, and hypothyroidism. Hypercholesterolemia associated with increased intake of fats and cholesterol-rich foods requires dietary changes and, possibly, medication to slow absorption of cholesterol.

A low serum cholesterol level (hypocholesterolemia) is commonly associated with malnutrition, cellular necrosis of the liver, or hyperthyroidism.

Getting to the heart of the matter

Abnormal cholesterol levels commonly require further testing to pinpoint the causative disorder, depending on the type of abnormality and the presence of overt signs. Abnormal levels associated with cardiovascular diseases, for example, may require lipoprotein phenotyping. (See *Total cholesterol test interference.*)

> Total cholesterol measurement helps assess the risk of atherosclerosis and coronary artery disease, evaluate fat metabolism, and analyze the efficacy of lipid-lowering drugs.

Warning!

Total cholesterol test interference

The following factors may alter total cholesterol test results:
• cholestyramine, clofibrate, colestipol, dextrothyroxine, haloperidol, neomycin, niacin, and chlortetracycline, which lower cholesterol levels; epinephrine, chlorpromazine, trifluoperazine, oral contraceptives, and trimethadione, which raise cholesterol levels; androgens, which may have a variable effect on cholesterol levels
• certain vitamins (such as vitamin E) that may cause false elevations
• pregnancy, which may increase levels
• emotional stress and the menstrual cycle
• myocardial infarction, which produces falsely low readings.

What needs to be done

• Fasting isn't needed for isolated cholesterol checks or screening, but fasting is required if part of a lipid profile. If fasting is required, instruct the patient to abstain from food and drink for 12 hours before the test.
• Perform a venipuncture, and collect the sample in a 7-ml tube containing EDTA. The patient should be in a sitting position for 5 minutes before the blood is drawn. Fingersticks can also be used for initial screening when using an automated analyzer. Document any drugs the patient is taking.
• Send the sample to the laboratory immediately.

Lipoprotein-cholesterol fractionation

Lipoprotein fractionation tests are used to isolate and measure the types of cholesterol in serum, low-density lipoproteins (LDLs), and high-density lipoproteins (HDLs). The HDL level is inversely related to the risk of coronary artery disease (CAD); the higher the HDL level, the lower the incidence of CAD. Conversely, the higher the LDL level, the higher the incidence of CAD.

The lipoprotein cholesterol fractionation test assesses the risk of CAD and the efficacy of lipid-lowering drugs.

What it all means

LDL cholesterol: For individuals who don't have CAD, desirable levels are less than 130 mg/dl (SI, less than 3.36 mmol/L), borderline high levels are in the range of 130 to 159 mg/dl (SI, 3.36 to 4.1 mmol/L), and high levels are more than 160 mg/dl (SI, more than 4.1 mmol/L). For individuals who have CAD, optimal levels are less than 100 mg/dl (SI, less than 2.6 mmol/L), and higher than optimal levels are more than 100 mg/dl (SI, more than 2.6 mmol/L).

HDL cholesterol: In males, these values range from 37 to 70 mg/dl (SI, 0.96 to 1.8 mmol/L); in females, from 40 to 85 mg/dl (SI, 1.03 to 2.2 mmol/L).

The lowdown on levels

Decreased LDL levels can occur during acute stress (illness, burns, myocardial infarction), inflammatory joint disease, chronic pulmonary disease, and myeloma. Decreased HDL levels are often seen in patients with hypertriglyceridemia. The HDL level may increase if the elevated triglyceride level is treated.

High LDL levels increase the risk of CAD. Elevated HDL levels generally reflect a healthy state, but they can also indicate chronic hepatitis, early stage primary biliary cirrhosis, or alcohol consumption. Rarely, a sharp rise (to as high as 100 mg/dl [SI, 2.58 mmol/L]) indicates a second type of HDL (alpha-HDL) that may signal CAD.

Normal levels but increased risk

Studies show that 3% of males in the United States have low HDL levels for unknown reasons even though their total cholesterol and triglyceride levels are normal. These males are at increased risk for CAD. Risk levels of CAD associated with HDL values are as follows:

• *dangerously high:* less than 25 mg/dl (SI, less than 0.64 mmol/L)
• *high:* 26 to 35 mg/dl (SI, 0.67 to 0.9 mmol/L)
• *moderate:* 36 to 44 mg/dl (SI, 0.93 to 1.1 mmol/L)
• *average:* 45 to 59 mg/dl (SI, 1.16 to 1.5 mmol/L)
• *below average:* 60 to 74 mg/dl (SI, 1.55 to 1.91 mmol/L)
• *probable protection:* greater than 75 mg/dl (SI, greater than 1.93 mmol/L). (See *Lipoprotein-cholesterol fractionation test interference.*)

What needs to be done

• Tell the patient to maintain a normal diet for 2 weeks before the test.
• Tell him to abstain from alcohol for 24 hours before the test, and to fast and avoid exercise for 12 to 14 hours before the test.
• As ordered, tell the patient to discontinue use of thyroid hormone, oral contraceptives, and antilipemic agents until after the test because they alter test results.
• Perform a venipuncture, and collect the sample in a 7-ml tube containing EDTA.
• Send the sample to the laboratory immediately to avoid spontaneous redistribution among the lipoproteins. If the sample can't be transported immediately, refrigerate it but don't allow it to freeze.

Warning!

Lipoprotein-cholesterol fractionation test interference

• Antilipemic medications, such as clofibrate, cholestyramine, colestipol, niacin, and gemfibrozil, lower values.
• Oral contraceptives, disulfiram, alcohol, miconazole, and high doses of phenothiazines increase values.
• Estrogens, bilirubin, hemoglobin, salicylates, iodine, vitamins A and D, and concurrent illness may alter test results.

Lipoprotein electrophoresis

Lipoprotein electrophoresis is used to determine levels of four major lipoproteins: chylomicrons, very low-density lipoproteins (VDLs), low-density lipoproteins (LDLs), and high-density lipoproteins (HDLs). Classification of patients by the pattern of their lipoprotein levels identifies hyperlipoproteinemias and hypolipoproteinemias.

What it all means

Lipoprotein electrophoresis reference values are as follows:
• *chylomicrons:* 0% to 2% (SI, 0 to 0.02)
• *beta or LDL:* 33% to 52% (SI, 0.33 to 0.52) mass fraction of total lipoprotein

Lipoprotein electrophoresis determines the classification of hyperlipoproteinemia.

Classifying familial hyperlipoproteinemias

Type	Causes and incidence	Laboratory findings
I	• Deficient lipoprotein lipase, resulting in increased chylomicrons • May be induced by alcoholism • Incidence: rare	• Increased chylomicron, total cholesterol, and triglyceride levels • Normal or slightly increased very low-density lipoprotein (VLDL) levels • Normal or decreased low-density lipoprotein (LDL) levels and high-density lipoprotein levels • Cholesterol-triglyceride ratio under 0.2
IIa	• Deficient cell receptor, resulting in increased LDL levels and excessive cholesterol synthesis • May be induced by hypothyroidism • Incidence: common	• Increased LDL levels • Normal VLDL levels • Cholesterol-triglyceride ratio over 2.0
IIb	• Deficient cell receptor, resulting in increased LDL levels and excessive cholesterol synthesis • May be induced by dysgammaglobulinemia, hypothyroidism, uncontrolled diabetes mellitus, or nephrotic syndrome • Incidence: common	• Increased LDL, VLDL, total cholesterol, and triglyceride levels
III	• Unknown cause, resulting in deficient VLDL-to-LDL conversion • May be induced by hypothyroidism, uncontrolled diabetes mellitus, or paraproteinemia • Incidence: rare	• Increased total cholesterol, VLDL, and triglyceride levels • Normal or decreased LDL levels • Cholesterol-triglyceride ratio of VLDL over 0.4 • Broad beta band observed on electrophoresis
IV	• Unknown cause, resulting in decreased levels of lipoprotein lipase • May be induced by uncontrolled diabetes mellitus, alcoholism, pregnancy, steroid or estrogen therapy, dysgammaglobulinemia, or hyperthyroidism • Incidence: common	• Increased VLDL and triglyceride levels • Normal LDL • Cholesterol-triglyceride ratio of VLDL under 0.25
V	• Unknown cause, resulting in defective triglyceride clearance • May be induced by alcoholism, dysgammaglobulinemia, uncontrolled diabetes mellitus, nephrotic syndrome, pancreatitis, or steroid therapy • Incidence: rare	• Increased VLDL total cholesterol and triglyceride levels • Chylomicrons present • Cholesterol-triglyceride ratio under 0.6

• *prebeta or VLDL:* 7% to 28% (SI, 0.07 to 0.28) mass fraction of total lipoprotein
• *alpha or HDL:* 10% to 30% (SI, 0.10 to 0.30) mass fraction of total lipoprotein.

Warning!

Lipoprotein electrophoresis interference

The following factors may alter lipoprotein electrophoresis results:
• failure to observe dietary and alcohol restrictions or recent use of antilipemics, which lower lipid levels
• administration of heparin (which activates the enzyme lipase, producing fatty acids from triglycerides) or collection of the sample in a heparinized tube, which may falsely elevate values
• hemolysis caused by rough handling of the sample.

The types of hyperlipoproteinemias or hypolipoproteinemias are identified by their characteristic electrophoretic patterns. The laboratory reports the type of lipoproteinemia present. Familial lipoprotein disorders are classified as either hyperlipoproteinemias or hypolipoproteinemias. (See *Classifying familial hyperlipoproteinemias*, page 79.)

Six types

The hyperlipoproteinemias break down into six types — I, IIa, IIb, III, IV, and V. Types IIa, IIb, and IV are relatively common. In contrast, all hypolipoproteinemias are rare; they include hypobetalipoproteinemia, abetalipoproteinemia (Bassen-Kornzweig syndrome), and alpha-lipoprotein deficiency (Tangier disease). (See *Lipoprotein electrophoresis interference*.)

What needs to be done

• Check the patient's drug history for use of heparin. Notify the laboratory if the patient is hospitalized for any other condition that might significantly alter lipoprotein metabolism, such as diabetes mellitus, nephrosis, or hypothyroidism.
• As ordered, withhold antilipemics, such as cholestyramine, for about 2 weeks before the test.
• Instruct the patient to abstain from alcohol for 24 hours before the test, eat a low-fat meal the night before the test, and then begin fasting at midnight.
• Perform a venipuncture, and collect the sample in a 7-ml tube containing EDTA.

- When drawing multiple samples, collect the sample for lipoprotein electrophoresis first, if possible, because venous obstruction by the tourniquet for 2 minutes (while other blood samples are being drawn) can affect test results.
- Fill the collection tube completely, and invert it gently several times to mix the sample and the anticoagulant adequately.

Other chemistry tests

Bilirubin

The serum bilirubin test measures serum levels of bilirubin. The main pigment in bile, bilirubin is the major product of hemoglobin catabolism. Serum bilirubin values are especially significant in neonates because excessive unconjugated bilirubin can accumulate in the brain, causing irreversible damage.

The bilirubin test evaluates liver function.

What it all means

In adults, indirect serum bilirubin measures 1.1 mg/dl (SI, 19 μmol/L) or less; direct serum bilirubin measures less than 0.5 mg/dl (SI, less than 6.8 μmol/L). In neonates, total serum bilirubin measures 2 to 12 mg/dl (SI, 34 to 205 μmol/L).

Abnormal indirect level

Elevated indirect serum bilirubin levels commonly indicate hepatic damage in which the cells can no longer conjugate bilirubin. Consequently, indirect bilirubin re-enters the bloodstream. High levels of indirect bilirubin are also common in patients with severe hemolytic anemia, when excessive indirect bilirubin overwhelms the liver's conjugating mechanism. If hemolysis continues, both direct and indirect bilirubin may rise. Other causes of elevated indirect bilirubin levels include congenital enzyme deficiency, such as Gilbert's disease and Crigler-Najjar syndrome.

Abnormal direct level

Elevated direct serum bilirubin levels usually indicate biliary obstruction, in which direct bilirubin, blocked from its normal pathway from the liver into the biliary tree, overflows into the bloodstream. If the obstruction continues, both direct and indirect bilirubin eventually may be elevated because of hepatic damage. In severe chronic hepatic damage, direct bilirubin concentrations may return to normal or near-normal levels, but elevated indirect bilirubin levels persist.

All about jaundice

In neonates, total bilirubin levels that reach or exceed 15 mg/dl (SI, 257 µmol/L) indicate the need for an exchange transfusion. Notify the doctor immediately of the results so prompt action can be taken.

What needs to be done

• Instruct the adult patient to fast for at least 4 hours before the test, although he may drink fluids. (Fasting isn't necessary for neonates.)
• If the patient is an adult, perform a venipuncture and collect the sample in a 7-ml clot-activator tube.
• If the patient is a neonate, perform a heelstick and fill the micro-capillary tube to the designated level with blood.
• Protect the sample from strong sunlight and ultraviolet light because bilirubin breaks down when exposed to light.
• Send the sample to the laboratory immediately.

Homocysteine

Homocysteine, a sulfur-containing amino acid, is a trans-methylation product of methionine. It's an intermediate in the synthesis of cysteine, which is produced by the enzymatic or acid hydrolysis of proteins. The test is useful for the biochemical diagnosis of inborn errors of methionine, folate, and vitamins B_6 and B_{12} metabolism.

What it all means

Normal total homocysteine levels are less than or equal to 13 µmol/L (SI, less than or equal to 13 µmol/L).

The lowdown on levels

Low homocysteine levels are associated with inborn or acquired folate or cobalamin deficiency and inborn vitamins B_6 or B_{12} deficiency.

Elevated homocysteine levels are associated with a higher incidence of atherosclerotic vascular disease. In patients with type 2 diabetes mellitus, studies have shown that homocysteine levels increase with even a modest deterioration in renal function.

What needs to be done

• Perform a venipuncture, and collect the sample in a 5-ml tube containing EDTA.

The homocysteine test diagnoses inborn errors of metabolism, detects acquired folate or cobalamin deficiency, and helps determine the risk of atherosclerosis and neural tube defects.

• Send the specimen to the laboratory immediately to be frozen in a plastic vial on dry ice.
• If a hematoma develops at the venipuncture site, apply warm soaks.

Quick quiz

1. Which of the following may suppress serum potassium levels?
  A. Penicillin G therapy
  B. Spironolactone therapy
  C. Insulin and glucose administration

Answer: C. Insulin and glucose administration, diuretic therapy, or I.V. infusions without potassium suppress serum potassium levels.

2. Your patient's serum sodium level is 130 mEq/L (SI, 130 mmol/L). You should interpret that result as:
  A. below normal.
  B. normal.
  C. above normal.

Answer: A. Normally, serum sodium levels range from 135 to 145 mEq/L (SI, 135 to 145 mmol/L).

3. Chloride levels relate inversely to which of the following?
  A. Bicarbonate
  B. Magnesium
  C. Potassium

Answer: A. Chloride levels relate inversely to those of bicarbonate and thus reflect acid-base balance.

4. Which of the following may cause a false decrease in serum bilirubin levels?
  A. Exposing the blood sample to room temperature
  B. Exposing the blood sample to direct sunlight
  C. Sulfonamide therapy

Answer: B. Exposing the sample to direct sunlight or ultraviolet light may depress the bilirubin serum level.

Scoring

☆☆☆ If you answered all four questions correctly, fantastic! Your blood-testing knowledge shows excellent bloodlines.

☆☆ If you answered two or three questions correctly, good job! You're more persistent than a bloodhound.

☆ If you answered fewer than two correctly, take heart and try again.

Hormone tests

Just the facts

In this chapter, you'll learn:

♦ about hormone tests and how they're performed

♦ what patient care is associated with hormone tests

♦ what factors can interfere with these tests

♦ what hormone test results may indicate.

A look at hormone tests

Hormones are substances that control activities of various tissues throughout the body. They act by altering the rate of synthesis and secretion of enzymes or other hormones, affecting the rate of enzymatic chemical reactions, and altering cell membrane permeability. Each hormone is important to the overall functioning of the body.

Taking care of business

When performing hormone tests, make sure that your patient is comfortable and that he understands the test to be performed. Use clear, simple language and avoid jargon. Inform him that the needle puncture might cause some brief discomfort and that he may feel brief pressure from the tourniquet.

After the test is over

Be sure to label blood samples clearly, and handle them gently to prevent hemolysis. Also, check the venipuncture site for bleeding and, if a hematoma develops, apply warm soaks. If the hematoma is large, check circulation in the extremity distal to the venipuncture site.

Pituitary hormones

The corticotropin test helps diagnose adrenal dysfunction.

Corticotropin

Corticotropin stimulates the adrenal cortex to secrete cortisol and, to a lesser degree, androgens and aldosterone. It increases the uptake of amino acids by muscle cells, promotes breakdown of fats, stimulates the pancreas to secrete insulin, and may contribute to the release of growth hormone. Corticotropin levels vary throughout the day; they typically peak between 6 a.m. and 8 a.m. and decline between 6 p.m. and 11 p.m.

The corticotropin test measures the plasma levels of corticotropin (also known as adrenocorticotropic hormone, or ACTH). The test may be ordered for patients with signs of adrenal hypofunction (insufficiency) or hyperfunction (Cushing's syndrome).

What it all means

Mayo Medical Laboratories sets baseline values at less than 120 pg/ml (SI, less than 26.4 pmol/L at 6 a.m. to 8 a.m.); these values may vary, however, depending on the laboratory.

The lowdown on levels

A higher-than-normal corticotropin level may indicate primary adrenal hypofunction (Addison's disease). In suspected Cushing's syndrome, an elevated corticotropin level suggests Cushing's disease. When corticotropin levels are moderately elevated, pituitary-dependent adrenal hyperplasia and nonadrenal tumors, such as oat cell carcinoma of the lungs, are suggested.

A low-normal corticotropin level suggests secondary adrenal hypofunction resulting from pituitary or hypothalamic dysfunction and implies adrenal hyperfunction due to adrenocortical tumor or hyperplasia. (See *Corticotropin test interference.*)

What needs to be done

• Withhold interfering medications for 48 hours or longer before the test. If they must be continued, note this on the laboratory slip.
• Provide a low-carbohydrate diet for 2 days before the test.
• The patient must fast and limit his physical activity for 10 to 12 hours before the test.
• For a patient with suspected adrenal hypofunction, perform the venipuncture for a baseline level between 6 a.m. and 8 a.m. (peak secretion).

• For a patient with suspected Cushing's syndrome, perform the venipuncture between 6 p.m. and 11 p.m. (low secretion).
• Collect the sample in a plastic tube or in a tube with EDTA.
• Make sure the tube is full because excess anticoagulant will affect the results.
• Pack the sample in ice and send it to the laboratory immediately.
• A temperature of 39.2° F (4° C) is necessary to retard enzyme activity. Immediate transfer of the sample, packed in ice, to the laboratory is essential for reliable test results.

Warning!

Corticotropin test interference

• Corticosteroids can lower levels.
• Estrogens, calcium gluconate, and ethanol can decrease levels.
• Lithium carbonate may interfere with corticotropin secretion.
• Menstrual cycle, pregnancy, a radioactive scan within 1 week before the test, or acute stress or depression may alter test results.

Rapid corticotropin

The rapid corticotropin test, also known as the rapid ACTH test or cosyntropin test, is gradually replacing the 8-hour corticotropin stimulation test as the most effective diagnostic tool for evaluating adrenal hypofunction. It provides faster results and causes fewer allergic reactions than the 8-hour test.

Back to baselines

This test requires baseline cortisol levels to evaluate the effect of cosyntropin administration on cortisol secretion. When morning cortisol levels are clearly high, adrenal hypofunction is ruled out and further testing isn't necessary.

What it all means

Normally, cortisol levels rise after 30 or 60 minutes to a peak of 18 µg/dl (SI, 500 nmol/L) or more 60 minutes after the cosyntropin injection. Generally, a doubling of the baseline cortisol value indicates a normal response and eliminates the possibility of adrenal hypofunction (insufficiency).

Hypofunction junction

In patients with primary adrenal hypofunction (Addison's disease), cortisol levels remain low.

If test results show below-normal increases in cortisol levels, stimulation of the adrenal cortex may be required for a longer period to determine whether the patient has primary or secondary adrenal hypofunction. (See *Rapid corticotropin test interference*, page 88.)

What needs to be done

• The patient may be required to fast for 10 to 12 hours before the test and must be relaxed and resting quietly for 30 minutes before the test. Tell the patient that the test will take at least 1 hour.

The rapid corticotropin test provides faster results to help identify primary and secondary adrenal hypofunction.

- Draw 5 ml of blood for a baseline value in a 5-ml heparinized tube labeled "preinjection," and send it to the laboratory.
- Inject 250 µg of cosyntropin I.V. (over 2 minutes).
- Draw another 5 ml of blood at 30 and 60 minutes after the cosyntropin injection in 5-ml heparinized tubes labeled with the exact draw time and "30 minutes postinjection" and "60 minutes postinjection," respectively. Send the samples to the laboratory immediately.
- Observe the patient for signs of allergic reaction to cosyntropin, such as hives, itching, and tachycardia.

Human growth hormone

Human growth hormone (hGH), also known as growth hormone and somatotropin, is a protein secreted by the anterior pituitary and is the primary regulator of human growth.

The hGH test, a quantitative analysis of plasma hGH levels, is usually performed as part of an anterior pituitary stimulation or suppression test. Such testing is crucial because clinical manifestations of an hGH deficiency can rarely be reversed by therapy.

What it all means

Normal hGH levels for men range from undetectable to 5 ng/ml (SI, 5 µg/L). Normal levels for women range from undetectable to 10 ng/ml (SI, 10 µg/L). Estrogen causes levels in women to be higher than levels in men. Children generally have higher hGH levels; these levels may range from undetectable to 16 ng/ml (SI, 16 µg/L).

The lowdown on levels

Increased hGH levels may indicate a pituitary or hypothalamic tumor (frequently an adenoma), which causes gigantism in children and acromegaly in adults and adolescents.

Patients with diabetes mellitus sometimes have elevated hGH levels without acromegaly. Suppression testing is necessary to confirm the diagnosis.

Pituitary infarction, metastatic disease, and tumors may reduce hGH levels. Dwarfism may be caused by low hGH levels, but confirmation of the diagnosis requires stimulation testing with arginine or insulin. (See *Growth hormone test interference*.)

What needs to be done

- Withhold all medications that affect hGH levels, such as pituitary-based steroids, as ordered. If these medications must be continued, note this on the laboratory request.

Warning!

Rapid corticotropin test interference

- Estrogens and amphetamines increase levels.
- Lithium carbonate decreases levels.
- Radioactive scan within 1 week before the test may alter results.
- Smoking and obesity may increase levels.

The hGH test helps diagnose dwarfism and pituitary or hypothalamic tumors and helps monitor hGH therapy.

Warning!

Growth hormone test interference

- Amphetamines, arginine, beta blockers, bromocriptine, dopamine, estrogens, glucagon, histamine, insulin, levodopa, methyldopa, and nicotinic acid may increase levels.
- Phenothiazines and corticosteroids may reduce levels.
- Radioactive scan within 1 week before the test may affect results.

- Make sure the patient is relaxed and recumbent for 30 minutes before the test because stress and physical activity elevate hGH levels. He needs to fast and limit physical activity for 10 to 12 hours before the test.
- Tell the patient that another sample may have to be drawn the following day for comparison and that the laboratory requires at least 2 days for analysis.
- Between 6 a.m. and 8 a.m. on 2 consecutive days, or as ordered, draw venous blood into a 7-ml clot-activator tube and send it to the laboratory.

Growth hormone suppression

Growth hormone suppression, also known as the glucose loading test, evaluates excessive baseline levels of human growth hormone (hGH) from the anterior pituitary by measuring the secretory response to a loading dose of glucose.

Secretion suppression

Normally, hGH raises plasma glucose and fatty acid concentrations; in response, insulin secretion increases to counteract these effects. A glucose load should suppress hGH secretion. In a patient with excessive hGH levels, the failure to suppress hGH indicates anterior pituitary dysfunction and confirms a diagnosis of acromegaly or gigantism.

What it all means

Normally, glucose suppresses hGH to levels ranging from undetectable to 3 ng/ml (SI, 3 µg/L) in 30 minutes to 2 hours. In a patient with active acromegaly, basal hGH levels are elevated to 75 ng/ml (SI, 75 µg/L) and aren't suppressed to less

The hGH suppression test helps assess elevated hGH levels and can confirm gigantism and acromegaly.

than 5 ng/ml (SI, 5 µg/L) during the test. In children, rebound stimulation may occur after 2 to 5 hours.

Suspicion and repetition

When the hGH levels are unchanged or increased in response to glucose loading, hGH hypersecretion is indicated and may confirm suspected acromegaly or gigantism. This response may be verified by repeating the test after a 1-day rest. (See *Growth hormone suppression test interference.*)

What needs to be done

• Withhold all steroids—including estrogens and progestogens—and other pituitary-based hormones. If these or other medications must be continued, note this on the laboratory request.
• Make sure the patient is relaxed and recumbent for 30 minutes before the test to prevent a false high reading. Tell him that he should fast for 10 to 12 hours before the test and that two blood samples will be drawn.
• Tell the patient that he may experience nausea after drinking the glucose solution and may feel some discomfort from the needle punctures. Tell him that the test takes about 1 hour.
• Between 6 a.m. and 8 a.m., draw 6 ml of venous blood (basal sample) into a 7-ml clot-activator tube. Label the tube, and send it to the laboratory immediately.
• Administer 100 g of glucose solution by mouth. To prevent nausea, advise the patient to drink the glucose slowly.
• About 1 hour later, draw venous blood into a second 7-ml clot-activator tube, label the tube, and send it to the laboratory immediately.

Warning!

Growth hormone suppression test interference

• Arginine, beta-adrenergic blockers, and estrogens increase hGH secretion and may affect test results.
• Amphetamines, bromocriptine, levodopa, dopamine, methyldopa, and histamine increase hGH secretion.
• Insulin, glucagon, and nicotinic acid raise hGH levels.
• Phenothiazines (chlorpromazine) and corticosteroids reduce hGH secretion.
• Radioactive scan within 1 week before the test may affect results.

Insulin tolerance

The insulin tolerance test measures serum levels of hGH and corticotropin after administration of a loading dose of insulin. It's more reliable than direct measurement of hGH and corticotropin. Normally, insulin-induced hypoglycemia stimulates hGH and corticotropin secretion. When stimulation fails, anterior pituitary or adrenal hypofunction is indicated and helps confirm an hGH or corticotropin insufficiency.

No-tolerance patients

Because the insulin tolerance test stimulates an adrenergic response, it isn't recommended for patients with cardiovascular or cerebrovascular disorders, epilepsy, or low basal plasma cortisol levels.

What it all means

Normally, blood glucose falls to 50% of the fasting level 20 to 30 minutes after insulin administration. This stimulates an increase of 10 to 20 ng/dl (SI, 10 to 20 µg/L) over baseline values in hGH and corticotropin, with peak levels occurring 60 to 90 minutes after insulin administration.

Reading responses

An increase in hGH levels of less than 10 ng/dl above baseline suggests hGH deficiency. However, a definitive diagnosis requires a supplementary stimulation test such as the arginine test. Additional testing is necessary to determine the site of the abnormality.

An increase in corticotropin levels of less than 10 ng/dl (SI, 10 µg/L) above baseline suggests adrenal insufficiency. The metyrapone or corticotropin stimulation test then confirms the diagnosis and determines whether insufficiency is primary or secondary. (See *Insulin tolerance test interference.*)

What needs to be done

• Instruct the patient to fast and restrict physical activity for 10 to 12 hours before the test.
• Tell the patient that he must remain relaxed and recumbent for 90 minutes before the test to prevent falsely elevated readings.
• Tell the patient that this test requires I.V. infusion of insulin and the collection of multiple blood samples.
• Warn the patient that he may experience an increased heart rate, diaphoresis, hunger, and anxiety after administration of insulin; these are transient but, if they become severe, the test will be discontinued.
• Between 6 a.m. and 8 a.m., collect three 5-ml samples of venous baseline samples — one in a tube with sodium fluoride and potassium oxalate for blood glucose (laboratory requirements may vary) and two in heparinized tubes for hGH and corticotropin.
• Next, administer an I.V. bolus of U-100 regular insulin (0.15 U/kg or as ordered) over 1 to 2 minutes.
• Using an indwelling venous catheter, draw additional blood samples (as described previously) at 15, 30, 45, 60, 90, and 120 minutes after administration of insulin.
• Label the tubes appropriately, note the collection time on the laboratory request, and send samples to the laboratory immediately.
• Have concentrated glucose solution available in case the patient has a severe hypoglycemic reaction to insulin.

The insulin tolerance test helps diagnose hGH or corticotropin deficiency, pituitary dysfunction, and adrenal hypofunction.

Warning!

Insulin tolerance test interference

• Corticosteroids elevate hGH levels; beta-adrenergic blockers and glucocorticoids depress hGH levels.
• Glucocorticoids, estrogens, calcium gluconate, amphetamines, methamphetamines, spironolactone, and ethanol depress corticotropin levels.

Serum follicle-stimulating hormone

A test of gonadal function that's performed more commonly in females than in males, the serum follicle-stimulating hormone (FSH) test is vital to infertility studies. To make a definitive diagnosis, FSH is typically combined with other hormone testing, such as luteinizing hormone, estrogen, or progesterone.

Flirtin' with follicles

In females, FSH spurs development of primary ovarian follicles into graafian follicles for ovulation. Secretion varies daily, and it fluctuates during the menstrual cycle, peaking at ovulation. In males, continuous secretion of FSH and testosterone stimulates and maintains spermatogenesis (formation of mature, functional sperm). Plasma levels fluctuate widely in females; to obtain a true baseline level, daily testing may be necessary (for 3 to 5 days), or multiple samples may be drawn on the same day.

What it all means

Reference values vary greatly, depending on the patient's age, stage of sexual development, and — for a female — the phase of her menstrual cycle. The following approximate values are for menstruating females:
- *follicular phase:* 5 to 20 mIU/ml (SI, 5 to 20 IU/L)
- *ovulatory phase:* 15 to 30 mIU/ml (SI, 15 to 30 IU/L)
- *luteal phase:* 5 to 15 mIU/ml (SI, 5 to 15 IU/L).

   Approximate values for adult males are 5 to 20 mIU/ml (SI, 5 to 20 IU/L); for menopausal females, 50 to 100 mIU/ml (SI, 50 to 100 IU/L).

The lowdown on levels

Decreased FSH levels may cause male or female infertility. Low FSH levels may indicate secondary hypogonadotropic states, which can result from anorexia nervosa, panhypopituitarism, or hypothalamic lesions.

   High FSH levels in females may indicate ovarian failure associated with Turner's syndrome (primary hypogonadism) or Stein-Leventhal syndrome (polycystic ovary syndrome). Elevated levels may occur in patients with precocious puberty (idiopathic or with central nervous system lesions) and in postmenopausal women. In males, abnormally high FSH levels may indicate destruction of the testes (from mumps orchitis or X-ray exposure), testicular failure, seminoma, or male climacteric. Congenital absence of the go-

> Essential in fertility studies, the FSH test can also help diagnose menstrual disorders and precocious puberty.

nads and early-stage acromegaly may cause FSH levels to rise in both sexes. (See *FSH test interference.*)

What needs to be done
• Withhold medications that may interfere with accurate determination of test results, such as estrogens and progestogen, for 48 hours before the test. If these medications must be continued, note this on the laboratory request.
• Make sure the patient is relaxed and recumbent for 30 minutes before the test.
• Perform a venipuncture using a 7-ml clot-activator tube, and send the sample to the laboratory immediately.
• If the patient is female, indicate the phase of her menstrual cycle on the laboratory request. If she's menopausal, note this as well.

Warning!

FSH test interference

• Ovarian steroid hormones, such as estrogen or progesterone, and related compounds, as well as phenothiazines (such as chlorpromazine), may inhibit the flow of releasing hormones from the hypothalamus and pituitary.
• Radioactive scan within 1 week before the test may alter results.

Plasma luteinizing hormone

The plasma luteinizing hormone test (or the interstitial-cell-stimulating hormone test) measures the amount of luteinizing hormone (LH) in the blood's serum. It's usually ordered for anovulation and infertility studies. For an accurate diagnosis, results must be evaluated in light of findings obtained from related hormone tests (FSH, estrogen, and testosterone levels, for example).

Cycling by

In females, cyclic LH secretion (with FSH) causes ovulation and transforms the ovarian follicle into the corpus luteum which, in turn, secretes progesterone. (See *Luteinizing hormone secretion cycle*, page 94.)

In males, continuous LH secretion stimulates the release of testosterone, which stimulates and maintains spermatogenesis (with FSH).

What it all means
Normal values vary widely, as follows:
• *adult females:* vary depending on the phase of the patient's menstrual cycle; follicular phase—5 to 15 mIU/ml (SI, 5 to 15 IU/L); ovulatory phase—30 to 60 mIU/ml (SI, 30 to 60 IU/L); luteal phase—5 to 15 mIU/ml (SI, 5 to 15 IU/L)
• *postmenopausal females:* 50 to 100 mIU/ml (SI, 50 to 100 IU/L)
• *adult males:* 5 to 20 mIU/ml (SI, 5 to 20 IU/L)
• *children:* 4 to 20 mIU/ml (SI, 4 to 20 IU/L).

LH testing can detect ovulation, help assess infertility, and help monitor ovulation induction therapy.

Now I get it!

Luteinizing hormone secretion cycle

The menstrual cycle has three distinct phases: menstrual phase (days 1 to 5); proliferative, or follicular, phase (days 6 to 13); and, after ovulation on day 14, secretory, or luteal, phase (days 15 to 28). In a normal cycle, the menstrual phase is characterized by endometrial sloughing, corpus luteum degeneration, and new follicle growth. Estrogen and progesterone levels are low, triggering increased secretion of follicle-stimulating hormone (FSH) and luteinizing hormone (LH).

During the follicular phase, the follicle stimulated by FSH reaches full size and increases its estrogen secretion. Simultaneously, FSH decreases while LH increases slowly but steadily.

During the late follicular phase, LH rises sharply and FSH rises slightly. On about the 14th day, within hours of this abrupt LH surge, plasma estrogen levels drop and ovulation occurs. After ovulation, levels of both LH and FSH fall rapidly.

During the final, or luteal, phase, the follicle reorganizes as the corpus luteum and secretes progesterone and estrogen. Within 7 or 8 days after ovulation, if fertilization hasn't occurred, the corpus luteum regresses and progesterone and estrogen levels decrease. The endometrium sloughs, and the menstrual cycle begins again.

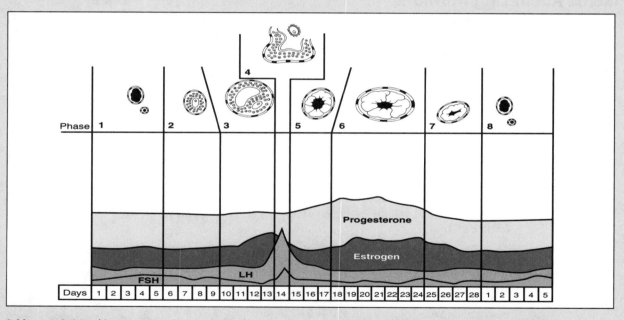

1. Menstrual phase (degeneration of corpus luteum)
2. Early follicular phase (development of follicle)
3. Late follicular phase (development of follicle)
4. Ovulation at midcycle (rupture of follicle)
5. Early luteal phase (development of corpus luteum)
6. Midluteal phase (development of corpus luteum)
7. Late luteal phase (development of corpus luteum)
8. Menstrual phase (degeneration of corpus luteum)

Trouble for the ovaries

In females, absence of a midcycle peak in LH secretion may indicate anovulation. Decreased or low-normal levels may indicate hypogonadism, findings that are commonly associated with amenorrhea. High LH levels may indicate congenital absence of ovaries or ovarian failure, which is associated with Stein-Leventhal syndrome (polycystic ovary syndrome), Turner's syndrome (ovarian dysgenesis), menopause, or early-stage acromegaly. Infertility can result from either primary or secondary gonadal dysfunction.

Dysfunction and failure

In males, low values may indicate secondary gonadal dysfunction (of hypothalamic or pituitary origin); high values may indicate testicular failure (primary hypogonadism) or destruction or congenital absence of testes. (See *Plasma LH test interference.*)

Warning!

Plasma LH test interference

• Radioactive scan within 1 week before the test
• Steroids (may decrease levels)

What needs to be done

• Withhold drugs that may interfere with plasma LH levels, such as steroids (including estrogens or progesterone), for 48 hours before the test. If these medications must be continued, note this on the laboratory request.
• Perform a venipuncture, collect the sample in a 7-ml clot-activator tube, and send it to the laboratory immediately.
• If the patient is a female, indicate the phase of her menstrual cycle on the laboratory request. If the patient is menopausal, note this on the laboratory request.

Thyroid-stimulating hormone

Thyroid-stimulating hormone (TSH) is a protein secreted by the anterior pituitary. It stimulates an increase in the size, number, and secretory activity of thyroid cells; heightens "iodine pump activity," commonly raising the ratio of intracellular to extracellular iodine as much as 350:1; and stimulates the release of triiodothyronine (T_3) and thyroxine (T_4). These hormones affect total body metabolism and are essential for normal growth and development.

Gettin' hip to hypothyroidism

This test, also known as the serum thyrotropin test, measures serum TSH levels by immunoassay. It can detect primary hypothyroidism and can determine whether it results from thyroid gland failure or from pituitary or hypothalamic dysfunction. Normal serum TSH levels rule out primary hypothy-

TSH levels can help diagnose primary hypothyroidism and distinguish it from secondary hypothyroidism. They also help monitor therapy for hypothyroidism.

roidism. This test may not distinguish between low-normal and subnormal levels, especially in secondary hypothyroidism.

The TRH challenge test evaluates thyroid function and can be performed after a baseline TSH reading has been obtained.

What it all means

Normal values for adults and children range from undetectable to 15 µIU/ml (SI, 15 mU/L). TSH levels that exceed 20 µIU/ml (SI, 20 mU/L) suggest primary hypothyroidism or, possibly, an endemic goiter (associated with dietary iodine deficiency). TSH levels may be slightly elevated in patients with normal thyroid function who have thyroid cancer.

Low TSH

Low or undetectable TSH levels may be normal but may occasionally indicate secondary hypothyroidism. Low TSH levels may also result from hyperthyroidism (Graves' disease) or thyroiditis. Testing with thyrotropin-releasing hormone is necessary to confirm the diagnosis.

What needs to be done

• Keep the patient relaxed and recumbent for 30 minutes before the test.
• As ordered, withhold steroids, thyroid hormones, aspirin, and other drugs that may influence test results. If these medications must be continued, note this on the laboratory request.
• Between 6 a.m. and 8 a.m., perform a venipuncture, collect the sample in a 5-ml clot-activator tube, and send it to the laboratory immediately.

Neonatal thyroid-stimulating hormone

The neonatal thyroid-stimulating hormone test, also known as the neonatal thyrotropin test, confirms congenital hypothyroidism after an initial screening test detects low thyroxine (T_4) levels.

The birth surge

Thyroid-stimulating hormone (TSH) levels normally surge after birth and trigger a rise in thyroid hormone, which is essential for neurologic development. In primary congenital hypothyroidism, the thyroid gland doesn't respond to TSH stimulation, which results in lower thyroid hormone levels and higher TSH levels. Early detection and treatment of congenital hypothyroidism are critical to prevent mental retardation and cretinism.

The neonatal TSH test can help diagnose congenital hypothyroidism. Early diagnosis and treatment can prevent permanent brain damage.

Peak technique

Collecting a filter paper sample

To collect a specimen for neonatal thyroid-stimulating hormone testing using the filter paper method, gather the following equipment: alcohol or povidone-iodine swabs • sterile lancet • specially marked filter paper • sterile 2″ × 2″ gauze pads • adhesive bandage • labels • gloves.

    Then follow the easy steps below.
- Assemble the necessary equipment, wash your hands thoroughly, and put on gloves.
- Wipe the infant's heel with an alcohol or povidone-iodine swab; then dry it thoroughly with a gauze pad.
- Perform a heelstick and squeeze the infant's heel gently, filling the circles on the filter paper with blood. Make sure the blood saturates the paper.
- Gently apply pressure with a gauze pad to ensure hemostasis at the puncture site.
- Allow the filter paper to dry, label it appropriately, and send it to the laboratory.

What it all means

At age 1 to 2 days, TSH levels are normally 25 to 30 µIU/ml (SI, 25 to 30 mU/L). Thereafter, levels are normally less than 25 µIU/ml (SI, 25 mU/L).

The lowdown on levels

Neonatal TSH levels must be interpreted in light of T_4 concentrations. Elevated TSH that's accompanied by decreased T_4 indicates primary congenital hypothyroidism. Depressed TSH and depressed T_4 may be present in secondary congenital hypothyroidism. When TSH is normal and is accompanied by depressed T_4, it may indicate hypothyroidism caused by a congenital defect or it may indicate transient congenital hypothyroidism caused by prematurity or prenatal hypoxia. A complete thyroid workup must be done to confirm the cause of hypothyroidism before treatment can begin. (See *Neonatal TSH test interference.*)

What needs to be done

This test can be performed using samples collected from serum or from filter paper. (See *Collecting a filter paper sample.*) For a serum sample, perform a venipuncture, and collect the sample in a 3-ml clot-activator tube. Label the sample, and send it to the laboratory immediately.

Warning!

Neonatal TSH test interference

- Corticosteroids, triiodothyronine, and thyroxine lower TSH levels.
- Lithium carbonate, potassium iodide, excessive topical resorcinol, and TSH injection raise TSH levels.

Thyroid-stimulating immunoglobulin

Thyroid-stimulating immunoglobulin (TSI), formerly called long-acting thyroid stimulator, appears in the blood of most patients with Graves' disease (thyrotoxicosis). This autoantibody reacts with the cell-surface receptors that usually combine with thyroid-stimulating hormone (TSH). TSI reacts with these receptors, activates intracellular enzymes, and promotes epithelial cell activity that functions outside the normal feedback regulation mechanism for TSH. It stimulates the thyroid gland to produce and excrete excessive amounts of thyroid hormones.

About 50% to 90% of people with thyrotoxicosis have elevated TSI levels. Positive test results strongly suggest Graves' disease, but they don't always correlate with overt signs of hyperthyroidism.

TSI testing helps evaluate for thyroid disease and monitor thyrotoxicosis treatment.

What it all means

TSI doesn't normally appear in serum. However, it may be present in 5% of people without hyperthyroidism or exophthalmos.

Increased TSI levels are associated with exophthalmos (abnormal protrusion of the eyeball), Graves' disease, and recurrence of hyperthyroidism. (See *TSI test interference.*)

What needs to be done

• Perform a venipuncture, and collect the sample in a 5-ml clot-activator tube.
• Note on the laboratory request if the patient had a radioactive iodine scan within 48 hours of the test.

Warning!

TSI test interference

Administration of radioactive iodine within 48 hours before the test may alter results.

Thyroid and parathyroid hormones

Thyroxine

Thyroxine (T_4) is an amine secreted by the thyroid gland in response to TSH from the pituitary and, indirectly, to thyrotropin-releasing hormone (TRH) from the hypothalamus. The rate of secretion is normally regulated by a complex system of negative and positive feedback involving three glands: the thyroid, anterior pituitary, and hypothalamus. The suspected precursor, or prohormone, of T_3 is T_4, which is converted to T_3 mainly in the liver and kidneys.

The T_4 that binds

Only a fraction of T_4 (about 0.3%) circulates freely in the blood; the rest binds strongly to plasma proteins, primarily to thyroxine-binding globulin (TBG). This minute fraction of free-circulating T_4 is responsible for the clinical effects of thyroid hormone. TBG binds so tenaciously that T_4 survives in the plasma for a relatively long time, with a half-life of about 6 days. This test measures the total circulating T_4 level when TBG is normal.

What it all means

Normal total T_4 levels range from 5 to 13.5 µg/dl (SI, 60 to 165 nmol/L). Normal T_4 levels don't guarantee normal thyroid functioning; for example, normal readings occur in T_3 thyrotoxicosis.

Results and further testing

Abnormally elevated levels of T_4 are consistent with primary and secondary hyperthyroidism, including excessive T_4 (levothyroxine) replacement therapy. Subnormal levels of T_4 suggest primary or secondary hypothyroidism or T_4 suppression by normal, elevated, or replacement levels of T_3. Overt signs of hyperthyroidism require further testing, and in doubtful cases of hypothyroidism, the TSH or TRH test may be indicated. (See *T_4 test interference.*)

What needs to be done

• As ordered, withhold any medications that may interfere with test results. If these medications must be continued, note this on the laboratory request. (If this test is being performed to monitor thyroid therapy, the patient continues to receive daily thyroid supplements.)
• Perform a venipuncture, collect the sample in a 7-ml clot-activator tube, and send the sample to the laboratory immediately.

Triiodothyronine

This highly specific immunoassay measures total serum content of triiodothyronine (T_3) to investigate clinical indications of thyroid dysfunction. T_3, the more potent thyroid hormone, is derived primarily from thyroxine (T_4). At least 50%, and as much as 90%, of T_3 is thought to be derived from T_4. The remaining 10% or more is secreted directly by the thyroid gland.

This test aids in the diagnosis of T_3 toxicosis, helps diagnose hypothyroidism or hyperthyroidism, and helps monitor the course of thyroid replacement therapy.

Warning!

T_4 test interference

• Estrogens, progestins, levothyroxine, and methadone increase thyroxine (T_4) levels.
• Free fatty acids, heparin, iodides, liothyronine sodium, lithium, phenylbutazone, phenytoin, propylthiouracil, salicylates (high doses), steroids, sulfonamides, and sulfonylureas decrease T_4.
• Clofibrate can increase or decrease T_4.

T_3 versus T_4

Like T_4 secretion, T_3 secretion occurs in response to TSH released by the pituitary and, secondarily, to thyrotropin-releasing hormone from the hypothalamus.

Although T_3 is present in the bloodstream in minute quantities and is metabolically active for only a short time, its impact on body metabolism dominates that of T_4. T_3 binds less firmly to TBG and therefore persists in the bloodstream for a short time—half of it disappears in about 1 day—whereas half of T_4 disappears in 6 days.

The triiodothyronine test helps diagnose hypo- and hyperthyroidism when thyroxine-binding globuin is normal.

What it all means

Normally, serum T_3 levels range from 80 to 200 ng/dl (SI, 1.2 to 3 nmol/l).

Serum T_3 and T_4 levels usually rise and fall in tandem. However, in T_3 toxicosis, only T_3 levels rise, while total and free T_4 levels remain normal. T_3 toxicosis occurs in patients with Graves' disease, toxic adenoma, or toxic nodular goiter. T_3 levels also surpass T_4 levels in patients receiving thyroid replacement containing more T_3 than T_4. In iodine-deficient areas, the thyroid may produce larger amounts of the more cellularly active T_3 than of T_4 in an effort to maintain the euthyroid state.

The lowdown on levels

Generally, T_3 levels appear to be a more accurate diagnostic indicator of hyperthyroidism than do T_4 levels. Although hyperthyroidism increases both T_3 and T_4 levels in about 90% of patients, it causes a disproportionate increase in T_3. In some patients with hypothyroidism, T_3 levels may fall within the normal range and may not be sufficient for diagnosis.

In pregnant patients, it's normal to see a rise in serum T_3 levels. Low T_3 levels may appear in euthyroid patients with systemic illness, during severe acute illness, or after trauma or major surgery; in such patients, however, TSH levels are within normal limits. Low serum T_3 levels are also sometimes found in euthyroid patients with malnutrition. (See T_3 test interference.)

What needs to be done

• As ordered, withhold medications that may influence thyroid function, such as steroids, propranolol, and cholestyramine. If such medications must be continued, record this information on the laboratory request.
• Perform a venipuncture, collect the sample in a 7-ml clot-activator tube, and send it to the laboratory immediately.

Warning!

T_3 test interference

• Heparin, iodides, lithium, methimazole, phenylbutazone, phenytoin, propranolol, salicylates, steroids, and sulfonamides
• Markedly increased or decreased TBG levels, regardless of cause
• Clofibrate, estrogen, liothyronine sodium, methadone, and progestins

• If a patient must receive thyroid preparations, such as T_3 (liothyronine), note the time of drug administration on the laboratory request.

Thyroxine-binding globulin

The thyroxine-binding globulin (TBG) test measures the serum level of TBG, the predominant protein carrier for circulating thyroxine (T_4) and triiodothyronine (T_3). TBG values may be identified by saturating the sample for TBG determination with radioactive T_4, then subjecting this sample to electrophoresis and quantitating the amount of TBG by the amount of radioactive T_4 bound or by radioimmunoassay.

The free Ts

Any condition that affects TBG levels and subsequent binding capacity also affects the amount of free T_4 (FT_4) and free T_3 (FT_3) in circulation. This can be clinically significant because only T_4 and FT_3 are metabolically active. If there is an underlying TBG abnormality, the tests for total T_3 and T_4 are rendered inaccurate; however, this doesn't alter results for FT_3 and FT_4.

What it all means

Normal values for serum TBG by immunoassay range from 16 to 32 µg/dl (SI, 120 to 180 mg/ml).

When TBGs are up...

Elevated TBG levels may indicate hypothyroidism and congenital (present at birth) excess, some forms of hepatic disease, or acute intermittent porphyria.

...and when they're down

Suppressed levels may indicate hyperthyroidism or congenital deficiency and can occur in active acromegaly, nephrotic syndrome, and malnutrition with hypoproteinemia, acute illness, or surgical stress.

Patients with TBG abnormalities require additional testing, such as the serum FT_3 and serum FT_4 tests, to evaluate thyroid function more precisely. (See *TBG test interference*.)

What needs to be done

• As ordered, withhold medications that may interfere with accurate testing, such as estrogens, anabolic steroids, phenytoin, salicylates, and thyroid preparations. If these medications must be continued, note this on the laboratory request.

The TBG test helps evaluate abnormal thyrometabolic states that don't correlate with thyroid hormone (triiodothyronine or thyroxine) values.

Warning!

TBG test interference

• Estrogens and phenothiazines (perphenazine) elevate TBG levels.
• Androgens, prednisone, phenytoin, and high doses of salicylates depress TBG levels.

- Perform a venipuncture, collect the sample in a 7-ml clot-activator tube, and send it to the laboratory immediately.

Triiodothyronine uptake

The T_3 uptake test helps diagnose hypothyroidism, hyperthyroidism, and primary disorders of TBG levels.

The triiodothyronine (T_3) uptake test measures free thyroxine (FT_4) levels. It does this indirectly by demonstrating the availability of serum protein-binding sites for thyroxine (T_4). The results of T_3 uptake are frequently combined with a T_4 radioimmunoassay or $T_4(D)$ (competitive protein-binding) test to determine the FT_4 index, a mathematical calculation that's thought to reflect FT_4 by correcting for thyroxine-binding globulin (TBG) abnormalities.

The T_3 uptake test has become less popular recently because rapid tests for T_3, T_4, and thyroid-stimulating hormone are readily available.

What it all means

Normal T_3 uptake values are 25% to 35%.

In primary thyroid disease, T_4 uptake and T_3 uptake vary in the same direction: A high T_3 uptake percentage in the presence of elevated T_4 levels indicates hyperthyroidism. A low uptake percentage, together with low T_4 levels, indicates hypothyroidism.

Reading the variance

Abnormality of TBG is suggested when the variance in T_4 and T_3 uptake are conflicting. For example, a high T_3 uptake percentage and a low or normal FT_4 level suggest decreased TBG levels. Such decreased levels may result from protein loss (as in nephrotic syndrome), decreased production (due to androgen excess or genetic or idiopathic causes), or competition for T_4 binding sites by certain drugs (salicylates, phenylbutazone, and phenytoin). Conversely, a low T_3 uptake percentage and a high or normal FT_4 level suggest increased TBG levels. Such increased levels may be caused by supplemental estrogen or estrogen produced by the body (pregnancy), or they may result from unknown causes. Thus, in primary disorders of TBG levels, measured T_4 and free sites change in the same direction. (See *T_3 uptake test interference.*)

What needs to be done

- Withhold medications, such as estrogens, androgens, phenytoin, salicylates, and thyroid preparations, that may interfere with test results. If they must be continued, note this on the laboratory request.
- Perform a venipuncture, collect the sample in a 7-ml clot-activator tube, and send it to the laboratory immediately.

Warning!

T_3 uptake test interference

- Steroids, clofibrate, and propranolol
- Markedly increased or decreased TBG levels, regardless of cause

Free thyroxine and free triiodothyronine

These tests measure serum levels of free thyroxine (FT_4) and free triiodothyronine (FT_3), the minute portions of thyroxine (T_4) and triiodothyronine (T_3) not bound to TBG and other serum proteins.

Boundless hormones

As the active components of T_4 and T_3, these unbound hormones enter target cells and are responsible for the thyroid's effects on cellular metabolism. Because levels of circulating FT_4 and FT_3 are regulated by a feedback mechanism that compensates for changes in binding protein concentrations by adjusting total hormone levels, measurement of free hormone levels is the best indicator of thyroid function. Of the two tests, FT_3 is the better indicator. This test may be useful in the 5% of patients in whom the standard T_3 or T_4 tests fail to produce diagnostic results.

What it all means

Normal range for FT_4 is 0.9 to 2.3 ng/dl (SI, 10 to 30 nmol/L); for FT_3, 0.2 to 0.6 ng/dl (SI, 0.003 to 0.009 nmol/L). Values vary depending on the laboratory.

The lowdown on levels

Elevated FT_4 and FT_3 levels typically indicate hyperthyroidism. T_3 toxicosis, a distinct form of hyperthyroidism, yields high FT_3 levels, with normal or low FT_4 values. Low FT_4 levels usually indicate hypothyroidism, except in patients receiving replacement therapy with T_3. Patients receiving thyroid hormone replacement therapy may have varying levels of FT_4 and FT_3, depending on the preparation used and the time of sample collection. (See *FT_4 and FT_3 test interference*.)

What needs to be done

• Perform a venipuncture, collect the sample in a 7-ml clot-activator tube, and send it to the laboratory immediately.

Plasma calcitonin

Plasma calcitonin, a radioimmunoassay, measures plasma levels of calcitonin (also known as thyrocalcitonin), a hormone secreted by specialized C cells of the thyroid gland in response to rising plasma calcium levels. While the exact role of calcitonin in normal human physiology hasn't been determined, calcitonin is known to inhibit bone resorption by osteoclasts and osteocytes and to in-

---

Advice from the experts

FT_4 and FT_3 test interference

Depending on the dosage, thyroid medication may increase levels. However, these medications shouldn't be withheld.

The plasma calcitonin test aids in the diagnosis of thyroid medullary carcinoma.

crease calcium excretion by the kidneys. Therefore, calcitonin acts as an antagonist to parathyroid hormone and lowers serum calcium levels.

This test is usually indicated in suspected medullary carcinoma of the thyroid, which causes hypersecretion of calcitonin without associated hypocalcemia. Uncertain results require further testing with I.V. pentagastrin or calcium to rule out this disease.

What it all means

Normal basal plasma calcitonin levels are as follows:
- *males:* 40 pg/ml (SI, 40 ng/L)
- *females:* 20 pg/ml (SI, 20 ng/L).

    Values after testing with 4-hour calcium infusion are as follows:
- *males:* 190 pg/ml (SI, 190 ng/L)
- *females:* 130 pg/ml (SI, 130 ng/L).

    Values after testing with pentagastrin infusion are as follows:
- *males:* 110 pg/ml (SI, 110 ng/L)
- *females*: 30 pg/ml (SI, 30 ng/L).

Calcitonin and carcinoma

Elevated plasma calcitonin levels in the absence of hypocalcemia usually indicate thyroid cancer. Occasionally, increased calcitonin levels may be associated with ectopic calcitonin production resulting from oat cell cancer of the lung or from breast cancer.

What needs to be done

- Tell the patient to fast overnight.
- Perform a venipuncture, collect the sample in a 7-ml heparinized tube, and send it to the laboratory immediately.

Parathyroid hormone

Parathyroid hormone (PTH), also known as parathormone, is secreted by the parathyroid glands and regulates plasma concentration of calcium and phosphorus.

Two tests are better than one

Currently, two tests are available to detect intact PTH and the N- and C-terminal fragments. Both tests can be used to confirm a diagnosis of hyperparathyroidism or hypoparathyroidism. The C-terminal PTH assay is more useful for diagnosing such chronic disturbances in PTH metabolism as secondary and tertiary hyperparathyroidism; it's also better for differentiating ectopic from pri-

The PTH test helps diagnose parathyroid disorders.

Advice from the experts

The ups and downs of PTH

Parathyroid hormone (PTH) levels vary depending on the disease process involved. The table below shows diseases and their causes as well as their effects on PTH levels.

Disorders	Causes	PTH levels	Calcium (ionized) levels
Primary hyperparathyroidism	• Parathyroid adenoma or carcinoma • Parathyroid hyperplasia	High	High to Normal
Secondary hyperparathyroidism	• Chronic renal disease • Vitamin D deficiency • Calcium malabsorption • Pregnancy and lactation	High	Low
Tertiary hyperparathyroidism	• Progressive secondary hyperparathyroidism	High	High to Normal
Hypoparathyroidism	• Accidental surgical removal of parathyroid glands • Autoimmune disease	Low	Low
Malignant tumors	• Squamous cell carcinoma of lung • Renal, pancreatic, or ovarian carcinoma	High to Normal	High

KEY: High ●   Normal ●   Low ○

mary hyperparathyroidism. The assay for intact PTH and the N-terminal fragment (both measured concomitantly) more accurately reflects acute changes in PTH metabolism and thus is useful in monitoring a patient's response to PTH therapy.

Measuring serum calcium, phosphorus, and creatinine levels with serum PTH is useful in identifying states of pathologic parathyroid function. Suppression or stimulation tests may confirm the diagnosis.

What it all means

Normal serum PTH levels vary depending on the laboratory and must be interpreted in relation to serum calcium levels. The following values are normal:
- *intact PTH:* 10 to 50 pg/ml (SI, 1.1 to 5.3 pmol/L)
- *N-terminal fraction:* 8 to 24 pg/ml (SI, 0.8 to 2.5 pmol/L)
- *C-terminal fraction:* 0 to 340 pg/ml (SI, 0 to 35.8 pmol/L).

Measured together with serum calcium levels, abnormally elevated PTH values may indicate primary, secondary, or tertiary hyperparathyroidism. Abnormally low PTH levels may result from hypoparathyroidism and from certain malignant diseases. (See *The ups and downs of PTH,* page 105.)

What needs to be done

- Tell the patient that he must fast for at least 8 hours before the test.
- Perform a venipuncture, draw 3 ml of blood into two separate 7-ml clot-activator tubes, and send them to the laboratory immediately so the serum can be separated and frozen for assay.

Adrenal and renal hormones

Serum aldosterone

The serum aldosterone test measures serum aldosterone levels. Aldosterone, secreted by the adrenal cortex, regulates ion transport across cell membranes in the renal tubules to promote reabsorption of sodium and chloride in exchange for potassium and hydrogen ions.

Consequently, aldosterone helps maintain blood pressure and blood volume and helps regulate fluid and electrolyte balance.

The serum aldosterone test identifies aldosteronism and, when supported by plasma renin levels, distinguishes between the primary and secondary forms of this disorder. Thus, it's helpful in identifying adrenal adenoma and adrenal hyperplasia, which are causes of primary aldosteronism. Secondary aldosteronism is commonly associated with salt depletion, potassium excess, heart failure with ascites, and other conditions that increase activity of the renin-angiotensin system.

The serum aldosterone test aids in the diagnosis of fluid and electrolyte imbalances.

What it all means

The following are normal serum aldosterone levels, which vary with the time of day and posture. Upright posture is accompanied by higher aldosterone levels, as indicated by these normal values:
- *upright individuals:* 7 to 30 ng/dl (SI, 190 to 832 pmol/L)
- *supine individuals:* 3 to 16 ng/dl (SI, 80 to 440 pmol/L).

Are we talkin' primary or secondary?

Excessive aldosterone secretion may indicate a primary or secondary disease. Primary aldosteronism (Conn's syndrome) may result from adrenocortical adenoma or carcinoma or from bilateral adrenal hyperplasia. Secondary aldosteronism can result from renovascular hypertension, heart failure, cirrhosis of the liver, nephrotic syndrome, cyclic edema with no known cause, or the third trimester of pregnancy.

Depressed serum aldosterone levels may indicate primary hypoaldosteronism, salt-losing syndrome, toxemia of pregnancy, or Addison's disease. (See *Serum aldosterone test interference.*)

What needs to be done

- As ordered, withhold all drugs that alter fluid, sodium, and potassium balance, especially diuretics, antihypertensives, corticosteroids, progesterone agents, and estrogens, for at least 2 weeks or, preferably, 30 days before the test.
- Also withhold all renin inhibitors, such as propranolol, for 1 week before the test. If these medications must be continued, note this on the laboratory request.
- Warn the patient that licorice produces an aldosterone-like effect and should be avoided for at least 2 weeks before the test.
- Tell the patient he needs to maintain a low-carbohydrate, normal-sodium diet for at least 2 weeks or, preferably, 30 days before the test.
- Before the patient rises from sleep, perform a venipuncture, collect the sample in a 7-ml clot-activator tube, and send it to the laboratory immediately.
- To evaluate the effect of postural change, draw another sample in a 7-ml clot-activator collection tube 4 hours later, with the patient in a standing position after he has been up and moving around.
- Alternatively, use a 24-hour urine collection.
- Record on the laboratory request whether the patient was in a supine position or stood during the venipuncture. If the patient is a premenopausal female, specify the phase of her menstrual cycle because aldosterone levels may fluctuate during the menstrual cycle.

Warning!

Serum aldosterone test interference

- Certain antihypertensives that promote sodium and water retention
- Diuretics, which promote sodium excretion
- Some corticosteroids, which mimic mineralocorticoid activity
- Radioactive scan within 1 week before the test

Plasma cortisol

Cortisol helps metabolize nutrients, mediate physiologic stress, and regulate the immune system. Cortisol secretion normally follows a diurnal (daily) pattern: Levels rise during the early morning hours and peak around 8 a.m., and then decline to very low levels in the evening and during the early phase of sleep. (See *Viewing the cortisol secretion cycle.*)

Measuring plasma cortisol levels can help diagnose Cushing's disease, Cushing's syndrome, and Addison's disease.

Signs of stress

Cortisol production is influenced by physical or emotional stress, which activates corticotropin. Thus, intense heat or cold, infection, trauma, exercise, obesity, and debilitating disease influence cortisol secretion.

The plasma cortisol is usually ordered for patients with signs of adrenal dysfunction, but dynamic tests, suppression tests for hyperfunction, and stimulation tests for hypofunction are generally required to confirm the diagnosis.

What it all means

Normally, plasma cortisol levels range from 9 to 24 µg/dl (SI, 250 to 690 nmol/L) in the morning and from 3 to 12 µg/dl (SI, 80 to 330 nmol/L) in the afternoon; the afternoon level is usually half the morning level.

Doin' the diurnal dance

Increased plasma cortisol levels may indicate adrenocortical hyperfunction in Cushing's disease or Cushing's syndrome. In patients with Cushing's syndrome, little or no difference in values is found between morning samples and afternoon samples. Diurnal variations may also be absent in otherwise healthy people who are under considerable emotional or physical stress.

Decreased cortisol levels may indicate primary adrenal hypofunction (Addison's disease). Tuberculosis, fungal invasion, and hemorrhage can cause adrenocortical destruction. Low cortisol levels resulting from secondary adrenal insufficiency may occur in conditions of impaired corticotropin secretion, such as hypophysectomy, postpartum pituitary necrosis, craniopharyngioma, or chromophobe adenoma. (See *Plasma cortisol test interference.*)

What needs to be done

• As ordered, withhold all medications that may interfere with plasma cortisol levels, such as estrogens, androgens, and phenytoin, for 48 hours before the test.

Warning!

Plasma cortisol test interference

• Levels are falsely elevated by estrogens (during pregnancy or in oral contraceptive use), obesity, stress, or severe hepatic or renal disease.
• Androgens and phenytoin may decrease levels.
• A radioactive scan within 1 week before the test may alter results.

Advice from the experts

Viewing the cortisol secretion cycle

Cortisol secretion rises in the early morning, peaking after the patient awakens. Levels decline sharply in the evening and during the early phase of sleep. They rise again during the night and peak by the next morning.

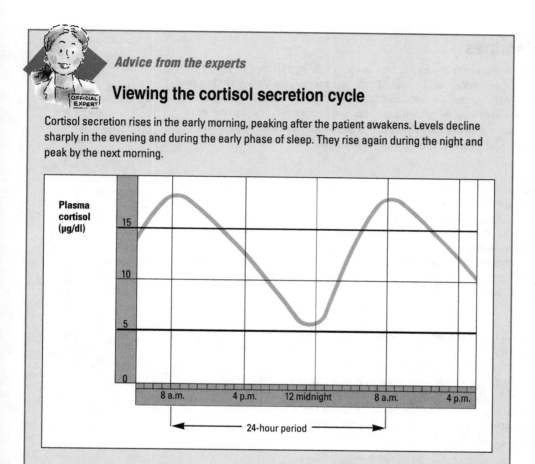

• If the patient is receiving replacement therapy and is dependent on exogenous steroids for survival, note this on the laboratory request as well as any other medications that must be continued.

• Make sure the patient is relaxed and recumbent for at least 30 minutes before the test.

• Tell the patient to maintain a normal-sodium diet for 3 days before the test and to fast and limit physical activity for 10 to 12 hours before the test.

• Perform a venipuncture, collect the sample in a 7-ml heparinized tube at approximately 8 a.m., label it appropriately, and send it to the laboratory immediately. For diurnal variation testing, draw another sample at approximately 4 p.m. Collect it in a heparinized tube, label it appropriately, and send it to the laboratory immediately.

• Record the collection time on the laboratory request.

Plasma catecholamines

The plasma catecholamine test is clinically significant in patients with hypertension and signs of adrenal medullary tumor and in patients with neural tumors that affect endocrine function. In patients with elevated plasma catecholamine levels, supportive confirmation by urinalysis that shows such catecholamine degradation products as metanephrine is needed.

Fight or flight

Major catecholamines include the hormones epinephrine and norepinephrine. When secreted into the bloodstream, adrenal medullary catecholamines prepare the body for the fight-or-flight reaction: They increase heart rate and contractility, constrict blood vessels, redistribute circulating blood toward the skeletal and coronary muscles, mobilize carbohydrate and lipid reserves, and sharpen alertness. (See *Fight-or-flight reaction: The protective response.*)

Sweating it out

The effects of the fight-or-flight reaction resemble those produced by direct stimulation of the sympathetic nervous system, but they're intensified and prolonged. Excessive catecholamine secretion by tumors causes hypertension, weight loss, episodic sweating, headache, palpitations, and anxiety.

Plasma levels commonly fluctuate in response to temperature, stress, postural change, diet, smoking, anoxia, volume depletion, renal failure, obesity, and use of certain drugs.

What it all means

The range of catecholamine levels is as follows:
- *supine*: epinephrine, undetectable to 110 pg/ml (SI, undetectable to 600 pmol/L); norepinephrine, 70 to 750 pg/ml (SI, 413 to 4,432 pmol/L)
- *standing*: epinephrine, undetectable to 140 pg/ml (SI, undetectable to 764 pmol/L); norepinephrine, 200 to 1,700 pg/ml (SI, 1,182 to 10,047 pmol/L).

High catecholamine levels may indicate pheochromocytoma, neuroblastoma, ganglioneuroblastoma, or ganglioneuroma. (See *Clonidine suppression test.*)

Elevations are possible with—but don't directly confirm— thyroid disorders, hypoglycemia, or cardiac disease. Electroconvulsive therapy or shock resulting from hemorrhage, endotoxins, or anaphylaxis also raises catecholamine levels.

Plasma catecholamine levels help rule out pheochromocytoma in patients with hypertension. They also help identify neural tumors, and diagnose autonomic nervous system dysfunction.

Fight-or-flight reaction: The protective response

The fight-or-flight reaction enables the body to confront a threat appropriately and resolve the situation. This innate stress reaction, which is automatic and immediate, helps us survive in dangerous situations. The events that take place during the fight-or-flight reaction are shown in the illustrations below.

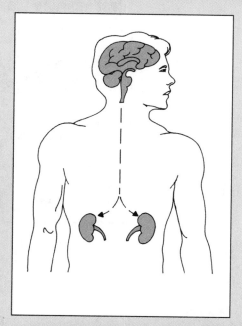

Stress triggers nerve impulse transmission by way of the sympathetic nervous system to the adenal medulla. The medulla releases epinephrine and norepinephrine.

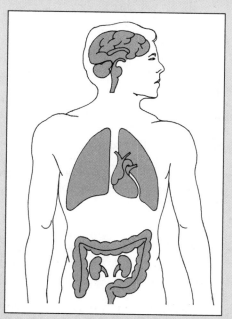

The fight-or-flight reaction increases the respiratory rate, cardiac output, blood pressure, and pulse rate; boosts blood supply to major organs; and decreases blood supply to the skin and intestines.

Peak technique

Clonidine suppression test

This test uses clonidine to help differentiate pheochromocytoma and essential hypertension. To perform the test, place the patient in the supine position. Collect a blood sample to obtain baseline catecholamine levels, and then administer 0.3 mg of oral clonidine. Collect a blood sample after 3 hours to measure catecholamine levels again and allow for comparison of findings.

Interpreting results
Patients with pheochromocytoma show no decrease in catecholamine levels after clonidine administration. In contrast, those with essential hypertension have normal catecholamine levels.

What's the cause?

Fractional analysis helps identify the cause of elevated catecholamine levels. For example, adrenal medullary tumors secrete epinephrine, whereas ganglioneuromas, ganglioblastomas, and neuroblastomas secrete norepinephrine.

In the patient with normal or low baseline catecholamine levels, failure to show an increase in the sample taken after standing suggests autonomic nervous system dysfunction. (See *Plasma catecholamine test interference*, page 112.)

What needs to be done

- If the patient is hospitalized, withhold medications that affect catecholamine levels, such as amphetamines, phenothiazines, sympathomimetics, and tricyclic antidepressants, as ordered.
- Insert an indwelling venous catheter (saline lock) 24 hours before the test as ordered. This may be needed because the stress of the venipuncture itself may significantly raise catecholamine levels.
- Make sure the patient is relaxed and recumbent for 45 to 60 minutes before the test.
- If necessary, provide blankets to keep him warm because low temperatures stimulate catecholamine secretion.
- Tell the patient that the test requires one or two blood samples.
- Tell the patient to strictly follow these pretest instructions: He must refrain from using self-prescribed medications, especially cold or allergy remedies that may contain sympathomimetics, for 2 weeks; he must exclude amine-rich foods and beverages, such as bananas, avocados, cheese, coffee, tea, cocoa, beer, and Chianti wine, from his diet for 48 hours; he must maintain vitamin C intake; he must abstain from smoking for 24 hours; and he must fast for 10 to 12 hours before the test.
- Perform a venipuncture between 6 a.m. and 8 a.m. Collect the sample in a 10-ml chilled tube containing EDTA.
- If a second sample is requested, have the patient stand for 10 minutes, and draw the sample into another tube exactly like the first. If a saline lock is used, you may need to discard the first 1 or 2 ml of blood.
- After collecting each sample, roll the tube slowly between your palms to distribute the EDTA without agitating the blood.
- Pack the tube in crushed ice to minimize deactivation of catecholamines, and send it to the laboratory immediately. Indicate on the laboratory request whether the patient was supine or standing and the time the sample was drawn.

 Warning!

Plasma catecholamine test interference

- Epinephrine, levodopa, amphetamines, phenothiazines, sympathomimetics, decongestants, and tricyclic antidepressants raise plasma catecholamine levels; reserpine lowers them.
- A radioactive scan within 1 week before the test may alter results.

Erythropoietin

This test of renal hormone production measures erythropoietin. It's used to evaluate anemia, polycythemia, and kidney tumors. It's also used to evaluate abuse of commercially prepared erythropoietin by athletes who use the drug to enhance their performance.

What it all means

The normal range by radioimmunoassay is 5 to 36 mU/ml (SI, 5 to 36 IU/L).

Low levels of erythropoietin appear in anemic patients with inadequate or absent hormone production and may occur in severe renal disease. Congenital absence of erythropoietin can also occur.

Elevated levels occur in anemias as a compensatory mechanism in the reestablishment of homeostasis. Inappropriate elevations (when the hematocrit, or HCT, is normal to high) are seen in polycythemia and erythropoietin-secreting tumors.

What needs to be done

• Keep the patient relaxed and recumbent for 30 minutes before the test.
• Explain to the patient that this test determines whether hormonal secretion is causing changes in his RBCs.
• Tell the patient that he must fast for 8 to 10 hours before the test.
• During and after the test
– Perform a venipuncture, collect the sample in a 5-ml clot-lactivator tube, and send it to the laboratory immediately.
– If requested, an HCT test may be performed at the same time by collecting an additional sample in a 2-ml tube with EDTA added.

> Erythropoietin testing can detect abuse of the substance and helps diagnose anemia, polycythemia, and kidney tumors. Erythropoietin use has been banned by the Tour de France and other athletic organizations.

Pancreatic and gastric hormones

Serum insulin

The serum insulin radioimmunoassay is a quantitative analysis of serum insulin levels, which are usually measured concomitantly with glucose levels because glucose is the primary stimulus for insulin release from pancreatic islet cells. The test helps evaluate patients suspected of having hyperinsulinemia resulting from pancreatic tumor or hyperplasia.

Efficient insulin

Insulin regulates the metabolism and transport or mobilization of carbohydrates, amino acids, proteins, and lipids. Stimulated by increased plasma levels of glucose, insulin secretion reaches peak levels after meals, when metabolism and food storage are greatest.

Warning!

Serum insulin test interference

- Corticotropin, corticosteroids, thyroid hormones, and epinephrine may raise levels.
- Use of insulin by type 2 diabetes patients may lower levels.
- High levels of insulin antibodies in type 1 diabetes patients may alter test results.

Measuring serum insulin can help diagnose hypoglycemia, glucocorticoid deficiency, severe hepatic disease, diabetes mellitus, and insulin resistance.

What it all means

Serum insulin levels normally range from 0 to 35 µU/ml (SI, 144 to 243 pmol/L).

Conjunction junction

Insulin levels are interpreted in conjunction with glucose concentration: A normal insulin level may be inappropriate for the glucose results. High insulin and low glucose levels after a significant fast suggest an islet cell tumor. Prolonged fasting or stimulation testing may be required to confirm the diagnosis. In insulin-resistant diabetic states, insulin levels are elevated; in non-insulin-resistant diabetes, they're low. (See *Serum insulin test interference.*)

What needs to be done

- As ordered, withhold corticotropin, corticosteroids (including oral contraceptives), thyroid supplements, epinephrine, and other medications that may interfere with test results. If they must be continued, note this on the laboratory request.
- Make sure the patient is relaxed and recumbent for 30 minutes before the test.
- Tell the patient that he must fast for 10 to 12 hours before the test and that a repeat test may be required.
- Tell the patient that, frequently, a simultaneous glucose tolerance test in which he must drink a glucose solution may be required.
- Perform a venipuncture, and collect one sample for insulin testing in a 7-ml tube with EDTA added; then collect a sample for glucose testing in a tube with sodium fluoride and potassium oxalate added, if requested.
- Pack the sample for insulin testing in ice, and immediately send it, along with the glucose sample, to the laboratory.

• In the patient with an islet cell tumor, fasting for this test may precipitate dangerously severe hypoglycemia. Keep glucose I.V. (50%) available to combat this reaction.

Plasma glucagon

Measuring glucagon levels helps diagnose glucagonoma, hypoglycemia, and idiopathic glucagon deficiency.

Glucagon, a polypeptide hormone, is secreted by alpha cells of the islets of Langerhans in the pancreas. It acts primarily on the liver to promote glucose production and control glucose. This test is a quantitative analysis of plasma glucagon by radioimmunoassay.

What it all means

Fasting glucagon levels are normally less than 60 pg/ml (SI, less than 60 ng/L).

The lowdown on levels

Elevated fasting glucagon levels (900 to 7,800 pg/ml [SI, 900 to 7,800 ng/L]) can occur in glucagonoma, diabetes mellitus, acute pancreatitis, and pheochromocytoma.

Abnormally low glucagon levels are associated with idiopathic glucagon deficiency and hypoglycemia due to chronic pancreatitis. (See *Plasma glucagon test interference*.)

What needs to be done

• As ordered, withhold insulin, catecholamines, and other drugs that could influence the test results. If they must be continued, note this on the laboratory slip.
• Have the patient lie down and relax for 30 minutes before the test.
• Tell the patient that he must fast for 10 to 12 hours before the test.
• Perform a venipuncture, and collect the sample in a chilled, 10-ml tube with EDTA added.
• Place the sample on ice, and send it to the laboratory immediately.

Warning!

Plasma glucagon test interference

• Exercise, stress, prolonged fasting, insulin, and catecholamines increase levels.
• Radioactive scans and tests within 48 hours before the test may alter results.

Gastrin

Gastrin is a polypeptide hormone produced and stored primarily in the antrum of the stomach and, to a lesser degree, in the islets of Langerhans. Gastrin's main function is to promote food digestion by triggering gastric acid secretion. Gastrin's secondary functions are to stimulate the release of pancreatic enzymes and the gastric enzyme pepsin, increase gastric and intestinal motility, and stimulate bile flow from the liver.

Abnormal gastrin secretion can result from tumors (gastrinomas) and from pathologic disorders affecting the stomach, pancreas and, less commonly, esophagus and small bowel. (See *Gastrin stimulation tests: The whys and hows.*)

Unclear ulcers

Gastrin analysis is useful in patients with suspected gastrinomas (Zollinger-Ellison syndrome). If the situation is doubtful, provocative testing may be necessary.

What it all means

Normal serum gastrin levels are 50 to 150 pg/ml (SI, 50 to 150 ng/L).

Strikingly high serum gastrin levels (over 1,000 pg/ml [SI, 1,000 ng/L]) confirm Zollinger-Ellison syndrome. Levels as high as 450,000 pg/ml [SI, 450,000 ng/L] have been reported.

Gastrin levels and pH

Gastrin levels may be high in various conditions, but the finding of very low gastric juice pH in conjunction with a very high serum gastrin level indicates autonomous hormone secretion not governed by a negative feed-

Analyzing gastrin levels helps confirm gastrinoma or the gastrin-secreting tumor in Zollinger-Ellison syndrome. It can also help distinguish between gastric and duodenal ulcers.

Peak technique

Gastrin stimulation tests: The whys and hows

Because some patients with duodenal or gastric ulcers have normal fasting gastrin levels, provocative testing is necessary to identify them; a protein-rich test meal serves this purpose. With duodenal gastric ulcers, gastrin levels increase markedly after such a meal.

Other indications

Provocative testing also distinguishes duodenal or gastric ulcers from Zollinger-Ellison syndrome, both of which may cause similar baseline gastrin levels. One test involves I.V. infusion of calcium gluconate (5 mg/kg of body weight over 3 hours). After the infusion, 10 ml of venous blood is drawn and sent to the laboratory. In Zollinger-Ellison syndrome, gastrin levels double, rising to about 500 pg/ml (SI, 500 ng/L); in duodenal or gastric ulcers, levels rise only moderately or don't change at all.

A third indication for provocative testing is an abnormally—but not strikingly—high fasting serum gastrin level, as in Zollinger-Ellison syndrome and pernicious anemia. To distinguish between the two, hydrochloric acid may be infused into the stomach through a nasogastric tube. Such infusion causes a sharp drop in gastrin levels in patients with pernicious anemia but not in those with Zollinger-Ellison syndrome.

back mechanism. Increased serum levels of gastrin may occur in a few patients with duodenal ulceration (less than 1%), in patients with achlorhydria (with or without pernicious anemia), or in patients with extensive stomach carcinoma (because of hyposecretion of gastric juices and hydrochloric acid). (See *Gastrin test interference.*)

What needs to be done

• As ordered, withhold all medications that may interfere with test results, especially anticholinergics—such as atropine and belladonna—and insulin. If these medications must be continued, note this on the laboratory request.
• Because stress can increase gastrin levels, make sure the patient is relaxed and recumbent for at least 30 minutes before the test.
• Tell the patient that he must abstain from alcohol for at least 24 hours and fast for 12 hours before the test (water is permitted).
• Perform a venipuncture, and collect the sample in a 10- to 15-ml clot-activator tube.
• To prevent destruction of serum gastrin by proteolytic enzymes, send the sample to the laboratory immediately to have the serum separated and frozen.

Warning!

Gastrin test interference

• Gastrin secretion is increased by amino acids (especially glycine), calcium carbonate, acetylcholine, calcium chloride, and ethanol; it's decreased by anticholinergics (atropine), hydrochloric acid, and secretin (a strongly basic polypeptide).
• Insulin-induced hypoglycemia increases gastrin secretion.

Gonadal hormones

Estrogens

Estrogens and progesterone are secreted by the ovaries. They're responsible for the development of secondary female sexual characteristics and for normal menstruation.

Estrogen through the years

Usually undetectable in children, these hormones are secreted by ovarian follicular cells during the first half of the menstrual cycle and by the corpus luteum during the luteal phase and during pregnancy. In menopause, estrogen secretion drops to a constant, low level. Three estrogens are present in the blood in measurable amounts: estrone, estradiol (which is the most potent), and estriol.

Radioimmunoassay measures serum levels of estradiol and estriol, which are used to evaluate abnormal ovarian function. (See *Predicting premature labor,* page 118.)

Tests of hypothalamic-pituitary function may be required to confirm the diagnosis.

Estrogen tests help determine fetal well-being, infertility, precocious or delayed puberty, and menstrual disorders.

Peak technique

Predicting premature labor

A simple salivary test can help determine whether a pregnant woman is at risk for premature labor. The test, known as SalEst, measures salivary levels of estriol, an estrogen that increases 1,000-fold during pregnancy. For at-risk women, the SalEst test is 98% accurate in ruling out premature labor and delivery.

Positive means premature
The test is performed on women between weeks 22 and 36 of gestation using their saliva and the SalEst test kit. Estriol has been found to increase 2 to 3 weeks before spontaneous onset of labor and delivery. A positive test confirms that the patient is at risk for premature labor.

What it all means

Normal serum estradiol levels for women vary widely during the menstrual cycle, ranging from 26 to 149 pg/ml (SI, 90 to 550 pmol/L). The range for postmenopausal women is 0 to 34 pg/ml (SI, 0 to 125 pmol/L).

Serum estradiol levels in men range from 12 to 34 pg/ml (SI, 40 to 125 pmol/L). In children under age 6, the normal level of serum estradiol is 3 to 10 pg/ml (SI, 10 to 36 pmol/L).

Estriol is secreted in large amounts by the placenta during pregnancy. Levels range from 2 ng/ml (SI, 7 nmol/L) by 30 weeks of pregnancy to 30 ng/ml (SI, 105 nmol/L) by week 40.

Estrogen effects

Decreased estrogen levels may indicate primary hypogonadism, or ovarian failure, such as in Turner's syndrome or ovarian agenesis; secondary hypogonadism such as in hypopituitarism; or menopause.

Abnormally high estrogen levels may occur with estrogen-producing tumors, in precocious puberty, and in severe hepatic disease, such as cirrhosis, that prevents clearance of plasma estrogens. High levels may also result from congenital adrenal hyperplasia (increased conversion of androgens to estrogen). (See *Estrogen test interference*.)

What needs to be done

- Withhold all steroid and pituitary-based hormones. If they must be continued, note this on the laboratory slip.

Warning!

Estrogen test interference

- Pregnancy and pretest use of estrogens such as oral contraceptives, which may increase estrogen levels
- Clomiphene, an estrogen antagonist
- Steroids and pituitary-based hormones such as dexamethasone.

- Perform a venipuncture, and collect the sample in a 10-ml clot-activator tube.
- If the patient is premenopausal, indicate the phase of her menstrual cycle on the laboratory slip.
- Send the sample to the laboratory immediately.

Plasma progesterone

Progesterone, an ovarian steroid hormone secreted by the corpus luteum, helps prepare the endometrium for implantation of the fertilized ovum. Progesterone levels peak during the midluteal phase of the menstrual cycle, and they may prolong the surge of luteinizing hormone after ovulation. If implantation doesn't occur, progesterone (and estrogen) levels drop sharply and menstruation begins about 2 days later.

Progesterone and pregnancy

During pregnancy, the placenta releases about 10 times the normal monthly amount of progesterone to maintain the pregnancy. Increased secretion begins toward the end of the first trimester and continues until delivery.

The plasma progesterone test measures plasma progesterone levels. It provides reliable information about corpus luteum function in fertility studies or placental function in pregnancy. Serial determinations are recommended. Although plasma levels provide accurate information, progesterone can also be monitored by measuring urine pregnanediol, a catabolite of progesterone.

What it all means

Normal values during menstruation are as follows:
- *follicular phase:* less than 150 ng/dl (SI, less than 5 nmol/L)
- *luteal phase:* 300 to 1,200 ng/dl (SI, 10 to 40 nmol/L).
    Normal values during pregnancy are as follows:
- *first trimester:* 1,500 to 5,000 ng/dl (SI, 50 to 160 nmol/L)
- *second and third trimesters:* 8,000 to 20,000 ng/dl (SI, 250 to 650 nmol/L).
    Normal values menopausal women are 10 to 22 ng/dl (SI, less than 2 nmol/L).

The lowdown on levels

Elevated progesterone levels may indicate ovulation, luteinizing tumors, ovarian cysts that produce progesterone, or adrenocortical

Plasma progesterone levels help assess placental function during pregnancy, confirm ovulation, and help assess corpus luteum function.

hyperplasias and tumors that produce progesterone along with other steroidal hormones.

Low progesterone levels are associated with amenorrhea, which can have several causes (such as panhypopituitarism or gonadal dysfunction), toxemia of pregnancy, threatened abortion, and fetal death. (See *Plasma progesterone test interference*.)

What needs to be done

• Tell the patient that this test may be repeated at specific times coinciding with phases of her menstrual cycle or at each prenatal visit.
• Perform a venipuncture, and collect the sample in a 7-ml heparinized tube.
• Completely fill the collection tube; then invert it gently at least 10 times to adequately mix the sample and the anticoagulant.
• Indicate the date of the patient's last menstrual period and the phase of her cycle on the laboratory request. If the patient is pregnant, indicate the month of gestation.
• Send the sample to the laboratory immediately.

Warning!

Plasma progesterone test interference

• Progesterone or estrogen therapy
• Radioisotopes or scans within 1 week before the test

Testosterone

The principal androgen secreted by the interstitial cells of the testes (Leydig's cells), testosterone induces puberty in the male and maintains male secondary sex characteristics.

Time for testosterone

Testosterone production begins to increase at the onset of puberty and continues to rise during adulthood. Production begins to taper off at about age 40, eventually dropping to approximately one-fifth the peak level by age 80. In females, the adrenal glands and the ovaries secrete small amounts of testosterone.

Testing testosterone

This test measures plasma or serum testosterone levels. When results are combined with measurements of plasma gonadotropin (follicle-stimulating hormone and luteinizing hormone) levels, it reliably aids evaluation of gonadal dysfunction in males and females.

What it all means

Normal levels of testosterone are as follows (laboratory values vary slightly):

> Testosterone levels help evaluate male infertility or other sexual dysfunction and diagnose hypogonadism.

- *males:* 300 to 1,200 ng/dl (SI, 10.4 to 41.6 nmol/L)
- *females:* 20 to 80 ng/dl (SI, 0.7 to 2.8 nmol/L)
- *prepubertal children:* values lower than adult levels.

Testosterone highs

Elevated testosterone levels in prepubertal males may indicate true sexual precocity (development occurs earlier than expected) caused by excessive gonadotropin secretion, or they may indicate pseudoprecocious puberty caused by male hormone production by a testicular tumor. They can also indicate congenital adrenal hyperplasia (excessive proliferation of normal cells), which results in precocious puberty in males (from ages 2 to 3) and pseudohermaphroditism and milder development of secondary sexual characteristics of females. Increased levels can occur with a benign or malignant adrenal tumor, hyperthyroidism, or beginning puberty. In females with ovarian tumors or polycystic ovarian syndrome, testosterone levels may rise, leading to hirsutism (excessive hair growth in unusual places).

Testosterone lows

Depressed testosterone levels can indicate primary hypogonadism (as in Klinefelter's syndrome) or secondary hypogonadism (hypogonadotropic eunuchoidism) from hypothalamic-pituitary dysfunction. Depressed testosterone levels can also follow orchiectomy, testicular or prostatic cancer, delayed male puberty, estrogen therapy, or cirrhosis. (See *Testosterone test interference.*)

What needs to be done

- Perform a venipuncture, and collect the sample in a 7-ml clot-activator tube. Use a heparinized tube if plasma is to be collected.
- Indicate the patient's age, sex, and history of hormone therapy on the laboratory request.
- The sample is stable and requires no refrigeration or preservative for up to 1 week. Frozen samples are stable for at least 6 months.

Warning!

Testosterone test interference

- Exogenous sources of estrogens or androgens, thyroid and growth hormones, and other pituitary-based hormones may alter results.
- Estrogens decrease free testosterone levels by increasing sex hormone–binding globulin, which binds testosterone; androgens can elevate these levels.

Placental hormone

Human chorionic gonadotropin

Human chorionic gonadotropin (hCG) is a hormone produced by the trophoblastic cells of the placenta. When conception occurs, the hCG assay may detect this hormone in the blood as early as

9 days after ovulation. This interval coincides with implantation of the fertilized ovum into the uterine wall.

hCG comes early

Although the precise function of this hormone is still unclear, hCG, along with progesterone, appears to maintain the corpus luteum during early pregnancy. Production of hCG increases steadily during the first trimester, peaking around the 10th week of gestation.

This serum immunoassay is more sensitive (and costly) than the routine pregnancy test using a urine specimen.

What it all means

Normal values for hCG are less than 4 mIU/L (SI, 4 IU/L). During pregnancy, hCG levels are quite variable and depend partially on the number of days since the last normal menstrual period.

The lowdown on levels

Elevated hCG levels indicate pregnancy; significantly higher concentrations are present in a multiple pregnancy. Increased levels may also suggest hydatidiform mole, trophoblastic neoplasm of the placenta, or nontrophoblastic carcinomas that secrete hCG (including gastric, pancreatic, and ovarian adenocarcinomas). Because levels are high in both conditions, hCG levels can't differentiate between pregnancy and tumor recurrence.

Low hCG levels can occur in ectopic pregnancy or pregnancy of fewer than 9 days. (See *Interference with hCG tests*.)

What needs to be done

- Perform a venipuncture, and collect the sample in a 7-ml clot-activator tube.
- Send the sample to the laboratory immediately.

> Testing hCG can detect pregnancy early and can also be used to monitor ovulation and conception, determine adequate hormone production in high-risk pregnancy, and help diagnose certain tumors.

Warning!

Interference with hCG tests

Heparin anticoagulants and EDTA depress plasma hCG.

Quick quiz

1. Which test assesses corpus luteum function?
   A. Plasma progesterone
   B. Estrogen
   C. Placental hormone

Answer: A. The plasma progesterone test assesses corpus luteum function as part of infertility studies.

2. Which drug can decrease hCG secretion?
   A. Estrogens
   B. Insulin
   C. Phenothiazines

Answer: C. Phenothiazines can reduce hCG secretion.

3. Which pretest precaution must the patient follow when preparing for a plasma catecholamine test?
   A. Limit vitamin C intake.
   B. Stay in a cool environment.
   C. Avoid amine-rich foods.

Answer: C. The patient must exclude amine-rich foods and beverages from the diet for 48 hours before a catecholamine test.

4. Which test helps diagnose anemia and polycythemia?
   A. Catecholamines
   B. Erythropoietin
   C. Plasma cortisol

Answer: B. An erythropoietin test can help diagnose anemia and polycythemia.

5. A serum gastrin level above 1,000 pg/ml (SI, 1,000 ng/L) confirms which disorder?
   A. Zollinger-Ellison syndrome
   B. Ganglioblastoma
   C. Addison's disease

Answer: A. A serum gastrin level above 1,000 pg/ml (SI, 1,000 ng/L) confirms Zollinger-Ellison syndrome.

Scoring

☆☆☆   If you answered all five questions correctly, wow! You're the Hercules of hormones!

☆☆   If you answered three or four questions correctly, excellent! You're cruisin' with cortisol!

☆   If you answered fewer than three correctly, hang in there. You'll be doing the hormone hoedown before you know it!

Immunologic tests

Just the facts

In this chapter, you'll learn:

♦ about immunologic tests and how they're performed

♦ what patient care is associated with immunologic tests

♦ what factors can interfere with these tests

♦ what immunologic test results may indicate.

A look at immunologic tests

Before immunologic testing, make sure that your patient understands the test to be performed. Use a clear, simple explanation. Inform him that the test requires a venipuncture that will cause some brief discomfort, and that he will feel brief pressure from the tourniquet. After you draw the blood samples, handle the specimens gently to prevent hemolysis, which can alter test results. Be sure to label the samples clearly. Monitor the venipuncture site for bleeding. If a hematoma develops, apply warm soaks. If the hematoma is large, monitor circulation in the extremity distal to the venipuncture site.

Easy does it! Be gentle with specimens.

Immunohematology

ABO blood typing

ABO blood typing classifies blood according to the presence of major antigens A and B on red blood cell (RBC) surfaces and according to the serum antibodies anti-A and anti-B. ABO blood typ-

Now I get it!

ABO blood types

Precise typing of donor blood and recipient blood helps avoid transfusing incompatible blood, which can be fatal. This illustration shows the recipient's blood type and the compatible donor type.

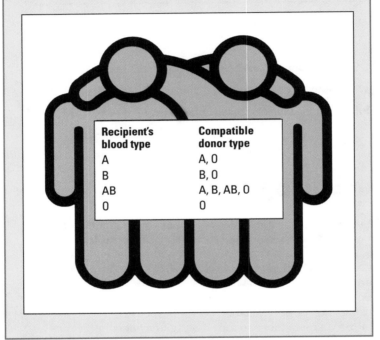

Recipient's blood type	Compatible donor type
A	A, O
B	B, O
AB	A, B, AB, O
O	O

ABO testing determines whether blood is type A, B, AB, or O, indicating whether a blood donor and recipient are compatible for transfusion.

ing is required before transfusions to prevent a lethal reaction—even if the patient is carrying an ABO blood group identification card.

There are four blood types in the ABO system: A, B, AB, and O.

Antigens

An antigen is a substance that can stimulate the formation of an antibody. RBCs carry antigens, which can initiate an immune response. Each blood group in the ABO system is named for antigens—A, B, both of these, or neither—that are carried on a person's RBCs. An antigen may induce formation of a corresponding antibody if given to a person who doesn't normally carry the antigen.

Antibodies

An antibody is an immunoglobulin molecule synthesized in response to a specific antigen. The ABO system includes two naturally occurring antibodies: anti-A and anti-B. One, both, or neither of these antibodies may be found in plasma. The interaction of corresponding antigens and antibodies of the ABO system can cause agglutination (clumping together).

O, you're everybody's type

Because group O lacks both A and B antigens, it can be transfused in limited amounts in an emergency to any patient — regardless of the recipient's blood type — with little risk of adverse reaction. (See *ABO blood types.*)

What it all means

Testing reveals blood type as type A, type B, type AB, or type O. (See *ABO blood typing interference.*)

What needs to be done

• Check the patient history for recent administration of blood, dextran, or I.V. contrast media.
• Perform a venipuncture, and collect the sample in a 10-ml tube without additives, as ordered.
• Label the sample with the patient's name, the hospital or blood bank number, the date, and the initials of the person who drew the specimen.
• Send the sample to the laboratory immediately with a properly completed laboratory request.

Warning!

ABO blood typing interference

• Recent administration of dextran or I.V. contrast media causes cellular aggregation that resembles agglutination.
• New antibodies may interfere with compatibility testing if the patient has received blood or has been pregnant in the past 3 months.

Rh typing

The Rhesus (Rh) system classifies blood by the presence or absence of the $Rh_0(D)$ antigen on the surface of RBCs. In this test, a patient's RBCs are mixed with serum containing anti-$Rh_0(D)$ antibodies and are observed for clumping. If clumping occurs, the $Rh_0(D)$ antigen is present, and the patient's blood is typed Rh-positive; if clumping doesn't occur, the antigen is absent, and the patient's blood is typed Rh-negative.

Rh typing establishes blood type according to the Rhesus system and helps determine donor-recipient blood compatibility.

What it all means

Classified as Rh-positive, Rh-negative, or Rh-positive Dᵘ, donor blood may be transfused only if it's compatible with the recipient's blood. (See *The ABCs of Rh₀[D] typing* and *An ounce of prevention*.)

What needs to be done

- Check the patient history for recent administration of dextran, I.V. contrast media, or drugs that may alter results.
- Perform a venipuncture, and collect the sample in a 7-ml tube with EDTA added, as ordered.
- Label the sample with the patient's name, the hospital or blood bank number, the date, and the initials of the person who drew the specimen.
- Send the sample to the laboratory immediately.
- If a transfusion is ordered, a transfusion request form must accompany the sample to the laboratory. (See *Rh typing interference*.)

Listen up!

An ounce of prevention

If an Rh-negative woman delivers an Rh-positive baby or aborts a fetus whose Rh-type is unknown, she should receive an injection of Rh₀(D) immune globulin within 72 hours to prevent future hemolytic disease of the neonate.

Now I get it!

The ABCs of Rh₀(D) typing

Classified as Rh₀(D)-positive, Rh₀(D)-negative, or Rh(Dᵘ)-positive, donor blood may be transfused only if it's compatible with the recipient's blood, as shown below.

Rh₀(D) recipient types	Compatible Rh₀(D) donor types	Incompatible Rh₀(D) donor types
Rh₀(D)-positive	Rh₀(D)-positive or Rh₀(D)-negative	None
Rh₀(D)-negative	Rh₀(D)-negative	Rh₀(D)-positive
Rh(Dᵘ)-positive	Rh(Dᵘ)-positive, Rh₀(D)-negative, or Rh₀(D)-positive (the least desirable choice because it may cause a mild hemolytic reaction)	None

Warning!

Rh typing interference

- Recent administration of dextran or I.V. contrast media may alter results.
- Methyldopa, cephalosporins, and levodopa may cause a false-positive result for the Dᵘ antigen.

Fetal-maternal erythrocyte distribution

Some transfer of red blood cells (RBCs) from fetal to maternal circulation occurs during most spontaneous or elective abortions and most normal deliveries. Fetal-maternal erythrocyte distribution measures the number of fetal RBCs in maternal circulation to allow calculation of the $Rh_0(D)$ immune globulin dosage needed for protection against maternal immunization to the $Rh_0(D)$ antigen, which can develop.

What it all means

Maternal whole blood should contain no fetal RBCs.

Elevated levels

An elevated fetal RBC volume in maternal circulation necessitates administration of more than one dose of $Rh_0(D)$ immune globulin. The number of vials needed is determined by dividing the calculated fetomaternal hemorrhage by 30 (a single vial of $Rh_0(D)$ immune globulin will provide protection against a 30-ml fetomaternal hemorrhage).

Don't delay

Administration of $Rh_0(D)$ immune globulin to an unsensitized Rh-negative mother as soon as possible (no later than 72 hours) after the birth of an Rh-positive infant or after a spontaneous or elective abortion prevents complications in subsequent pregnancies. Most clinicians now administer $Rh_0(D)$ immune globulin preventively at 28 weeks' gestation to women who are Rh-negative but have no detectable Rh antibodies.

Who needs the screen?

The following patients should be screened for Rh isoimmunization or irregular antibodies: all Rh-negative mothers during their first prenatal visit and at 28 weeks' gestation, and all Rh-positive mothers with a history of transfusion, a jaundiced infant, stillbirth, cesarean delivery, or induced or spontaneous abortion.

What needs to be done

• Explain to the patient that this blood test determines blood group and helps determine how many doses of $Rh_0(D)$ immune globulin she'll require to prevent immunization as a result of this pregnancy.
• Check the patient history for recent administration of dextran, I.V. contrast media, or drugs that may alter results.

Testing for fetal-maternal erythrocyte distribution measures fetal-maternal blood transfer and helps determine the amount of $Rh_0(D)$ immune globulin needed to prevent maternal immunization to the $Rh_0(D)$ antigen.

• Perform a venipuncture, and collect the sample in a 10-ml tube with EDTA added, as ordered.
• Label the sample with the patient's name, the hospital or blood bank number, the date, and the initials of the person who drew the specimen.
• Send the sample to the laboratory immediately with a properly completed laboratory request.

Crossmatching

Crossmatching establishes the compatibility or incompatibility of a donor's and a recipient's blood. It's the best antibody detection test available for avoiding lethal transfusion reactions.

Major matching

After the donor's and the recipient's ABO blood type and Rh factor type are determined, major crossmatching tests for compatibility between the donor's red blood cells (RBCs) and the recipient's serum. They're compatible if the recipient's serum has no antibodies that would destroy transfused cells and possibly cause an acute hemolytic reaction.

Minor matching

Minor crossmatching tests for compatibility between the donor's serum and the recipient's RBCs. This crossmatch is less important, however, because the donor's antibodies are greatly diluted in the recipient's plasma. Because the antibody-screening test is routinely performed on all blood donors, minor crossmatching is often omitted.

What it all means

Absence of clumping indicates compatibility between the donor's and the recipient's blood, which means that the transfusion of donor blood can proceed.

Positive = no match

A positive crossmatch indicates incompatibility between the donor's blood and the recipient's blood, which means the donor's blood can't be transfused to the recipient. The sign of a positive crossmatch is clumping after the donor's RBCs and the recipient's serum are correctly mixed and in-

Crossmatching, which prevents deadly transfusion reactions, is the final check for compatibility between donor and recipient blood.

cubated. Clumping indicates an undesirable antigen-antibody reaction. The donor's blood must be withheld and the crossmatch continued to determine why the blood is incompatible and to identify the antibody.

Negative = probable compatibility

A negative crossmatch—the absence of clumping—indicates probable compatibility between the donor's blood and the recipient's blood, which means the transfusion of donor blood can proceed. It doesn't guarantee a safe transfusion, but it's the best method available to prevent an acute hemolytic reaction. (See *Crossmatching test interference.*)

What needs to be done

• Check the patient history for recent administration of blood, dextran, or I.V. contrast media.
• Perform a venipuncture, and collect the sample in a 10-ml tube without additives or with EDTA added. ABO typing, Rh typing, and crossmatching are all done together.
• Label the sample with the patient's name, the hospital or blood bank number, the date, and the initials of the person who drew the specimen.
• Indicate on the laboratory request the amount and type of blood component needed.
• Send the sample to the laboratory immediately. Crossmatching must be performed on the sample within 72 hours.
• If more than 72 hours have elapsed since a previous transfusion, previously crossmatched donor blood must be crossmatched again with a new recipient serum sample to detect newly acquired incompatibilities before the transfusion.

Direct antiglobulin

Also known as the direct Coombs' test, the direct antiglobulin test detects antibodies on the surfaces of red blood cells (RBCs). These antibodies coat RBCs when they become sensitized to an antigen such as Rh factor.

One step direct

In this test, antiglobulin (Coombs') serum added to saline-washed RBCs results in clumping if antibodies or complement is present. This test is "direct" because it requires only one step: the addition of Coombs' serum to washed cells.

Warning!

Crossmatching test interference

• Previous administration of dextran or I.V. contrast media causes clumping. A previous blood transfusion may produce antibodies to donor blood.
• Administration of certain drugs may produce antibodies.

What it all means

A negative test, in which neither antibodies nor complement appears on the RBCs, is normal.

Crossed and coated

A positive test on umbilical cord blood indicates that maternal antibodies have crossed the placenta and have coated fetal RBCs, causing hemolytic disease of the newborn (HDN).

I beg to differ

In other patients, a positive test result may indicate hemolytic anemia and may help differentiate between autoimmune and secondary hemolytic anemia, which can be drug-induced or associated with an underlying disease such as lymphoma. A positive test result can also indicate sepsis.

Borderline

A borderline or slightly positive test result may suggest a transfusion reaction in which the patient's antibodies react with transfused RBCs containing the corresponding antigen. (See *Direct antiglobulin test interference*.)

What needs to be done

• If the patient is a neonate, explain to the parents that this blood test helps diagnose HDN.
• If the patient is suspected of having hemolytic anemia, explain that this test determines whether it's caused by an immune system abnormality, from the use of certain drugs, or from some unknown cause.
• As ordered, withhold medications that may induce autoimmune hemolytic anemia.

> The direct antiglobulin test can do a lot! It helps diagnose hemolytic disease of the neonate and congenital anemias. It can also be used to investigate hemolytic transfusion reactions.

Warning!

Direct antiglobulin test interference

Positive results may occur with use of quinidine, methyldopa, cephalosporins, sulfonamides, chlorpromazine, diphenylhydantoin, ethosuximide, hydralazine, levodopa, mefenamic acid, melphalan, penicillin, procainamide, rifampin, streptomycin, tetracyclines, or isoniazid.

- For an adult, perform a venipuncture, and collect the sample in two 5-ml tubes with EDTA added.
- For a neonate, draw 5 ml of cord blood into a tube with EDTA or no additives, as ordered, after the cord is clamped and cut.
- The test must be performed within 24 hours; send the specimen to the laboratory immediately.
- Label the sample with the patient's full name, the facility or blood bank number, the date, and the initials of the person who drew the specimen.

Antibody screening

The antibody screening test, also known as the indirect Coombs' test and the indirect antiglobulin test, detects unexpected circulating antibodies in the patient's serum. After incubating the serum with group O RBCs, which are unaffected by anti-A or anti-B antibodies, an antiglobulin (Coombs') serum is added. Clumping occurs if the patient's serum contains an antibody to one or more antigens on the RBCs.

Checkin' ID

The antibody screening test detects 95% to 99% of the circulating antibodies. Then the antibody identification test determines the specific identity of the antibodies. (See *What the antibody identification test shows.*)

By detecting unexpected antibodies in circulation, the antibody screening test prevents conflicts between the blood of donors and recipients.

Now I get it!

What the antibody identification test shows

The antibody identification test identifies unexpected circulating antibodies detected by the antibody screening test (indirect Coombs' test). In this test, group O red blood cells (RBCs)—at least three with and three without a specific antigen—are combined with serum containing unknown antibodies and are observed for clumping. If the serum contains the corresponding antibody to the RBC antigen, a positive reaction occurs with RBCs that have the antigen but not with those that lack the antigen. For example, serum that reacts with Rh-positive cells but not Rh-negative cells probably contains the anti-Rho(D) antibody.

At least three RBCs containing the antigen and three without it are used in each test to reduce error. Serum that contains rare or multiple antibodies requires more complicated procedures.

What it all means

A negative test result is normal. That is, clumping doesn't occur, indicating that the patient's serum contains no circulating antibodies (other than anti-A and anti-B).

Positively unexpected

A positive result indicates the presence of unexpected circulating antibodies to RBC antigens, which demonstrates donor and recipient incompatibility.

Antibody presence

A positive result in a pregnant patient with Rh-negative blood may indicate the presence of antibodies to the Rh factor from a previous transfusion with incompatible blood or from a previous pregnancy with an Rh-positive fetus.

Pregnancy may necessitate repetition

A positive result above a titer of 1:8 indicates that the fetus may develop hemolytic disease of the newborn. As a result, repeated testing throughout the patient's pregnancy is necessary to evaluate progressive development of circulating antibody levels. (See *Antibody screening interference.*)

What needs to be done

- Check the patient history for recent administration of blood, dextran, or I.V. contrast media, and note any such administration on the laboratory request.
- Label the sample with the patient's name, the hospital or blood bank number, the date, and the initials of the person who drew the specimen. Include the patient's diagnosis and any history of transfusions, pregnancy, or drug therapy on the laboratory request.
- Send the sample to the laboratory immediately. The antibody screening must be done within 72 hours after the sample is drawn.

Warning!

Antibody screening interference

- Previous administration of blood, dextran, or I.V. contrast media causes clumping.
- If the patient has received a transfusion or has been pregnant within the past 3 months, antibodies may alter test results.

> Testing for leukoagglutinins can differentiate between hemolytic and febrile non-hemolytic transfusion reactions.

Leukoagglutinins

The leukoagglutinin test detects leukoagglutinins (also known as white cell antibodies or human leukocyte antigen [HLA] antibodies) — antibodies that react with white blood cells (WBCs) and may cause a transfusion reaction. These antibodies usually develop after exposure to foreign WBCs through transfusions, pregnancies, or allografts.

What it all means

A negative test result is normal. That is, clumping doesn't occur, indicating that the patient's serum contains no antibodies. There are no known factors that interfere with the leukoagglutinin test.

Heated reaction

A positive result in a blood recipient indicates the presence of agglutinins, identifying his transfusion reaction as a febrile non-hemolytic reaction to these antibodies. Recipients who test positive for HLA antibodies may need HLA-matched platelets to control bleeding episodes caused by thrombocytopenia. (See *Precautions before the next transfusion.*)

What needs to be done

• Check the patient history for recent administration of blood, dextran, or I.V. contrast media, and note any such administration on the laboratory request.
• Perform a venipuncture, and collect the sample in a 10-ml clot-activator tube. The laboratory needs 3 to 4 ml of serum for testing.
• Label the sample with the patient's name, the hospital or blood bank number, the date, and the initials of the person who drew the specimen. Be sure to include on the laboratory request the patient's suspected diagnosis and any history of blood transfusions, pregnancies, and drug therapy.

Advice from the experts

Precautions before the next transfusion

If a patient who received a transfusion has a positive leukoagglutinin test, he should receive acetaminophen 1 to 2 hours before the next transfusion. To prevent further reactions, he should also receive specially prepared leukocyte-poor blood, or a leukocyte removal blood filter should be used during administration.

General cellular function

T- and B-lymphocyte assays

Lymphocytes — key cells in the immune system — have the capacity to recognize antigens through special receptors found on their surfaces. The two primary kinds of lymphocytes, T and B cells, originate in the bone marrow. T cells mature under the influence of the thymus gland; B cells evolve without thymic influence.

No difference

T- and B-lymphocyte assays recover approximately 80% of the lymphocytes but don't differentiate between T and B cells. The percentage of T and B cells is determined by attaching a label or marker and using different identification techniques. Null cells are usually determined by subtracting the sum of T and B cells from total lymphocytes.

T- and B-lymphocyte assays can help diagnose immunodeficiency diseases and monitor immunotherapy.

What it all means

T-cell and B-cell values may differ from one laboratory to another, depending on test technique. Generally, T cells constitute 68% to 75% of total lymphocytes; B cells, 10% to 20%; and null cells, 5% to 20%.

Suggestive material

An abnormal T-cell or B-cell count suggests but doesn't confirm specific diseases. The B-cell count is elevated in chronic lymphocytic leukemia, multiple myeloma, Waldenström's macroglobulinemia, and DiGeorge syndrome (a congenital T-cell deficiency). The B-cell count decreases in acute lymphocytic leukemia and in certain congenital or acquired immunoglobulin deficiency diseases. In other immunoglobulin deficiency diseases, especially if only one immunoglobulin class is deficient, the B-cell count remains normal.

T-cells on the rise

The T-cell count rises occasionally in infectious mononucleosis; it rises more often in multiple myeloma and acute lymphocytic leukemia. T cells decrease in congenital T-cell deficiency diseases, such as DiGeorge, Nezelof, and Wiskott-Aldrich syndromes, and in chronic lymphocytic leukemia, Waldenström's macroglobulinemia, and acquired immunodeficiency syndrome. (See *T- and B-lymphocyte assay interference.*)

What needs to be done

- Perform a venipuncture, and collect the sample in a 7-ml heparinized tube.
- Fill the collection tube completely, and invert it gently several times.
- Transport the sample to the laboratory immediately; keep it at room temperature.
- If antilymphocyte antibodies are suspected, notify the laboratory.

> **Uh oh!   Warning!**
>
> ## T- and B-lymphocyte assay interference
>
> - Changes in health status, stress, surgery, chemotherapy, steroid or immunosuppressive therapy, and radiography can rapidly change T- and B-cell counts.
> - Immunoglobulins that sometimes occur in autoimmune disease, can alter test results.

> Lymphocyte transformation testing helps assess immunodeficiency states, provides histocompatibility typing of tissue transplant recipients and donors, and determines exposure to certain pathogens.

Lymphocyte transformation

Transformation tests evaluate the ability of lymphocytes to change into actively multiplying cells without injection of antigens into the patient's skin. These in vitro tests eliminate the risk of adverse effects but can still accurately assess the ability of lymphocytes to reproduce and to recognize and respond to antigens.

Long division

The mitogen assay evaluates the cell division response of T-lymphocytes and B-lymphocytes to a foreign antigen. The antigen

Now I get it!

Insight into lymphocyte marker assays

A normal immune response requires a balance between the regulatory activities of several interacting cell types — primarily T-helper and T-suppressor cells. By using highly specific antibodies, levels of lymphocyte differentiation can be defined, and both normal and malignant cells can be analyzed.

Lymphocyte marker assay	Why it's done
CD3	• To measure mature T cells when the immune system malfunctions
CD4	• To identify and characterize the proportion of T-helper cells in autoimmune or immunoregulatory disorders • To detect immunodeficiency disorders such as acquired immunodeficiency syndrome • To differentiate T-cell acute lymphoblastic leukemia from T-cell lymphomas and other lymphoproliferative disorders
CD8	• To identify and characterize the proportion of T-suppressor cells in autoimmune and immunoregulatory disorders
CD2	• To characterize lymphoproliferative disorders
CD20	• To differentiate lymphoproliferative disorders of T-cell origin such as B-cell chronic lymphocytic leukemia
CD19	• To identify B-cell lymphoproliferative disorders such as B-cell chronic lymphocytic leukemia
CALLA (common acute lymphocytic leukemia antigen) marker, CD10	• To identify bone marrow regeneration • To identify non-T-cell acute lymphocytic leukemia
Lymphocyte subset panel (CD3/CD4/CD8/CD19)	• To evaluate immunodeficiencies • To identify immunoregulation associated with autoimmune disorders • To characterize lymphoid malignancies
Lymphocytic leukemia marker panel (CD3/CD4/CD8/CD19/CD10)	• To characterize lymphocytic leukemias as T, B, non-T, non-B, regardless of the stage of the malignant cells

assay uses specific substances — such as purified protein derivative, *Candida*, mumps, tetanus toxoid, and streptokinase — to stimulate lymphocyte transformation. The mixed lymphocyte culture (MLC) assay helps match transplant recipients and donors and tests immunocompetence. (See *Insight into lymphocyte marker assays.*)

What it all means

Results depend on the mitogens used. Reference ranges accompany test results. In general, a positive test is normal; a negative test indicates deficiency.

An impression of depression

In the mitogen and antigen assays, a low stimulation index or unresponsiveness indicates a depressed or defective immune system. Serial testing can monitor the effectiveness of therapy in a patient with an immunodeficiency disease.

Are we compatible?

In the MLC test, the stimulation index is a measure of compatibility. A high index indicates poor compatibility; conversely, a low stimulation index indicates good compatibility.

A high stimulation index in response to the relevant pathogen can also demonstrate exposure to malaria, hepatitis, mycoplasmal pneumonia, periodontal disease, and certain viral infections in patients who no longer have detectable serum antibodies. (See *Lymphocyte transformation test interference*.)

What needs to be done

- If a radioisotope scan is scheduled, make sure the serum sample for this test is drawn first.
- Perform a venipuncture. For an adult, collect the sample in a 7-ml heparinized tube; for a child, use a 5-ml heparinized tube.
- Fill the collection tube completely, and invert it gently several times to mix the sample and anticoagulant adequately. Send the sample to the laboratory immediately.

Warning!

Lymphocyte transformation interference

- Pregnancy or the use of oral contraceptives causes a low stimulation index.
- Chemotherapy may affect the accuracy of test results unless pretherapy baseline values are available for comparison.
- A radioisotope scan performed within 1 week before the test or failure to send the sample to the laboratory immediately can affect the accuracy of test results.

General humoral function

Immunoglobulins G, A, and M

Immunoglobulins, proteins that can function as specific antibodies in response to antigen stimulation, account for humoral immunity. Deviations from normal immunoglobulin percentages occur in many immune disorders, including cancer, hepatic disorders, rheumatoid arthritis, and systemic lupus erythematosus.

Immunoelectrophoresis identifies immunoglobulin (IgG), IgA, and IgM in a serum sample; levels are measured by radial immunodiffusion or nephelometry. Some laboratories detect imunoglobulin by indirect immunofluorescence and radioimmunoassay.

What it all means

Serum Ig levels for adults range as follows:
- *IgG:* 800 to 1,800 mg/dl (SI, 8 to 18 g/L)
- *IgA:* 100 to 400 mg/dl (SI, 1 to 4 g/L)
- *IgM:* 55 to 150 mg/dl (SI, 0.55 to 1.5 g/L).

The lowdown on levels

IgG, IgA, and IgM levels change in various disorders. (See *Serum immunoglobulin levels in various disorders.*) In congenital and acquired hypogammaglobulinemias (decreased levels of gamma-globulin in the blood), myelomas, and macroglobulinemia, the findings confirm the diagnosis. (See *IgG, IgA, and IgM test interference,* page 140.)

Measuring immunoglobulins helps diagnose multiple myeloma and Waldenström's macroglobulinemia as well as cirrhosis and hepatitis. It can also monitor the effectiveness of chemotherapy or radiation therapy.

Serum immunoglobulin levels in various disorders

The chart below shows the changes in serum levels of immunoglobulins (Ig) G, A, and M associated with certain diseases.

Disorder	IgG	IgA	IgM
Acute lymphocytic leukemia	Normal	Decreased	Normal
Chronic lymphocytic leukemia	Decreased	Decreased	Decreased
Acute myelocytic leukemia	Normal	Decreased	Normal
Chronic myelocytic leukemia	Normal	Normal	Normal
Hodgkin's disease	Normal	Decreased	Normal
Hepatitis	Increased	Normal	Increased
Biliary cirrhosis	Normal	Increased	Increased
Rheumatoid arthritis	Increased	Normal	Increased
Systemic lupus erythematosus	Increased	Increased	Increased
Nephrotic syndrome	Decreased	Increased	Normal

Warning!

IgG, IgA, and IgM test interference

- Radiation therapy or chemotherapy may reduce Ig levels.
- Anticonvulsants, asparaginase, hydralazine, hydantoin derivatives, oral contraceptives, and phenylbutazone may raise levels.
- Methotrexate and severe hypersensitivity to bacille Calmette-Guérin vaccine may lower levels.
- Dextrans, phenytoin, and high methylprednisolone doses lower IgG and IgA levels; dextrans and methylprednisolone lower IgM levels.
- Methadone raises IgA levels; addiction to narcotics may raise IgM levels.

What needs to be done

- Tell the patient to restrict food and fluids, except for water, for 12 to 14 hours before the test.
- Perform a venipuncture, and collect the sample in a 7-ml clot-activator tube.
- Send the sample to the laboratory immediately to prevent deterioration of immunoglobulins.

Immune complex assays

When immune complexes are produced faster than they can be cleared by the lymph system, immune complex disease, such as postinfectious syndromes, serum sickness, drug sensitivity, rheumatoid arthritis, and systemic lupus erythematosus (SLE), may occur.

Diplomatic immunity

Histologic examination of tissue obtained by biopsy and the use of fluorescence or staining with antibodies specific for immunologic types generally detect immune complexes. However, because tissue biopsies can't provide information about titers of complexes still in circulation, serum assays, which detect circulating immune complexes indirectly, may be required. Because of the inherent variability of these complexes, several serum test methods may be appropriate, using C1, rheumatoid factor, or cellular substrates such as Raji cells as reagents.

> Immune complex assays detect immune complexes in serum. They help monitor response to therapy and assess disease severity.

What it all means

Normally, immune complexes aren't detectable in serum.

Complex presence

Immune complexes may be present in serum in many autoimmune diseases, such as SLE and rheumatoid arthritis. However, for a definitive diagnosis, the presence of these complexes must be considered with other test results. For example, in SLE, immune complexes are associated with high titers of antinuclear antibodies and circulating antinative deoxyribonucleic acid antibodies. (See *Immune complex assay interference.*)

What needs to be done

• If the patient is scheduled for a C1q (a component of C1) assay, check his history for recent heparin therapy. Report such therapy to the laboratory because it may affect test results.
• Perform a venipuncture, and collect the sample in a 7-ml clot-activator tube.
• Send the sample to the laboratory immediately to prevent deterioration of immune complexes.

Warning!

Immune complex assay interference

Cryoglobulins in the serum can alter results.

Raji cell assay

Raji cell assay, which is performed to detect the presence of circulating immune complexes, studies the Raji lymphoblastoid cell line. Identifying these cells, which have receptors for immunoglobulin G (IgG) complement, is helpful in evaluating autoimmune disease.

What it all means

No Raji cells should be present.

Rage, rage against the Raji

The Raji cell assay can detect immune complexes found in viral, microbial, and parasitic infections; metastasis; autoimmune disorders; and drug reactions. This test may also detect immune complexes associated with celiac disease, cirrhosis, Crohn's disease, cryoglobulinemia, dermatitis herpetiformis, sickle cell anemia, and ulcerative colitis.

What needs to be done

• Perform a venipuncture, and collect the sample in a clot-activator tube. Send the sample to the laboratory promptly.

The Raji cell assay analyzes the progress of autoimmune disease.

Complement assays

Complement is a collective term for a system of at least 15 serum proteins designed to destroy foreign cells and to help remove foreign materials.

Complement deficiency can increase susceptibility to infection and predispose a patient to other diseases. Complement assays are indicated in patients with known or suspected immune-mediated disease or repeatedly abnormal response to infection.

Various laboratory methods are used to evaluate and measure total complement and its components; hemolytic assay, laser nephelometry, and radial immunodiffusion are the most common.

Not all of the story

Although complement assays provide valuable information about a patient's immune system, the results must be considered in light of serum immunoglobulin and autoantibody tests for a definitive diagnosis of immune-mediated disease or abnormal response to infection.

What it all means

Normal values for complement range as follows:
- *total complement:* 40 to 90 U/ml (SI, 0.4 to 0.9 g/L)
- *C3:* men, 80 to 180 mg/dl (SI, 0.8 to 1.8 g/L); women, 76 to 120 mg/dl (SI, 0.76 to 1.2 g/L)
- *C4:* men, 15 to 60 mg/dl (SI, 0.15 to 0.6 g/L); women, 15 to 52 mg/dl (SI, 0.15 to 0.52 g/L).

Short on complement

Complement abnormalities may be genetic or acquired; acquired abnormalities are most common. Depressed total complement levels (which are clinically more significant than elevations) may result from excessive formation of antigen-antibody complexes, insufficient synthesis of complement, inhibitor formation, or increased complement catabolism; decreased levels are characteristic in such conditions as systemic lupus erythematosus (SLE), acute poststreptococcal glomerulonephritis, and acute serum sickness. Low levels may also occur in some patients with advanced cirrhosis of the liver, multiple myeloma, hypogammaglobulinemia, and rapidly rejecting allografts.

Too complementary

Elevated total complement may occur in obstructive jaundice, thyroiditis, acute rheumatic fever, rheumatoid arthritis, acute myocardial infarction, ulcerative colitis, and diabetes.

Complement assays help detect immune-mediated disease or genetic complement deficiency. They also help monitor the effectiveness of therapy.

C3 deficiency is characteristic in recurrent pyogenic infection, and C4 deficiency is characteristic in SLE. (See *Complement assay interference.*)

What needs to be done

• Perform a venipuncture, and collect the sample in a 7-ml tube without additives.
• Send the sample to the laboratory immediately because complement is heat labile and deteriorates rapidly.

Warning!

Complement assay interference

Recent heparin therapy can alter test results.

Radioallergosorbent test

The radioallergosorbent test (RAST) measures immunoglobulin E (IgE) antibodies in serum by radioimmunoassay and identifies specific allergens that cause rashes, asthma, hay fever, drug reactions, or other atopic complaints. RAST is easier to perform and more specific than skin testing; it's also less painful for and less dangerous to the patient. However, careful selection of specific allergens, based on the patient's clinical history, is crucial for effective testing.

Skin testing is preferred

Although skin testing is still the preferred means of diagnosing IgE-mediated hypersensitivities, RAST may be more useful when a skin disorder makes accurate reading of skin tests difficult, when a patient requires continual antihistamine therapy, or when skin tests are negative but the patient's clinical history supports IgE-mediated hypersensitivity.

What it all means

RAST results are interpreted in relation to a control or reference serum, which differs among laboratories.

Overly sensitive

Elevated serum IgE levels suggest hypersensitivity to the specific allergen or allergens used. (See *Radioallergosorbent test interference*, page 144.)

What needs to be done

• If the patient is scheduled for a radioactive scan, make sure the sample is collected before the scan.

The radioallergosorbent test helps identify allergens to which the patient has immediate (IgE-mediated) hypersensitivity.

• Perform a venipuncture, and collect the sample in a 7-ml clot-activator tube. Generally, 1 ml of serum is sufficient for five allergen assays. Be sure to note on the laboratory request the specific allergens tested.

Warning!

Radioallergosorbent test interference

A radioactive scan within 1 week before sample collection may alter test results.

Human leukocyte antigen

The human leukocyte antigen (HLA) test identifies a group of antigens that are present on the surfaces of all nucleated cells but are most easily detected on lymphocytes.

Antiserum breakup

Three types of HLA (HLA-A, HLA-B, and HLA-C) are measured with a lymphocyte microcytotoxicity assay. A lymphocyte sample is mixed with known antisera to these antigens and complement. Lymphocytes react with a specific antiserum, which causes the cells to break up and allow a dye to enter; they may then be detected by phase microscopy.

Mixed reaction

A fourth type of HLA, HLA-D, is measured by a mixed leukocyte reaction. Leukocytes from the recipient and the donor are combined in culture to determine HLA-D compatibility.

What it all means

In HLA-A, HLA-B, and HLA-C testing, lymphocytes that react with the test antiserum break up and are detected by phase microscopy. In HLA-D testing, leukocyte incompatibility is marked by blast formation, DNA synthesis, and reproduction.

Incompatible HLA-A, HLA-B, HLA-C, or HLA-D groups may cause unsuccessful tissue transplantation.

Strong association

Many diseases have a strong association with certain types of HLA. For example, HLA-DR5 is associated with Hashimoto's thyroiditis. HLA-B8 and HLA-Dw3 are associated with Graves' disease, whereas HLA-B8 alone is associated with chronic autoimmune hepatitis, celiac disease, and myasthenia gravis. HLA-Dw3 alone is associated with Addison's disease, Sjögren's syndrome, dermatitis herpetiformis, and systemic lupus erythematosus.

Fatherly ID

In paternity testing, an alleged father who presents a phenotype (two haplotypes: one from the father and one from the mother) with no haplotype or antigen pair identical to one of the child's is

The HLA test helps provide histocompatibility typing of tissue recipients and donors and can aid genetic counseling and paternity testing.

excluded as the father. An alleged father with one haplotype identical to one of the child's may be the father; the probability varies with the incidence of the haplotype in the population. (See *HLA test interference*.)

What needs to be done

• Check the patient history for recent blood transfusions, and report them to the doctor, who may want to postpone HLA testing.
• Perform a venipuncture, and collect the sample in a tube with ACD (acid citrate dextrose) added.

Warning!

HLA test interference

HLA from blood transfused with 72 hours before sample collection may alter test results.

Autoantibodies

Antinuclear antibodies

In such conditions as systemic lupus erythematosus (SLE), scleroderma, and certain infections, the body's immune system may perceive portions of its own cell nuclei as foreign and may produce antinuclear antibodies (ANA). Specific types of ANA include antibodies to deoxyribonucleic acid (DNA), nucleoprotein, histones, nuclear ribonucleoprotein, and other nuclear constituents.

Guilty by association

Although ANA are harmless on their own because they don't penetrate living cells, they sometimes form antigen-antibody complexes that cause damage, as in SLE. Because of multi-organ involvement, test results aren't diagnostic and can only partially confirm clinical evidence. (See *ANA incidence in various disorders*, page 146.)

What it all means

Using Hep-2 cells, the test for ANA is negative at a titer of 1:40 or below. If mouse kidney substrate is being used, the test is negative at a titer of less than 1:20. Results are reported as positive, with pattern and serum titer noted, or negative.

Sensitive but nonspecific

Although this test is a sensitive indicator of ANA, it isn't specific for SLE. Low titers may occur in patients with viral diseases, chronic hepatic

ANA testing helps to screen for SLE and can monitor the effectiveness of your treatment.

ANA incidence in various disorders

This chart shows the percentage of patients with certain disorders whose serum contains antinuclear antibodies (ANA). About 40% of elderly people and 5% of the general population also have positive ANA findings.

Disorder	Positive ANA
Systemic lupus erythematosus (SLE)	95% to 100%
Lupoid hepatitis	95% to 100%
Felty's syndrome	95% to 100%
Progressive systemic sclerosis (scleroderma)	75% to 80%
Drug-associated SLE-like syndrome (hydralazine, procainamide, isoniazid)	Approximately 50%
Sjögren's syndrome	40% to 75%
Rheumatoid arthritis	25% to 60%
Healthy family member of SLE patient	Approximately 25%
Chronic discoid lupus erythematosus	15% to 50%
Juvenile arthritis	15% to 30%
Polyarteritis nodosa	15% to 25%
Miscellaneous diseases	10% to 50%
Dermatomyositis, polymyositis	10% to 30%
Rheumatic fever	Approximately 5%

disease, collagen vascular disease, or autoimmune diseases as well as in some healthy adults; incidence increases with age. The higher the titer, the more specific the test is for SLE, for which the titer often exceeds 1:256. (See *ANA test interference.*)

What needs to be done

- If appropriate, inform the patient that the test will be repeated to monitor response to therapy.
- Check the patient history for drugs that may affect test results. Note such drug use on the laboratory request.
- Perform a venipuncture, and collect the sample in a 7-ml tube with no additives.
- Keep a clean, dry bandage over the site for at least 24 hours.

 Warning!

ANA test interference

Certain drugs—most commonly isoniazid, hydralazine, and procainamide—can produce a syndrome resembling systemic lupus erythematosus.

A long list
Other drugs with this effect include chlorpromazine, clofibrate, phenytoin, griseofulvin, ethosuximide, gold salts, methyldopa, oral contraceptives, penicillin, phenylbutazone, methysergide, streptomycin, sulfonamides, tetracyclines, mephenytoin, quinidine, primidone, reserpine, and trimethadione.

Antithyroid antibodies

In such autoimmune disorders as Hashimoto's thyroiditis and Graves' disease (hyperthyroidism), thyroglobulin, the major colloidal storage compound, is released into blood. Antithyroglobulin antibodies are produced to attack this foreign substance; the ensuing autoimmune response damages the thyroid gland.

> Measuring antithyroid antibodies helps confirm Hashimoto's thyroiditis, Graves' disease, and other thyroid disorders.

What it all means

The normal titer is less than 1:100 for both antithyroglobulin and antimicrosomal antibodies. Low levels of these antibodies are normal in 10% of the general population and in 20% or more of people age 70 and older. There are no known factors that interfere with the antithyroid antibody test.

Suggestive titers

The presence of antithyroglobulin or antimicrosomal antibodies in serum can indicate subclinical autoimmune thyroid disease, Graves' disease, or idiopathic myxedema. High titers (1:400 or more) strongly suggest Hashimoto's thyroiditis.

These antibodies may also occur in patients with other autoimmune disorders, such as systemic lupus erythematosus, rheumatoid arthritis, or autoimmune hemolytic anemia.

What needs to be done

• Perform a venipuncture, and collect the sample in a 7-ml tube with no additives.

> Measuring TSI helps diagnose thyroid disease and monitor treatment of thyrotoxicosis.

Thyroid-stimulating immunoglobulin

Thyroid-stimulating immunoglobulin (TSI), formerly called long-acting thyroid stimulator, appears in the blood of most patients with Graves' disease. This autoantibody reacts with the cell-surface receptors that usually combine with thyroid-stimulating hormone (TSH). TSI stimulates the thyroid gland to produce and excrete excessive amounts of thyroid hormones.

What it all means

TSI doesn't normally appear in serum. However, it may be present in 5% of people without hyperthyroidism or exophthalmos.

TSI on the rise

Increased TSI levels are associated with exophthalmos, Graves' disease (thyrotoxicosis), and recurrence of hyperthyroidism. (See *TSI test interference.*)

What needs to be done

• Perform a venipuncture, and collect the sample in a 5-ml clot-activator tube.
• Note on the laboratory request whether the patient had a radioactive iodine scan within 48 hours before the test.

Warning!

TSI test interference

Administration of radioactive iodine within 48 hours before the test may affect the accuracy of results.

Rheumatoid factor

The rheumatoid factor (RF) test is the most useful immunologic test for confirming rheumatoid arthritis (RA). In this disease, "renegade" immunoglobulin (Ig)G antibodies, produced by lymphocytes in the synovial joints, react with other IgG or IgM molecules to produce immune complexes, complement activation, and tissue destruction. How IgG molecules become antigenic is still unknown, but they may be altered by aggregating with viruses or other antigens. These immune complexes can migrate from the synovial fluid to other areas of the body, causing vasculitis, subcutaneous nodules, or lymphadenopathy. The IgG or IgM molecules that react with altered IgG are called rheumatoid factors.

What it all means

Normal RF titer is less than 1:20; normal rheumatoid screening test is nonreactive.

RF positive

Positive RF titers are found in 80% of patients with RA. Titers above 1:80 strongly suggest a diagnosis of RA; titers between 1:20 and 1:80 are difficult to interpret because they occur in many other diseases, such as systemic lupus erythematosus, scleroderma, polymyositis, tuberculosis, infectious mononucleosis, leprosy, syphilis, sarcoidosis, chronic hepatic disease, subacute bacterial endocarditis, and chronic pulmonary interstitial fibrosis. In addition, 5% of the general population, including as many as 25% of elderly people, have positive RF titers.

RF negative

Conversely, a negative RF titer doesn't rule out RA; 20% to 25% of patients with RA lack reactive RF titers, and RF itself isn't reac-

Testing for RF is the best way to confirm that you have rheumatoid arthritis.

Warning!

RF test interference

- Inadequately activated complement may cause false-positive results.
- Serum with high lipid or cryoglobulin levels may cause false-positive results, requiring test repetition after fat intake restriction.
- Serum with high immunoglobulin (Ig) G levels may cause false-negative results through competition with IgG on the surface of latex particles or sheep red blood cells used as substrate.

tive until 6 months after the onset of active disease. Repeating the test is sometimes useful. However, a correlation between RF and RA is inconclusive, and positive diagnosis always requires correlation with clinical status. (See *RF test interference.*)

What needs to be done

- Perform a venipuncture, and collect the sample in a 7-ml clot-activator tube.
- Because a patient with RA may be immunocompromised from the disease or from corticosteroid therapy, keep the venipuncture site covered with a clean, dry bandage for 24 hours. Check regularly for signs of infection.

Cold agglutinins

Cold agglutinins are antibodies (usually of the immunoglobulin M [IgM] type) that cause RBCs to aggregate at low temperatures. Transient elevations of these antibodies develop during certain infectious diseases, notably primary atypical pneumonia. Small amounts may also occur in healthy people. The test for cold agglutinins reliably detects such pneumonia within 1 to 2 weeks after onset.

What it all means

Results are reported as positive or negative. Positive results are titered. Normal titers are less than 1:64, but they may be higher in elderly persons.

Riding high with infection

High titers may occur as primary phenomena or secondary to infections or lymphoreticular malignancy (cancer involving the phagocytic cells in the lymph system). Levels may be elevated in infectious mononucleosis, cytomegalovirus infection, hemolytic anemia, multiple myeloma, scleroderma, malaria, cirrhosis, congenital syphilis, peripheral vascular disease, pulmonary embolism, trypanosomiasis, tonsillitis, staphylococcemia, scarlatina, influenza and, occasionally, pregnancy.

Chronically high with pneumonia

Chronically elevated titers are most commonly associated with pneumonia and lymphoreticular malignancy; an acute transient elevation commonly accompanies many viral infections.

Positive, peak, then disappear

In primary atypical pneumonia, cold agglutinins appear in serum in one-half to two-thirds of all patients during the 1st week of acute infection. Titers usually become positive at 7 days, peak above 1:32 in 4 weeks, and disappear rapidly after 6 weeks. When sequential titers verify this pattern and clinical evidence of pneumonia exists, the diagnosis is confirmed.

Testing for cold agglutinins helps confirm pneumonia and viral infection.

Sounding the alarm on lymphoma

Extremely high titers (1:2,000 or higher) can occur with idiopathic cold agglutinin disease that precedes development of lymphoma. Patients with titers this high are susceptible to intravascular agglutination, which causes significant clinical problems. (See *Cold agglutinins test interference.*)

What needs to be done

• If appropriate, inform the patient that the test will be repeated to monitor his response to therapy.
• If the patient is receiving antimicrobial drugs, note this on the laboratory request because these drugs may interfere with the development of cold agglutinins.
• Perform a venipuncture, and collect the sample in a 7-ml tube without additives that has been *prewarmed* to 98.6° F (37° C).
• Send the sample to the laboratory immediately.
• Don't refrigerate the sample; cold agglutinins will coat the RBCs, leaving none in the serum.

 Warning!

Cold agglutinins test interference

Antimicrobials can interfere with development of cold agglutinins.

Acetylcholine receptor antibodies

The acetylcholine receptor (AChR) antibodies test is the most useful test for confirming myasthenia gravis (MG), a disorder of neuromuscular transmission. In normal muscle contraction, acetylcholine (ACh) is released from the terminal end of the nerve and binds to AChR sites on the muscle motor end plate. In MG, antibodies block and destroy AChR sites, causing muscle weakness that can be either generalized or localized to the ocular muscles.

Two test methods — a binding assay and a blocking assay — are available to determine the relative concentration of AChR antibodies in serum. AChR-binding antibodies are found in about 90% of patients with generalized MG and in about 50% of those with localized MG. When the AChR-binding assay is negative in a patient with MG symptoms, the AChR-blocking assay may be performed.

Presence of AChR antibodies confirms MG. Further testing can monitor MG therapy.

What it all means

Normal serum is negative for AChR-binding antibodies and is negative for AChR-blocking antibodies.

Confirming results

Positive AChR antibodies in symptomatic adults confirm the diagnosis of MG. Patients with only ocular symptoms tend to have lower antibody titers than those with generalized symptoms. (See *AChR antibody test interference.*)

What needs to be done

• Check the patient history for immunosuppressive drugs that may affect test results, and note their use on the laboratory request.

Warning!

AChR antibody test interference

• Patients undergoing thymectomy, thoracic duct drainage, immunosuppressive therapy, or plasmapheresis may show reduced AChR antibody levels.
• Patients with amyotrophic lateral sclerosis may show false-positive results.

- Perform a venipuncture, and collect the sample in a 7-ml tube without additives.
- Check the venipuncture site for infection, and promptly report any change because patients with autoimmune disease have compromised immune systems. Keep a clean, dry bandage over the site for at least 24 hours.
- Keep the sample at room temperature, and send it to the laboratory immediately.

Anti-insulin antibodies

Some diabetic patients form antibodies to the insulin they take. These antibodies bind with some of the insulin, making less insulin available for glucose metabolism and necessitating increased insulin dosages. This phenomenon is known as insulin resistance.

> Testing for anti-insulin antibodies confirms insulin resistance.

Detective work

Performed on the blood of a diabetic patient receiving insulin, the anti-insulin antibody test detects insulin antibodies. Insulin antibodies are immunoglobulins, called anti-insulin Ab. The most common type of anti-insulin Ab is immunoglobulin (Ig) G, but anti-insulin Ab is also found in the other four classes of Ig — A, D, E, and M. IgM may cause insulin resistance, and IgE has been associated with allergic reactions.

What it all means

Less than 3% of the patient's serum should bind with labeled human and pork insulin.

Abnormal response or resistance?

Elevated levels may occur in insulin allergy or resistance and in factitious hypoglycemia. (See *Anti-insulin antibody test interference.*)

What needs to be done

- If the patient has recently had a radioactive test, note this on the laboratory request.
- Perform a venipuncture, and collect the sample in a 7-ml tube with no additives.

UH-OH   *Warning!*

Anti-insulin antibody test interference

Radioactive test within 1 week before the test may alter results.

Anti-double-stranded DNA antibodies

About two-thirds of patients with active systemic lupus erythematosus (SLE) have measurable levels of autoantibodies to double-stranded (native) deoxyribonucleic acid (known as anti-ds-DNA). These antibodies are rarely detected in patients with other connective tissue diseases.

The anti-ds-DNA antibody test measures and differentiates these antibody levels in a blood sample. If anti-ds-DNA antibodies are present, they combine with native DNA and form complexes that are too large to pass through a membrane filter. The test counts these oversized complexes.

Testing for anti-double-stranded DNA antibodies helps confirm SLE and monitor its therapy.

What it all means

An anti-ds-DNA antibody level less than 25 IU is considered negative for SLE.

The lowdown on levels

Elevated anti-ds-DNA antibody levels may indicate SLE. Values of 25 to 30 IU are considered borderline positive. Values of 31 to 200 IU are positive, and those greater than 200 IU are strongly positive.

Depressed anti-ds-DNA antibody levels may follow immunosuppressive therapy, demonstrating effective treatment of SLE. (See *Anti-ds-DNA antibody test interference*.)

What needs to be done

• If the patient has recently had a radioactive test, note this on the laboratory request.
• Perform a venipuncture, and collect the sample in a 7-ml tube with no additives. Some laboratories may specify a tube with either EDTA or sodium fluoride and potassium oxalate added.

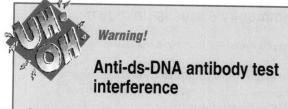

Warning!

Anti-ds-DNA antibody test interference

Radioactive scan within 1 week before collection of a sample may alter results.

Viruses

Rubella antibodies

Although rubella (German measles) is generally a mild viral infection in children and young adults, it can produce severe infection in a fetus, resulting in spontaneous abortion, stillbirth, or congenital rubella syndrome. Because rubella infection normally induces immunoglobulin (Ig) G and IgM antibody production, measuring rubella antibodies can determine present infection and immunity resulting from past infection. (See *When immunity status is unknown.*)

What it all means

Titer of 1:8 or less indicates little or no immunity against rubella; titer greater than 1:10 indicates adequate protection against rubella.

The lowdown on levels

Antibody levels normally appear 2 to 4 days after the onset of the rash, peak in 3 to 4 weeks, then slowly decline but remain detectable for life. In rubella infection, acute serum titers range from 1:8 to 1:16; convalescent serum titers, from 1:64 to 1:1,024+. A fourfold rise or greater from the acute to the convalescent titer indicates a recent rubella infection.

The presence of rubella-specific IgM antibodies indicates recent infection in an adult and congenital rubella in an infant.

Testing for rubella antibodies is pretty important to me. It can diagnose rubella infection and determine susceptibility in women of childbearing age and in children.

Peak technique

When immunity status is unknown

Rubella exposure risk may be evaluated using two serum samples, as follows:
• The first sample should be drawn in the acute phase of clinical symptoms. If clinical symptoms aren't apparent, the sample should be drawn as soon as possible after the suspected exposure.
• The second sample should be drawn 3 to 4 weeks later, during the convalescent phase.

What needs to be done

• Explain to the patient that if a current infection is suspected, a second blood sample will be needed in 3 to 4 weeks to identify a rise in the titer.
• Perform a venipuncture, and collect the sample in a 7-ml clot-activator tube.

Hepatitis B surface antigen

Hepatitis B surface antigen (HBsAg) appears in the serum of patients with hepatitis B virus, formerly called serum hepatitis or long-incubation hepatitis. This antigen, also known as hepatitis-associated antigen and Australia antigen, can be detected during the extended incubation period and usually during the first 3 weeks of acute infection or if the patient is a carrier.

Grave complication

Because transmission of hepatitis is one of the gravest complications associated with blood transfusions, all donors must be screened for hepatitis B before their blood is stored. This test, required by the Food and Drug Administration, has helped reduce the incidence of hepatitis, but it doesn't screen for hepatitis A (infectious hepatitis). (For information on related test, see *Understanding the viral hepatitis test panel*, pages 156 and 157.)

What it all means

Serum should be negative for HBsAg.

Retest if positive

The presence of HBsAg in a patient with hepatitis confirms hepatitis B. In chronic carriers and persons with chronic active hepatitis, HBsAg may be present in serum several months after the onset of acute infection. If the antigen is found in donor blood, the blood must be discarded because of the high risk of transmitting hepatitis. Blood samples that test positive should be retested because inaccurate results occur. (See *HBsAg test interference.*)

What needs to be done

• Check the patient history for hepatitis B vaccine.
• If the patient is giving blood, explain the donation procedure to him.
• Perform a venipuncture, and collect the sample in a 10-ml clot-activator tube.

> The HBsAg test screens blood donors as well as people at risk for contracting the disease.

Warning!

HBsAg test interference

Patients who have received the hepatitis B vaccine may test positive.

Now I get it!

Understanding the viral hepatitis test panel

The three types of viral hepatitis produce similar symptoms but differ in the way they're transmitted, the course of treatment, prognosis, and carrier status. When the patient's clinical history is insufficient to determine the hepatitis type, blood tests can aid diagnosis. Hepatitis A, B, and C antigens produce type-specific antibodies detectable by a variety of methods. Timing of the appearance and disappearance of these antibodies, along with the patient's symptoms, helps diagnose and stage acute and chronic forms of these distinct diseases.

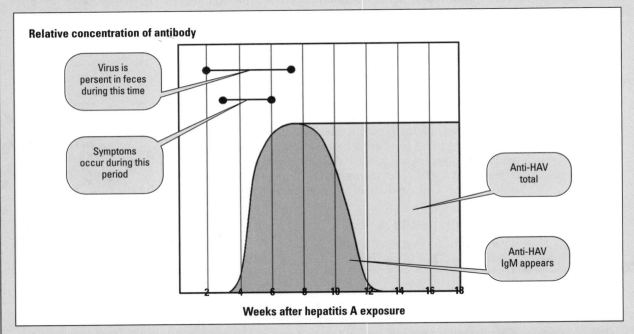

Relative concentration of antibody

Virus is persent in feces during this time

Symptoms occur during this period

Anti-HAV total

Anti-HAV IgM appears

Weeks after hepatitis A exposure

Typical sequence of hepatitis A markers after exposure
Hepatitis A is present in blood and feces only briefly before symptoms appear; hepatitis A virus (HAV) may elude detection. However, anti-HAV, the antibody to hepatitis A virus, appears early in the acute disease phase, persists for many years after recovery, and ultimately provides immunity. A single positive anti-HAV test may indicate previous exposure to the virus, but because this antibody persists so long in the bloodstream, only evidence of rising anti-HAV titers confirms hepatitis A as the cause of current or recent infection. Determining recent infection relies on identifying the antibody as immunoglobulin M (IgM; associated with recent infection). A negative anti-HAV test rules out hepatitis A.

Typical sequence of hepatitis B and C markers after exposure
Hepatitis B viral particles contain a surface protein and a core protein. The surface antigen (HBsAg) appears in blood during the long incubation period (up to 26 weeks) or during the early

Understanding the viral hepatitis test panel *(continued)*

acute phase of infection (2 to 3 weeks) and normally peaks after symptoms begin. High HBsAg levels continuing 6 months after the onset of acute infection suggest chronic hepatitis or carrier status. Potential blood donors are screened for this antigen to prevent transmission of hepatitis B to recipients.

Another antibody that develops after exposure to hepatitis B is anti-HBc, caused by the core component of the virus. An early indicator of acute infection, antibody (IgM) to core antigen (anti-HBc IgM) is rarely detected in chronic infection. Thus, it's also useful in distinguishing acute infection from chronic infection.

Anti-HBs, antibody to the surface antigen, appears after the HBsAg has disappeared from blood. Detection of this antibody signals late recovery from infection. Anti-HBs remains in the blood to provide immunity.

Testing for hepatitis C

A single-stranded RNA virus causes hepatitis C (formerly called non-A, non-B hepatitis). Antibody tests have been designed to detect anti-HCV. Anti-HCV can appear relatively late in the infection, usually 16 to 24 weeks after initial elevation of liver enzyme levels. Progress of the infection can be monitored by periodic analysis of alanine aminotransferase and anti-HCV levels. Clinical symptoms and disease spread are similar to that of hepatitis B, but the chronic infection rate is much higher. Plasma of chronically infected HCV patients remains infectious.

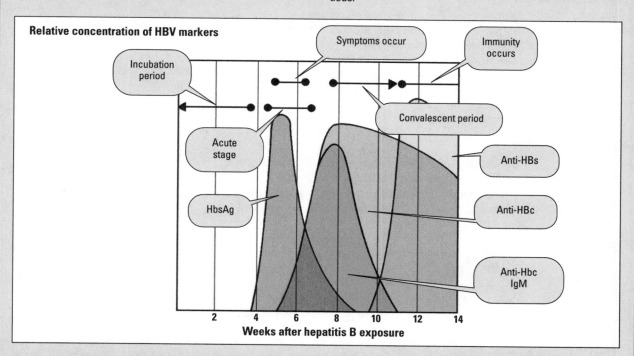

Relative concentration of HBV markers

Incubation period / Symptoms occur / Immunity occurs / Acute stage / Convalescent period / Anti-HBs / HbsAg / Anti-HBc / Anti-Hbc IgM

Weeks after hepatitis B exposure
2   4   6   8   10   12   14

Graphs adapted with permission from Serodiagnostic Assessment of Acute Viral Hepatitis. Abbott Park, Ill.: Abbott Laboratories, 1992.

• Because hepatitis B is easily transmitted, wash your hands carefully after the procedure. Remember to wear gloves when drawing blood and to dispose of the needle properly.

Heterophil antibodies

Heterophil antibody tests detect and identify two immunoglobulin M antibodies in human serum that react against foreign RBCs: Epstein-Barr virus (EBV) antibodies and Forssman antibodies.

What it all means

Normally, the titer is less than 1:56 but may be higher in elderly people. Some laboratories refer to a normal titer as "negative" or as having "no reaction."

Abnormal results

Although heterophil antibodies are present in the sera of about 80% of patients with infectious mononucleosis (IM) 1 month after onset, a positive finding—a titer higher than 1:56—doesn't confirm this disorder; a high titer can also result from systemic lupus erythematosus, syphilis, cryoglobulinemia, or the presence of antibodies to nonsyphilitic treponematosis, such as yaws, pinta, and bejel. A gradual increase in titer during week 3 or 4 followed by a gradual decrease during weeks 4 to 8 proves most conclusive for IM.

Delayed reaction

A negative titer doesn't always rule out this disorder; occasionally, the titer becomes reactive 2 weeks later. Therefore, if symptoms persist, the test should be repeated in 2 weeks. Confirmation of IM depends on het-

Heterophil antibody tests aid in the diagnosis of IM.

Listen up!

Explaining mononucleosis

If your patient's heterophil antibody titer is positive and infectious mononucleosis (IM) is confirmed, explain the treatment plan.

If the titer is positive but IM isn't confirmed, or if the titer is negative but symptoms persist, explain that additional testing will be necessary in a few days or weeks to confirm the diagnosis and plan effective treatment.

erophil agglutination tests and hematologic tests. (See *Explaining mononucleosis* and *Heterophil antibody test interference*.)

What needs to be done

Perform a venipuncture, and collect the sample in a 7-ml clot-activator tube.

Warning!

Heterophil antibody test interference

• Narcotics and phenytoin therapy can produce false-positive results.
• Patients with lymphoma, hepatitis, or leukemia may have false-positive results.

Epstein-Barr virus antibodies

Epstein-Barr virus (EBV), a member of the herpesvirus group, is the causative agent in infectious mononucleosis, Burkitt's lymphoma, and nasopharyngeal carcinoma. Although the virus doesn't reproduce in standard cell cultures, most EBV infections can be recognized by testing the patient's serum for antibodies (monospot test), which usually appear within the first 3 weeks of illness and then decline rapidly within a few weeks. (See *Monospot test for infectious mononucleosis*, page 160.)

Alternatively, EBV-specific antibodies, which develop to several antigens, can be measured with high sensitivity and specificity by indirect immunofluorescence tests. The test profile can help determine whether the patient was infected recently or in the remote past.

What it all means

Serum from patients who have never been infected with EBV will have no detectable antibodies to the virus measured by either the monospot or indirect immunofluorescence test. The monospot test is positive only during the acute phase of EBV infection; the indirect immunofluorescence test will detect and discriminate between acute and past infection.

What needs to be done

• Perform a venipuncture, and collect 5 ml of sterile blood in a clot-activator tube. Allow the blood to clot for at least 1 hour at room temperature.
• Transfer the serum to a sterile tube or vial, and send it to the laboratory promptly. If transfer must be delayed, store the serum at 39.2° F (4° C) for 1 or 2 days or at –4° F (–20° C) for longer periods to prevent bacterial contamination.

Just call me Epstein-Barr. Testing for antibodies to me helps diagnose heterophil-negative infectious mononucleosis.

Now I get it!

Monospot test for infectious mononucleosis

The monospot test detects the infectious mononucleosis (IM) antibody. Heterophil antibodies, normally present in the blood, are produced in large amounts in patients with IM. These antibodies quickly clump together with horse red blood cells (RBCs).

The monospot test is performed by adding the patient's serum to horse RBCs on a slide. If clumping occurs, heterophil antibodies are present confirming IM.

Respiratory syncytial virus antibodies

Respiratory syncytial virus (RSV) is the major viral cause of severe lower respiratory tract disease in infants, but it may cause infections in persons of any age. RSV infections are most common and produce the most severe disease during the first 6 months of life.

Immunoglobulin (Ig) G and IgM class antibodies can be easily measured using the indirect immunofluorescence test. Specific results for IgM are obtained only after separating this class of antibody from IgG. Prevalence of IgG antibodies to RSV is extremely high (greater than 95%), especially in adults.

What it all means

Serum from patients who have never been infected with RSV will have no detectable antibodies to the virus (less than 1:5). In infants, serologic diagnosis of RSV infections is difficult because of the presence of maternal IgG antibodies; thus, the presence of IgM antibodies is most significant.

Ruling out RSV

RSV infection can be ruled out in patients whose serum samples have no detectable antibodies to the virus. The presence of IgM or a fourfold or greater increase in IgG antibodies indicates active RSV infection.

The RSV test diagnoses infections caused by RSV.

What needs to be done

• Perform a venipuncture, and collect 5 ml of sterile blood in a clot-activator tube. Allow the blood to clot for at least 1 hour at room temperature.
• Transfer the serum to a sterile tube or vial, and send it to the laboratory at once. If transfer must be delayed, store the serum at 39.2° F (4° C) for 1 to 2 days or at –4° F (–20° C) for longer periods to avoid bacterial contamination.

Herpes simplex antibodies

Herpes simplex virus (HSV), a member of the herpesvirus group, causes severe signs and symptoms, including genital lesions, keratitis or conjunctivitis, generalized dermal lesions, and pneumonia.

Two types

The HSV antibodies test confirms infections caused by HSV.

Of the two closely related types, type 1 usually causes infections above the waistline; type 2 primarily involves the external genitalia. Primary contact with this virus occurs in early childhood as acute stomatitis or, more commonly, as an inapparent infection. More than 50% of adults have antibodies to HSV.

Sensitive tests are used to demonstrate immunoglobulin (Ig) M class antibodies to HSV or to detect a fourfold or greater increase in IgG class antibodies between acute- and convalescent-phase serum.

What it all means

Serum from patients who have never been infected with HSV will have no detectable antibodies (less than 1:5). Patients with primary HSV infection develop IgM and IgG class antibodies. Reportedly, more than 50% of adults have IgG class antibodies to HSV because of prior infection. Reactivated infections caused by HSV can be recognized serologically only by an increase in IgG class antibodies between acute- and convalescent-phase serum.

Fourfold or greater = HSV

HSV infection can be ruled out in patients whose serum shows no detectable antibodies to the virus. The presence of IgM antibodies or a fourfold or greater increase in IgG antibodies indicates active HSV infection.

What needs to be done

• Perform a venipuncture, and collect 5 ml of sterile blood in a tube (color of top to be designated by the laboratory). Allow the blood to clot for at least 1 hour at room temperature.

• Transfer the serum to a sterile tube or vial, and promptly send it to the laboratory. If transfer must be delayed for 1 or 2 days, store the serum at 39.2° F (4° C); if it must be delayed longer, store at –4° F (–20° C) to avoid bacterial contamination.

Human immunodeficiency virus antibodies

A number of test methods are used to detect antibodies to human immunodeficiency virus (HIV) in serum. Among the most common are enzyme immunoassay, fluorescence immunoassay, and enzyme-linked immunosorbent assay (ELISA). Each of these methods requires a blood sample. Patient care, normal findings, and posttest care are the same for all. (See *Quick check: The rapid HIV test.*)

The HIV test can be used to screen patients and donated blood for HIV.

What it all means

Test results should be nonreactive. No known factors interfere with HIV antibodies.

Earlier exposure

This test detects previous exposure to HIV. A negative result doesn't necessarily mean that HIV antibodies aren't present. For example, the tests don't identify individuals who have been exposed to the virus but who haven't yet developed antibodies. A positive test for the HIV antibody can't determine whether the person

harbors actively replicating virus or when he'll present signs and symptoms of acquired immunodeficiency syndrome (AIDS).

Western blot — highly recommended

A false-positive result may reflect a lack of specificity of the test method used. As a result, the Western blot test for HIV is recommended for all persons with positive antibody tests. The Western blot test for HIV confirms HIV because it detects specific viral proteins present in HIV. (See *When test results are positive.*)

Quick check: The rapid HIV test

For the estimated 700,000 people a year who don't check back for test results, a rapid human immunodeficiency virus (HIV) test may be done. The SUDS HIV-1 is currently the only rapid HIV test with FDA approval. The results are obtained in less than 10 minutes, using a color indicator similar to a home pregnancy test. If it's positive, a confirmatory test must be done to validate the results.

Listen up!

When test results are positive

If your patient tests positive for human immunodeficiency virus (HIV), follow these guidelines:
• Keep your patient's HIV antibody test results confidential. When he receives the results, give him another opportunity to ask you questions.
• Encourage your patient with a positive result to seek medical follow-up care. Tell him to report early signs of AIDS, such as fever, weight loss, axillary or inguinal lymphadenopathy, rash, and persistent cough or diarrhea. Females should also report gynecologic symptoms.
• To prevent the spread of HIV, teach him safe sex precautions. Instruct him not to share razors, toothbrushes, or utensils that may be contaminated with blood and to clean such items with household bleach diluted 1:10 in water. Advise him not to donate blood, tissues, or organs.
• Urge the patient to inform his doctor and dentist about his condition so they can take precautions.

What needs to be done

• Perform a venipuncture, and collect the sample in a 10-ml barrier tube, which helps prevent contamination when pouring the serum.

Cytomegalovirus antibody screen

After primary infection, cytomegalovirus (CMV) remains latent in white blood cells (WBCs). The presence of CMV antibodies indicates past infection with this virus.

Screening tests for CMV antibodies are qualitative; they detect the presence of antibody at a single low dilution. In quantitative methods, several dilutions of the serum sample are tested to indicate acute infection with CMV.

What it all means

Patients who have never been infected with CMV have no detectable antibodies to the virus. Immunoglobulin IgG and IgM are normally negative.

A serum sample collected early during the acute phase or late in the convalescent stage may not contain detectable IgG or IgM antibodies to CMV. Therefore, a negative result doesn't preclude recent infection. More than a single sample is needed to ensure accurate results.

> *Presence of CMV antibodies indicates infection. The test screens organ donors and helps detect prior CMV infection in immunocompromised patients.*

Seronegative recipient needs seronegative donor

A serum sample that tests positive for antibodies at this single dilution indicates that the patient has been infected with CMV and that his WBCs contain latent virus capable of being reactivated in an immunocompromised host. Immunosuppressed patients who lack antibodies to CMV should receive blood products or organ transplants from donors who are also seronegative. Patients with CMV antibodies don't require seronegative blood products.

What needs to be done

• Perform a venipuncture, and collect the sample in a 5-ml tube without additives.
• Allow the blood to clot for at least 1 hour at room temperature.
• Transfer the serum to a sterile tube or vial, and send it to the laboratory.
• If transfer must be delayed, store the serum at 39.2° F (4° C) for 1 to 2 days or at –4° F (–20° C) for longer periods to avoid contamination.

Bacteria and fungi

Fungal serology

Most fungal organisms enter the body as spores inhaled into the lungs or infiltrated through wounds in the skin or mucosa. If the body's defenses can't destroy the organisms initially, the fungi multiply to form lesions; blood and lymph vessels may then spread the mycoses (diseases caused by a fungus) throughout the body. Mycosis may be deep-seated or superficial. Deep-seated mycosis occurs primarily in the lungs; superficial mycosis occurs in the skin or the mucosal linings.

Presence of antifungal antibodies indicates a fungal infection. Testing can monitor the effectiveness of mycosis therapy.

Culture club

Although cultures are usually performed to diagnose mycosis by identifying the causative organism, serologic tests occasionally provide the sole evidence of mycosis. These tests are used to detect blastomycosis, coccidioidomycosis, histoplasmosis, aspergillosis, sporotrichosis, and cryptococcosis. Fungal serologic tests use immunodiffusion, complement fixation, precipitin, latex agglutination, or agglutination methods to demonstrate the presence of mycotic antibodies.

What it all means

Depending on the test method, a negative finding or normal titer usually indicates the absence of mycosis. Elevated titers indicate that mycosis is present. (See *Fungal serology interference.*)

What needs to be done

• If appropriate, explain to the patient that the test monitors his response to therapy, and that it may be repeated during the course of his illness.
• Instruct the patient to restrict food and fluids for 12 to 24 hours before the test.
• Perform a venipuncture, and collect the sample in a 10-ml, sterile clot-activator tube.
• Send the sample to the laboratory immediately. If transport must be delayed, store the sample at 39.2° F (4° C).

Bacterial meningitis antigen

The bacterial meningitis antigen test can detect specific antigens of *Streptococcus pneumoniae*, *Neisseria meningitidis*, and *Haemophilus influenzae* type b, the principal organisms that cause meningitis. This test can be performed on samples of serum, cerebrospinal fluid (CSF), urine, pleural fluid, or joint fluid; however, the preferred specimen is CSF or urine.

What it all means

Normal results are negative for bacterial antigens.

A positive ID

Positive results identify the specific bacterial antigen: *S. pneumoniae*, *N. meningitidis*, *H. influenzae* type b, or group B streptococci in infants younger than 3 months. (See *Bacterial meningitis antigen test interference*, page 166.)

What needs to be done

• Explain the purpose of the test to the patient, and inform him that a urine or CSF specimen is required.
• If a CSF specimen is needed, describe how it will be obtained.
• Explain who will perform the lumbar puncture and when, and that transient discomfort may be felt from the needle puncture.
• Advise the patient that a headache is the most common adverse effect of lumbar puncture, but that cooperation during the test minimizes this effect.

Warning!

Fungal serology interference

• Some antigens, such as the blastomycosis and histoplasmosis antigens, may cross-react to produce false-positive results or high titers.
• Recent skin testing with fungal antigens may elevate titers.
• Many mycoses depress the immune system, causing low titers or false-negative results.

Testing for the bacterial meningitis antigen can identify the causative agent in meningitis.

- Make sure the patient or a family member has signed a consent form (if a CSF specimen is being obtained).
- As required, collect a 10-ml urine specimen or a 1-ml CSF specimen in a sterile container.
- Promptly send the specimen to the laboratory on a refrigerated coolant.

Warning!

Bacterial meningitis antigen test interference

Previous antimicrobial therapy may alter test results.

Lyme disease serology

Lyme disease is a multisystem disorder characterized by dermatologic, neurologic, cardiac, and rheumatic manifestations in various stages. Studies point to a commonly tickborne spirochete, *Borrelia burgdorferi*, as the causative agent.

50% early versus 100% late

Serologic tests for Lyme disease measure antibody response to this spirochete and indicate current infection or past exposure. These tests can identify 50% of patients with early-stage Lyme disease; nearly 100% of patients with later complications of carditis, neuritis, or arthritis; and 100% of patients in remission.

What it all means

Normal serum values are nonreactive.

Suggestive but not definite

A positive Lyme serologic test strongly suggests the diagnosis but isn't definitive because other treponemal diseases and high rheumatoid factor titers can cause false-positive results. Patients with other treponemal diseases demonstrate considerable cross-reactivity; up to 20% of patients with high rheumatoid factor titers may have positive Lyme disease reactions.

Don't be misled

In addition, a negative result doesn't rule out Lyme disease, because more than 15% of patients with Lyme disease fail to develop antibodies. (See *Lyme disease serology interference.*)

What needs to be done

- Instruct the patient to fast for 12 hours before the blood sample is drawn but to drink fluids as usual.

Lyme disease serology testing measures antibody response to the spirochete that causes Lyme disease.

- Perform a venipuncture, and collect the sample in a 7-ml clot-activator tube.
- Send the specimen to the laboratory immediately.

Helicobacter pylori antibodies

Helicobacter pylori is a spiral, gram-negative bacterium associated with chronic gastritis and idiopathic chronic duodenal ulceration. Although a gastric specimen can be obtained by endoscopy and cultured for *H. pylori*, the *H. pylori* antibody blood test is a more useful noninvasive screening procedure and may be performed using the enzyme-linked immunosorbent assay (ELISA) test.

What it all means

Normally, no antibodies to *H. pylori* are revealed. Test results are reported as negative or positive. There are no known factors that interfere with *H. pylori* antibodies.

Bacterium antibodies

A positive *H. pylori* test result indicates that the patient has antibodies to the bacterium. The serologic results should be interpreted in light of the clinical findings.

What needs to be done

- Perform a venipuncture, and collect the sample in a 7-ml clot-activator tube.
- Send the sample to the laboratory immediately.

Warning!

Lyme disease serology interference

Analysis of serum with high lipid levels may cause inaccurate results and requires test repetition after a period of restricted fat intake.

Because you have GI symptoms, we're testing for H. pylori antibodies to diagnose an ulcer.

Miscellaneous tests

Venereal Disease Research Laboratory test

The Venereal Disease Research Laboratory test, commonly known as the VDRL test, is widely used to screen for primary and secondary syphilis.

The VDRL test uses a serum sample but may also be performed on cerebrospinal fluid (CSF) to test for tertiary syphilis. However, the VDRL test of CSF is less sensitive than the fluorescent treponemal antibody absorption test. The rapid plasma reagin test can also be used to diagnose syphilis. (See *Rapid plasma reagin test*, page 168.)

What it all means

Absence of flocculation is reported as a nonreactive test.

Ifs, ands, or lesions

Definite flocculation is reported as a reactive test; slight floccula-tion is reported as a weakly reactive test. A reactive VDRL test oc-curs in about 50% of patients with primary syphilis and in nearly all patients with secondary syphilis. If syphilitic lesions exist, a re-active VDRL test is diagnostic. If no lesions are evident, a reactive VDRL test necessitates repeated testing. However, biologic false-positive reactions can be caused by conditions unrelated to syph-ilis, such as infectious mononucleosis, malaria, leprosy, hepatitis, systemic lupus erythematosus, rheumatoid arthritis, and such nonsyphilitic treponemal diseases as pinta or yaws.

On to the next stage

A reactive VDRL test using a CSF specimen indicates neurosyph-ilis, which can follow the primary and secondary stages in untreat-ed persons. (See *What to tell the patient with suspected syphilis.*)

A nonreactive test doesn't rule out syphilis because *T. pal-lidum* causes no detectable immunologic changes in the serum for 14 to 21 days after infection. However, dark-field microscopic examination of exudate from suspicious lesions can provide early diagnosis by identifying causative spirochetes. (See *VDRL test in-terference.*)

What needs to be done

- Tell the patient to abstain from alcohol for 24 hours before the test.

The VDRL test screens for primary and secondary syphilis and can monitor the patient's response to treatment.

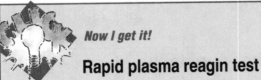

Now I get it!

Rapid plasma reagin test

The rapid plasma reagin (RPR) test, a rapid serologic test, is an accept-able substitute for the Venereal Disease Research Laboratory (VDRL) test in diagnosing syphilis. Available as a kit, the RPR test uses a cardi-olipin antigen to detect reagin, the antibody relatively specific for *Tre-ponema pallidum,* the agent that causes syphilis.

In the RPR test, like the VDRL test, normal serum shows no floccula-tion.

Listen up!

What to tell the patient with suspected syphilis

If your patient's VDRL test is nonreactive or borderline but syphilis hasn't been ruled out, instruct the patient to return for follow-up testing. Explain that borderline test results don't necessarily mean he's free from the disease.

If the test is reactive, explain the importance of proper treatment. Teach the patient about venereal disease and how it's spread, and stress the need for antibiotic therapy. Also, prepare him for mandatory inquiries from public health authorities. If the test is reactive but the patient shows no signs of syphilis, explain that many uninfected persons show false-positive reactions. Stress the need for further specific tests to rule out syphilis.

Warning!

VDRL test interference

- Ingestion of alcohol within 24 hours before the test can produce transient nonreactive results.
- A faulty immune system can cause nonreactive results.

- Perform a venipuncture, and collect the sample in a 7-ml clot-activator tube.

Carcinoembryonic antigen

Carcinoembryonic antigen (CEA) is a protein normally found in embryonic endodermal epithelium and fetal tissue. CEA production usually stops before birth but may begin again later if a neoplasm develops.

Because CEA levels are raised by biliary obstruction, alcoholic hepatitis, chronic heavy smoking, and other conditions as well as by benign or malignant neoplasms, the CEA test can't be used as a general indicator of cancer. Measurement of CEA levels is useful for staging and monitoring treatment of certain cancers. Other tests are used to diagnose certain types of cancer. (See *Using CEA tests to monitor cancer treatment*, page 170.)

CEA testing is a good way to monitor the effectiveness of cancer therapy. It can also help stage cancer and test for recurrence.

What it all means

Normal serum CEA values are less than 5 ng/ml (SI, 5 mg/L) in healthy nonsmokers. Approximately 5% of the population has above-normal CEA levels.

On the trail to success

If serum CEA levels are above normal before surgical resection, chemotherapy, or radiation

Advice from the experts

Using CEA tests to monitor cancer treatment

Because many patients in the early stages of colorectal cancer have normal or low levels of carcinoembryonic antigen (CEA), the CEA test doesn't screen successfully for early malignancy. However, it's a good tool for monitoring response to cancer therapy. After a patient's serum CEA level has decreased following surgery, chemotherapy, or other treatment, any increase suggests cancer recurrence or diminished effectiveness of treatment.

Both charts below show CEA levels in patients during and after colorectal cancer treatment. In the top chart, initial results show the usual dramatic drop in response to treatment; the subsequent rise in CEA indicates a diminishing response to chemotherapy. In the bottom chart, the progressive CEA rise signals cancer recurrence 8 months before clinical symptoms or radiologic evidence.

therapy, a return to normal within 6 weeks after therapy suggests successful treatment. Persistent elevation of CEA levels, however, suggests residual or recurrent tumor.

Beware of heights

High CEA levels are characteristic in various malignant conditions, particularly endodermally derived neoplasms of the GI organs and the lungs and in certain nonmalignant conditions, such as benign hepatic disease, hepatic cirrhosis, alcoholic pancreatitis, and inflammatory bowel disease. Elevated CEA levels may also result from nonendodermal cancers, such as breast cancer and ovarian cancer. (See *CEA test interference.*)

What needs to be done

• If appropriate, inform the patient that the test will be repeated to monitor the effectiveness of therapy.
• Perform a venipuncture, and collect the sample in a 7-ml tube without additives.
• Send the sample to the laboratory immediately.

Warning!

CEA test interference

• Chronic cigarette smoking may elevate CEA antigen levels, altering test results.
• Alcohol ingestion may alter results.

Alpha-fetoprotein

Alpha-fetoprotein (AFP) is a glycoprotein produced by fetal tissue and tumors that differentiate from midline embryonic structures. During fetal development, AFP levels in serum and amniotic fluid rise; because this protein crosses the placenta, it appears in maternal serum. In late stages of pregnancy, AFP levels in fetal and maternal serum and in amniotic fluid begin to diminish. During the 1st year of life, serum AFP levels continue to decline and usually remain low thereafter.

What it all means

When testing by immunoassay, AFP values are less than 15 ng/ml (SI, 15 mg/L) in males and nonpregnant females. Values in maternal serum are less than 2.5 multiples of median for fetal gestational age.

Elevations in pregnant patients...

Elevated maternal serum AFP levels may suggest a neural tube defect or other neural tube anomalies after 14 weeks' gestation. AFP levels rise sharply in approximately 90% of fetuses with anencephaly and in 50% of those with spina bifida. Definitive diagnosis requires ultrasonography and amniocentesis. High AFP levels may indicate intrauterine death or such anom-

AFP levels can help determine the need for amniocentesis or high-resolution ultrasound in a pregnant woman. They can also monitor the effectiveness of therapy in some malignant diseases.

alies as duodenal atresia, omphalocele, tetralogy of Fallot, or Turner's syndrome.

...and in nonpregnant patients

Elevated serum AFP levels in 70% of nonpregnant persons may indicate hepatocellular carcinoma (although low AFP levels don't rule it out) or germ cell tumor of gonadal, retroperitoneal, or mediastinal origin. Serum AFP level rises in patients with ataxia-telangiectasia and in patients with cancer of the pancreas, stomach, or biliary system. Transient modest elevations can occur in nonneoplastic hepatocellular disease, such as alcoholic cirrhosis and acute or chronic hepatitis. Elevation of AFP levels after remission suggests tumor recurrence.

Favorable response

In patients with hepatocellular carcinoma, a gradual decrease in serum AFP levels indicates a favorable response to therapy. In patients with germ cell tumors, serum AFP and human chorionic gonadotropin levels should be measured at the same time. (See *AFP test interference.*)

What needs to be done

• Advise the patient that she may need further testing.
• Perform a venipuncture, and collect the sample in a 7-ml clot-activator tube. Record the patient's age, race, weight, and gestational period on the laboratory request.

TORCH test

The TORCH test detects exposure to pathogens involved in congenital and neonatal infections. These pathogens are commonly associated with congenital or neonatal infections that aren't clinically apparent and may cause severe central nervous system impairment. This test confirms such infection serologically by detecting specific antibodies in infant blood.

What it all means

Test results should be negative for TORCH agents.

Exams in sequence

Toxoplasmosis is diagnosed by sequential examination that shows rising antibody titers, changing titers, and serologic conversion from negative to positive; a titer of 1:256 suggests recent *Toxoplasma* infection. Approximately two-thirds of infected infants are

---

Warning!

AFP test interference

Multiple pregnancy may cause false-positive results.

The TORCH test aids diagnosis of acute, congenital, and intrapartum infections.

asymptomatic at birth; one-third show signs of cerebral calcification and choroidoretinitis.

Hereditary factor

In infants less than 6 months old, rubella infection is associated with a marked and persistent rise in complement-fixing antibody titer over time. Persistence of rubella antibody in an infant after age 6 months strongly suggests congenital infection. Congenital rubella is associated with cardiac anomalies, neurosensory deafness, growth retardation, and encephalitic symptoms. Detection of herpes antibodies in cerebrospinal fluid with signs of herpetic encephalitis and persistent herpes simplex virus type 2 antibody levels confirms herpes simplex infection in a neonate without obvious herpetic lesions.

What needs to be done

• Obtain a 3-ml sample of venous or cord blood. Send it to the laboratory promptly for serologic testing.

Tuberculin skin tests

Tuberculin skin tests are used to screen patients for previous infection by the tubercle bacillus. They're routinely performed in children, young adults, and people with radiographic findings that suggest this infection.

In both the old tuberculin (OT) and the purified protein derivative (PPD) tests, intradermal injection of the tuberculin antigen causes a delayed hypersensitivity reaction in patients with active or dormant tuberculosis; sensitized lymphocytes gather at the injection site, causing erythema, vesiculation, and induration that peaks within 24 to 48 hours and persists for at least 72 hours.

Accurate or easy?

The most accurate tuberculin test method, the Mantoux test, uses a single-needle intradermal injection of PPD, which permits precise measurement of dosage. Multipuncture tests, such as the tine test, Mono-Vacc test, and Aplitest, involve intradermal injections using tines impregnated with OT or PPD. Because multipuncture tests require less skill and are more rapidly administered than the Mantoux test, they're generally used for screening. However, a positive multipuncture test usually requires a Mantoux test for confirmation. (See *Performing tuberculin skin tests*, page 174, and *Tuberculin skin test follow-up*, page 174.)

Tuberculin skin tests help determine whether a patient has been exposed to TB.

What it all means

For the Mantoux test, induration less than 5 mm in diameter or no induration indicates a negative reaction.

For the tine test and Aplitest, no induration or induration less than 2 mm in diameter indicates a negative reaction. No induration indicates a negative reaction for the Mono-Vacc test. (See *Reading tuberculin skin test results.*)

Equal opportunity test

A positive tuberculin reaction indicates previous infection by tubercle bacilli. It doesn't distinguish between an active and dormant infection; nor does it provide a definitive diagnosis. If a positive reaction occurs, sputum smear and culture and chest X-rays are necessary to provide more information.

Listen up!

Tuberculin skin test follow-up

If you're performing a tuberculin test on an outpatient, instruct him to return at the specified time so test results can be read. Tell him that a positive reaction to a skin test appears as a red, hard, raised area at the injection site.

If it itches, don't scratch
Although the area may itch, instruct the patient not to scratch it. Stress that a positive reaction doesn't always indicate active tuberculosis.

Peak technique

Performing tuberculin skin tests

Before you perform tuberculin skin testing, gather the following equipment: alcohol swabs, a vial of purified protein derivative (intermediate strength)—5 tuberculin units (TU) per 0.1 ml, a 1-ml tuberculin syringe with a ½″ (1.3-cm) or ⅝″ (1.6-cm) 25G or 26G needle for the Mantoux test, and a commercially available device (tine, Mono-Vacc, or Aplitest) for multipuncture tests. Be sure to have epinephrine (1:1,000) and a 3-ml syringe available to treat an anaphylactic or acute hypersensitivity reaction.

Next, have the patient sit with his arm extended and supported on a flat surface. Clean the volar surface of the upper forearm with alcohol, and let the area dry completely.

Test procedures
The procedure depends on which test you conduct:
• *Mantoux test*—Perform an intradermal injection.
• *Multipuncture tests*—Remove the protective cap on the injection device to expose the four tines. Hold the patient's forearm in one hand, stretching the forearm skin tightly. With your other hand, firmly depress the device into the skin (without twisting it). Hold the device in place for at least 1 second before removing it. If you have applied sufficient pressure, you'll see four puncture sites and a circular depression on the patient's skin.

After the test
Record where the test was given, the date and time, and when it's to be read. Tuberculin skin tests generally are read 48 to 72 hours after injection. However, the Mono-Vacc test can be read 48 to 96 hours after the test.

Advice from the experts

Reading tuberculin skin test results

Read the Mantoux, tine, and Aplitest skin tests 48 to 72 hours after injection. Read the Mono-Vacc test 48 to 96 hours afterward.

In a well-lighted room, flex the patient's forearm slightly. Observe the injection site for erythema and vesiculation; then gently rub your finger over the site to detect induration. If induration is present, measure the diameter in millimeters, preferably using a plastic ruler marked in concentric circles of specific diameter.

In multipuncture tests, you may find separate areas of induration around individual punctures or induration involving more than one puncture site. If so, measure the diameter of the largest single area of induration or coalesced induration.

Warning!

Tuberculin skin test interference

• Corticosteroids, other immunosuppressants, or live vaccine viruses (measles, mumps, rubella, or polio) given within the previous 4 to 6 weeks may suppress skin reactions.
• Elderly people and patients with viral infection, malnutrition, febrile illness, uremia, immunosuppressive disorders, or miliary tuberculosis (TB) may have suppressed skin reactions.
• If less than 10 weeks have elapsed since TB infection, the skin reaction may be suppressed.

Borderline

In the Mantoux test, induration of 5 to 9 mm in diameter indicates a borderline reaction; larger induration, a positive reaction. Because patients with atypical mycobacteria other than tubercle bacilli may have borderline reactions, repeat testing is necessary.

Vesicular presence

In the tine test or Aplitest, vesicles indicate a positive reaction; induration of 2 mm in diameter without vesicles requires confirmation by the Mantoux test. Any induration in the Mono-Vacc test indicates a positive reaction but requires confirmation by the Mantoux test. (See *Tuberculin skin test interference.*)

What needs to be done

• Check the patient's history for active TB, the results of previous skin tests, and hypersensitivities. If the patient has had TB, don't perform a skin test; if he's had a positive reaction to previous skin tests, consult the doctor or follow your facility's policy.
• Tuberculin skin tests are contraindicated in patients with active TB, a current reaction to smallpox vaccinations, any type of rash, or a skin disorder.
• Don't perform a skin test in areas with excessive hair, acne, or insufficient subcutaneous tissue, such as over a tendon or bone.

Quick quiz

1. Which blood type can be transfused in limited amounts in an emergency to any patient regardless of the recipient's blood type?

A. Type O
B. Type A
C. Type B

Answer: A. Because type O blood lacks both A and B antigens, it can be transfused in limited amounts in an emergency to any recipient—with little risk of adverse reaction.

2. Within which period must crossmatching be performed on a blood sample?

A. 24 hours
B. 36 hours
C. 72 hours

Answer: C. Crossmatching, which establishes the compatibility of donor and recipient blood, must be performed on a blood sample within 72 hours.

3. Infection by RSV can be ruled out when:

A. serum samples have no detectable antibodies to the virus.
B. IgM is present in the serum sample.
C. IgG antibodies increase fourfold.

Answer: A. In patients whose serum samples have no detectable antibodies to the virus, RSV can be ruled out.

4. Which instruction should you give a patient before Lyme disease serology testing?

A. Avoid alcohol for 24 hours before the test.
B. Fast for 12 hours before the test.
C. Don't take phenytoin within 8 hours of testing.

Answer: B. Instruct the patient to fast for 12 hours before the test but to drink fluids as usual.

Scoring

☆☆☆ If you answered all four questions correctly, hooray! You're the Sultan of Serum Samples!

☆☆ If you answered two or three questions correctly, great! You're an immunologic icon!

☆ If you answered fewer than two correctly, don't worry. These assays will become easy in no time!

5

Urine tests

Just the facts

In this chapter, you'll learn:

♦ about urine tests

♦ what patient care is associated with these tests

♦ what factors can interfere with test results

♦ what urine test results may indicate.

A look at urine tests

Urine formation is one of the primary functions of the urinary system. When formed, normal urine consists of sodium, chloride, potassium, calcium, magnesium, sulfates, phosphates, bicarbonate, uric acid, ammonium ions, creatinine, and urobilinogen (a bilirubin derivative resulting from the action of intestinal bacteria). A few leukocytes and red blood cells (and in males, some spermatozoa) may enter urine as it passes from the kidney to the ureteral orifice. The urine of a person receiving drugs normally excreted in urine contains drug substances as well. Because urine tests can reveal much about a patient's overall well-being, these tests are valuable tools for diagnosing many disorders. Before urine testing begins, explain the procedure to the patient.

Urinalysis screens for renal or urinary tract disease and helps detect metabolic and systemic disease.

Urinalysis

Routine urinalysis serves many functions. It can be used to screen patients for kidney and urinary tract disease and can help detect metabolic or systemic disease.

During the course of a routine urinalysis, you'll:
• evaluate the color, odor, and opacity of urine
• determine urine's specific gravity and pH
• detect and measure protein, glucose, and ketone bodies
• examine urine sediment for blood cells, casts, and crystals.

What it all means

Results of urine tests are based on the elements that make up urine. Even with normal findings, these elements have certain characteristics. (See *Normal findings in routine urinalysis*.)

Normal findings in routine urinalysis

Element	Findings
Macroscopic	
Color	Straw to dark yellow
Odor	Slightly aromatic
Appearance	Clear
Specific gravity	1.005 to 1.035
pH	4.5 to 8.0
Protein	None
Glucose	None
Ketones	None
Bilirubin	None
Urobilinogen	Normal
Hemoglobin	None
Red blood cells (RBCs)	None
Nitrite (bacteria)	None
White blood cells (WBCs)	None
Microscopic	
RBCs	0 to 2 per high-power field
WBCs	0 to 5 per high-power field
Epithelial cells	0 to 5 per high-power field
Casts	None, except 1 to 2 hyaline casts per low-power field
Crystals	Present
Bacteria	None
Yeast cells	None
Parasites	None

Specific gravity is a weighty issue! It measures the weight of a substance, such as urine, and compares it with the weight of an equal volume of another substance.

Pondering the pathologic

Abnormal findings show an alteration in the normal characteristics of urine. The following abnormal findings typically suggest a pathologic condition:

• *color change*—from diet, drugs, or disease
• *unusual odor*—due to ketone bodies, infection, or disease
• *turbidity* (cloudiness)—from kidney infection
• *low specific gravity* (less than 1.005)—from diabetes insipidus, acute tubular necrosis, or pyelonephritis
• *fixed specific gravity* (1.010 regardless of fluid intake)—from chronic glomerulonephritis with severe kidney damage
• *high specific gravity* (greater than 1.035)—from nephrotic syndrome, dehydration, acute glomerulonephritis, heart failure, liver failure, or shock
• *high pH* (alkaline urine)—from Fanconi's syndrome, urinary tract infection, or metabolic or respiratory alkalosis
• *low pH* (acidic urine)—from renal tuberculosis, pyrexia, phenylketonuria, alkaptonuria, or acidosis
• *proteinuria* (excess serum proteins in urine)—from renal failure or, possibly, multiple myeloma
• *sugars in urine*—usually from diabetes mellitus but possibly from pheochromocytoma (brain tumor), Cushing's syndrome, impaired tubular reabsorption, advanced kidney disease, increased intracranial pressure, or I.V. solutions containing glucose and total parenteral nutrition containing from 10% to 50% glucose
• *ketone bodies* (used as fuel by muscle and brain tissue)—from diabetes mellitus, starvation, pregnancy and lactation, or diarrhea or vomiting
• *bilirubin*—from liver disease or from fibrosis of the biliary canaliculi (as in cirrhosis)
• *increased urobilinogen*—liver damage, hemolytic disease, or severe infection (increased values)
• *decreased urobilinogen*—biliary obstruction, inflammatory disease, antimicrobial therapy, severe diarrhea, or renal insufficiency
• *blood cells*—infection, obstruction, inflammation, trauma, tumors, or other causes
• *excessive casts*—renal disease
• *calcium oxalate crystals*—hypercalcemia
• *cystine crystals*—inborn error of metabolism
• *bacteria, yeast cells, parasites*—genitourinary tract infection or contamination of external genitalia.

> Turbidity refers to the cloudiness of a solution caused by particles or sediment.

Advice from the experts

Drugs that influence routine urinalysis results

The table below lists some commonly used drugs and their effects on routine urinalysis results.

Drugs that change urine color
amitriptyline (blue-green)
Iron salts (black)
levodopa (dark)
methylene blue (blue-green)
metronidazole (dark)
Oral anticoagulants (orange)
Phenothiazines (dark)
phenytoin (red to reddish brown or pink)
rifampin (red-orange)

Drugs that cause proteinuria
Aminoglycosides
amphotericin B
bacitracin
Cephalosporins
cisplatin
Nonsteroidal anti-inflammatory drugs
Sulfonamides

Drugs that cause true glycosuria
ammonium chloride
carbamazepine
Corticosteroids

Estrogens
lithium carbonate
phenytoin
Thiazide diuretics

Drugs that cause true ketonuria
insulin (excessive doses)
isoniazid (intoxication)

Drugs that increase white blood cell count
allopurinol
ampicillin
aspirin (toxicity)
methicillin

Drugs that cause hematuria
amphotericin B
aspirin
bacitracin
caffeine
Coumarin derivatives
indomethacin
methicillin
Sulfonamides

What needs to be done

- Tell the patient to avoid stress and strenuous exercise before the test.
- Check for drugs that influence urinalysis. (See *Drugs that influence routine urinalysis results.*)
- Collect a random urine specimen of at least 15 ml, preferably a first-voided morning specimen.
- If the patient is being evaluated for renal colic, strain the specimen to catch stones or stone fragments.
- Refrigerate the specimen if analysis will be delayed longer than 1 hour.

Enzymes

Urine amylase

Amylase is a starch-splitting enzyme produced primarily in the pancreas and salivary glands. It's usually secreted into the alimentary tract and then absorbed into the blood. Small amounts of amylase are also absorbed into the blood directly from the pancreas and salivary glands. After glomerular filtration, amylase is excreted in the urine.

What it all means

Urinary excretion of 10 to 80 amylase U/hour (SI, 265 to 680 U/day) is generally considered normal.

A variety of conditions can cause elevated amylase levels, including acute pancreatitis; obstruction of the pancreatic duct, intestines, or salivary duct; carcinoma of the head of the pancreas; mumps; acute injury to the spleen; renal disease with impaired absorption; perforated peptic or duodenal ulcers; and gallbladder disease. (See *Urine amylase test interference*, page 182.)

When amylase is lookin' low

Depressed levels occur in association with chronic pancreatitis, cachexia, alcoholism, cancer of the liver, cirrhosis, hepatitis, and hepatic abscess.

What needs to be done

- If a female patient is menstruating, the test may have to be rescheduled.
- The test requires urine collection for 2, 6, 8, or 24 hours, and certain steps should be followed when collecting a specimen. (See *Teaching the patient to collect a timed urine specimen*, page 182.)
- The following medications may raise urine amylase levels and should be withheld for 24 hours before the test: morphine, meperidine, codeine, pentazocine, bethanechol, thiazide diuretics, indomethacin, and ethyl alcohol. Fluoride may decrease levels. If any of the medications must be continued, note this on the laboratory request.
- Collect a 2-, 6-, 8-, or 24-hour specimen.
- Cover and refrigerate the specimen during the collection period. If the patient is catheterized, keep the collection bag on ice.

Teaching the patient to collect a timed urine specimen

Explain the following process to the patient to make sure he properly collects a timed urine specimen:
- Provide a container for patient to void into.
- Have the patient void and then discard this specimen.
- Following this discarded specimen, instruct him to pour every voided specimen into the collection bottle.
- If required, keep the specimen on ice or refrigerated (if collecting at home, keep the specimen in a brown paper bag separated from other refrigerated contents).
- Warn the patient not to void directly into the specimen container, especially if it contains a preservative.
- Ask the patient to void just before the collection period ends, if possible, and add it to the collection bottle.
- Seal the specimen bottle, attach a label, and send it to the laboratory.

Urine amylase test interference

- Use of morphine, meperidine, codeine, pentazocine, bethanechol, thiazide diuretics, indomethacin, or alcohol within 24 hours of the test may raise levels.
- Fluoride may lower levels.
- High levels of bacterial contamination of the specimen or blood in the urine may alter results.
- Coughing or talking over the sample may result in salivary amylase in the urine.

Hormones

Urine aldosterone

Aldosterone promotes retention of sodium and excretion of potassium by the renal tubules, thereby helping regulate blood pressure and fluid and electrolyte balance.

The urine aldosterone test measures urine levels of aldosterone, the principal mineralocorticoid secreted by the zona glomerulosa of the adrenal cortex.

What it all means

Normally, urine aldosterone levels range from 2 to 20 µg/24 hours (SI, 5.6 to 7.2 nmol/24 day).

Primarily speaking...

Increased urine aldosterone levels suggest primary or secondary aldosteronism. The primary form usually arises from an aldosterone-secreting tumor of the adrenal cortex, but it may also result from adrenocortical hyperplasia (abnormal reproduction of normal cells). Patients with primary aldosteronism have increased aldosterone and decreased renin levels.

Warning!

Urine aldosterone test interference

- Excess intake of licorice or glucose
- Some antihypertensive and corticosteroid drugs
- Radioactive scan performed 1 week before the test

> Urine aldosterone testing aids diagnosis of primary and secondary aldosteronisms.

...and a secondary opinion

Secondary aldosteronism, the more common form, results from external stimulation of the adrenal cortex. The major systemic disorders that result in secondary aldosteronism are malignant hypertension, heart failure, cirrhosis of the liver, nephrotic syndrome, and idiopathic cyclic edema.

The lowdown on levels

Low urine aldosterone levels may result from Addison's disease, hypernatremia, overhydration, and toxemia of pregnancy. Aldosterone levels normally rise during pregnancy but rapidly decline following parturition. (See *Urine aldosterone test interference.*)

What needs to be done

- Check the patient's history for drugs that may affect aldosterone levels.
- The patient should maintain a normal sodium diet (3 g/day) before the test, avoid sodium-rich foods, and avoid strenuous physical exercise and stressful situations during the collection period.
- The test requires collection of a 24-hour urine specimen.
- Collect a 24-hour specimen in a bottle containing a preservative, such as boric acid, to keep the specimen at a pH of 4.0 to 4.5.
- Refrigerate the specimen or place it on ice during the collection period.

Urine free cortisol

The urine free cortisol test measures urine levels of the portion of cortisol not bound to the corticosteroid-binding globulin transcortin.

Free and easy, unbound and active

Only about 10% of free cortisol is unbound and physiologically active. Urine cortisol concentrations increase significantly when the amount secreted exceeds the binding capacity of transcortin, which is normally almost saturated.

What it all means

Normally, free cortisol values range from 20 to 90 μmol/24 hours (SI, 55 to 230 μmol/day). Elevated free cortisol levels may indicate Cushing's syndrome resulting from adrenal hyperplasia, an adrenal or pituitary tumor, or ectopic corticotropin production. (See *Urine free cortisol test interference.*)

What needs to be done

• Check the patient's history for medications that may interfere with test results, such as reserpine, phenothiazines, morphine, amphetamines, and prolonged steroid use.
• The patient should avoid stressful situations and excessive physical exercise during the collection period.
• The test requires collection of a 24-hour urine specimen, and the proper collection technique should be used.
• Collect a 24-hour specimen in a bottle containing a preservative to keep the specimen at a pH of 4.0 to 4.5.
• Refrigerate the specimen or place it on ice during the collection period.

The urine free cortisol test helps diagnose Cushing's syndrome.

Urine catecholamines

The urine catecholamine test measures urine levels of the major catecholamines—dopamine, epinephrine, and norepinephrine. Dopamine is secreted by the central nervous system; epinephrine, by the adrenal medulla; and norepinephrine, by both.

Catecholamines help regulate metabolism and prepare the body for the fight-or-flight response to stress. Certain tumors can also secrete catecholamines. One of the most common of these is a pheochromocytoma, which causes intermittent or persistent hypertension.

Conditions for collection

A 24-hour urine specimen is preferred for this test because catecholamine secretion fluctuates diurnally and in response to pain, heat, cold, emotional stress, physical exercise, hypoglycemia, injury, hemorrhage, asphyxia, and drugs.

Warning!

Urine free cortisol test interference

• Reserpine, phenothiazines, morphine, amphetamines, oral contraceptives, danazol, aldactone, and prolonged corticosteroid therapy may alter levels.
• Dexamethasone, ethacrynic acid, thiazides, and ketoconazole may decrease levels.
• Pregnancy causes increased levels.

What it all means

Normally, urine epinephrine values range from undetectable to 10 ng/24 hours (SI, 55 nmol/day); norepinephrine, from undetectable to 100 ng/24 hours (SI, 591 nmol/day); and metanephrines, from 0.1 to 1.6 mg/24 hours (SI, 0.5 to 8.7 μmol/day).

Abnormal findings

In a patient with undiagnosed hypertension, elevated urine catecholamine levels following a hypertensive episode usually indicate a pheochromocytoma.

Elevated catecholamine levels without marked hypertension may be caused by a neuroblastoma or a ganglioneuroma. Elevated catecholamine levels may also be seen in severe systemic situations, cor pulmonale, manic depressive disorders, or depressive neurosis.

Consistently low-normal catecholamine levels may indicate dysautonomia (a rare autonomic nervous system disease with mental retardation), marked by orthostatic hypotension. (See *Urine catecholamine test interference.*)

Measuring urine catecholamine levels aids pheochromocytoma diagnosis in patients with unexpained hypertension. It also aids diagnosis of neuroblastoma, ganglioneuroma, and dysantonia.

What needs to be done

• Check the patient's drug history for medications that may affect catecholamine levels.
• Stressful situations and excessive physical activity should be avoided during the collection period.
• The test may require a 24-hour specimen or a random specimen.

UH-OH!

Warning!

Urine catecholamine test interference

• Caffeine, insulin, nitroglycerin, aminophylline, ethanol, sympathomimetics, methyldopa, tricyclic antidepressants, chloral hydrate, quinidine, quinine, tetracycline, B-complex vitamins, isoproterenol, levodopa, and monoamine oxidase inhibitors may raise levels.
• Clonidine, guanethidine, reserpine, and iodine-containing contrast media may lower levels.
• Phenothiazines, erythromycin, and methenamine compounds may raise or lower levels.

- For a 24-hour urine specimen, collect it in a bottle containing a preservative to keep the specimen acidified to a pH of 3.0 or less; for a random specimen, collect it immediately after a hypertensive episode.
- Refrigerate a 24-hour specimen or place it on ice during the collection period.

Total urine estrogens

The total urine estrogens test is a quantitative analysis of total urine levels of estradiol, estrone, and estriol—the major estrogens present in significant amounts in urine.

What it all means

Total estrogen levels range as follows:
- *nonpregnant females:* 5 to 80 µg/24 hours (SI, 5 to 80 µg/day)
- *pregnant females:* first trimester: 0 to 800 µg/24 hours (SI, 0 to 800 µg/day); second trimester: 800 to 5,000 µg/24 hours (SI, 800 to 5,000 µg/day); third trimester: 5,000 to 50,000 µg/24 hours (SI, 5,000 to 50,000 µg/day)
- *postmenopausal females:* less than 10 µg/24 hours (SI, less than 10 µg/day)
- *males:* levels range from 4 to 24 µg/24 hours (SI, 4 to 24 µg/day).

Ebb and flow

In nonpregnant females, total urine estrogen levels rise and fall during the menstrual cycle.

Estrogen's suggestions

Decreased total urine estrogen levels may reflect ovarian agenesis; primary ovarian insufficiency, which can be caused by Stein-Leventhal syndrome, for example; or secondary ovarian insufficiency, which can be caused by pituitary or adrenal hypofunction or metabolic disturbances.

Elevated total estrogen levels in nonpregnant females may indicate tumors of ovarian or adrenocortical origin, adrenocortical hyperplasia, or a metabolic or hepatic disorder. In males, elevated total estrogen levels are associated with testicular tumors. (See *Total urine estrogen test interference.*)

What needs to be done

- Collect the urine over a 24-hour period, using a bottle containing a preservative to keep the specimen at a pH of 3.0 to 5.0.

Measuring total urine estrogens helps establish fetoplacental status and can help diagnose ovarian, adrenocortical, and testicular tumors.

- If the patient is pregnant, note the approximate week of gestation on the laboratory slip.
- If the patient is a nonpregnant female, note the stage of her menstrual cycle.
- Refrigerate the specimen or keep it on ice during the collection period.

Urine human chorionic gonadotropin

As a qualitative analysis of urine levels of human chorionic gonadotropin (hCG), this test can detect pregnancy as early as 14 days after ovulation. Quantitative measurements can evaluate suspected hydatidiform mole or hCG-secreting tumors.

The hCG life cycle

Levels of hCG rise steadily and rapidly during the first trimester, peak around the 10th week of gestation, and subsequently taper off to less than 10% of peak levels.

What it all means

In qualitative analysis, if agglutination fails to occur, the test results are positive, which indicates pregnancy.

In quantitative analysis, urine hCG levels in the first trimester of a normal pregnancy may be as high as 500,000 IU/24 hours (SI, up to 500,000 IU/L[6]); / in the second trimester, they range from 10,000 to 25,000 IU/24 hours (SI, 10,000 to 25,000 IU/L[6]); and in the third trimester, from 5,000 to 15,000 IU/24 hours (SI, 5,000 to 15,000 IU/L[6]). Levels decline rapidly after delivery and are undetectable within a few days.

When a baby is on the way

During pregnancy, elevated urine hCG levels may indicate multiple pregnancy or erythroblastosis fetalis (hemolytic disease of the newborn characterized by anemia, jaundice, and enlargement of the liver and spleen); low levels may indicate threatened abortion or ectopic pregnancy.

Nonpregnant patients

Measurable hCG levels in males and nonpregnant females may indicate choriocarcinoma, ovarian or testicular tumors, melanoma, multiple myeloma, or gastric, hepatic, pancreatic, or breast cancer. (See *Urine hCG test interference*, page 188.)

Warning!

Total urine estrogen test interference

Drugs that may influence total urine estrogen levels include:
- steroid hormones
- methenamine mandelate
- phenazopyridine hydrochloride
- phenothiazines
- tetracyclines
- phenolphthalein
- ampicillin
- meprobamate
- senna
- cascara sagrada
- hydrochlorothiazide.

The hCG test is a reliable way to confirm pregnancy.

What needs to be done

- Check the patient's recent medication history for use of drugs that may affect hCG levels.
- The patient should restrict fluids for 8 hours before the test.
- The test requires a first-voided morning specimen or a 24-hour urine collection.
- For qualitative analysis, collect a first-voided morning specimen. If this isn't possible, collect a random specimen.
- For quantitative analysis of hCG, collect a 24-hour urine specimen.
- Specify the date of the patient's last menstrual period on the laboratory request. The test should be performed at least 5 days after a missed period.
- Refrigerate the 24-hour specimen or keep it on ice.

Warning!

Urine hCG test interference

- Phenothiazine use may result in false-negative or false-positive results.
- Gross proteinuria (more than 1 g/24 hours), hematuria, or an elevated erythrocyte sedimentation rate may produce false-positive results.
- Early pregnancy, ectopic pregnancy, or threatened abortion may produce false-negative results.

Metabolites

Urine 17-hydroxycorticosteroids

This test measures urine levels of 17-hydroxycorticosteroids (17-OHCS) — metabolites of the hormones that regulate glyconeogenesis. More than 80% of all urinary 17-OHCS are metabolites of cortisol, the primary adrenocortical steroid. Because cortisol secretion varies diurnally and in response to stress and many other factors, urine 17-OHCS levels are most accurately determined from a 24-hour specimen.

What it all means

The following are reference values:
- *males:* 5.5 to 14.4 mg/24 hours (SI, 15.2 to 39.7 µmol/day)
- *females:* 4.9 to 12.9 mg/24 hours (SI, 13.5 to 35.6 µmol/day)
- *children ages 8 to 12:* less than 4.5 mg/24 hours (SI, less than 11 µmol/day)
- *children under age 8:* less than 1.5 mg/24 hours (SI, less than 4.1 µmol/day).

The lowdown on levels

Levels normally increase slightly during the first trimester of pregnancy. Patients who are obese or very muscular may excrete slightly higher amounts of 17-OHCS because of increased cortisol catabolism. Elevated urine 17-OHCS levels may indicate Cushing's syndrome, adrenal carcinoma or adenoma, or a pituitary tumor.

The urine 17-OHCS test assesses adrenocortical function.

Warning!

Urine 17-OHCS test interference

- Drugs that may elevate levels include meprobamate, phenothiazines, spironolactone, ascorbic acid, chloral hydrate, colchicine, erythromycin, paraldehyde, glutethimide, chlordiazepoxide, penicillin G, hydroxyzine, quinidine, quinine, iodides, and methenamine.
- Drugs that may suppress levels include estrogens, oral contraceptives, phenothiazines, hydralazine, phenytoin, thiazide diuretics, nalidixic acid, and reserpine.

Increased levels may also occur in patients with virilism, hyperthyroidism, or severe hypertension. Extreme stress induced by such conditions as acute pancreatitis and eclampsia also increases urine 17-OHCS levels.

Low urine 17-OHCS levels may indicate Addison's disease, hypopituitarism, or myxedema. (See *Urine 17-OHCS test interference.*)

What needs to be done

- Check the patient's history for drugs that may affect 17-OHCS levels.
- Tell the patient he should avoid excessive physical exercise and stressful situations during the testing period.
- Collect a 24-hour urine specimen in a bottle containing a preservative.
- Tell the patient that he can resume activities restricted during the test as well as administration of medications withheld for testing.
- Refrigerate the specimen or place it on ice during the collection period.

Urine 17-ketosteroids

This test measures urine levels of 17-ketosteroids (17-KS), which are steroids and steroid metabolites characterized by a ketone

Hey, man... don't stress out! High-stress situations cause 17-OHCS levels to vary.

group on carbon 17 in the steroid nucleus. They originate primarily in the adrenal glands but can also originate in the testes, which produce one-third of 17-KS in males, and the ovaries, which produce a minimal amount of 17-KS in females.

Androgenic activity

Although not all 17-KS are androgens, all cause androgenic effects. For example, excessive secretion of 17-KS may result in hirsutism (excessive hair growth) and increased clitoral or phallic size; in utero, elevated 17-KS levels may cause a female fetus to develop a male urogenital tract.

Because 17-KS don't include all the androgens, such as testosterone (the most potent androgen), this test provides only a rough estimate of androgenic activity.

What it all means

The following are reference values:
• *men:* 8 to 25 mg/24 hours (SI, 27 to 85 µmol/day)
• *women:* 5 to 15 mg/24 hours (SI, 17 to 52 µmol/day)
• *children:* less than 3 mg/24 hours (SI, 3 to 10 µmol/day).

The lowdown on levels

Elevated urine 17-KS levels may result from adrenal hyperplasia, carcinoma or adenoma, or adrenogenital syndrome. In women, elevated levels may also indicate ovarian dysfunction or androgenic arrhenoblastoma. In men, elevated 17-KS levels may indicate interstitial cell tumor of the testis. Characteristically, 17-KS levels also rise during pregnancy, severe stress, chronic illness, or debilitating disease.

Depressed urine 17-KS levels may result from Addison's disease, panhypopituitarism, eunuchoidism, or castration and may occur in cretinism, myxedema, and nephrosis. When this test is used to monitor cortisol therapy for adrenogenital syndrome, 17-KS levels typically return to normal with adequate cortisol administration. (See *Urine 17-KS test interference.*)

What needs to be done

• Check the patient's history for drugs that may affect test results.
• If the patient is menstruating, urine collection may have to be postponed.
• The patient should avoid excessive physical exercise and stressful situations during the collection period.

The 17-KS test helps diagnose adrenal and gonadal dysfunction and adrenogenital syndrome. It can also monitor the effects of cortisol therapy in the treatment of adrenogenital syndrome.

- Collect a 24-hour urine specimen in a bottle containing a preservative to keep the specimen at a pH of 4.0 to 4.5.
- Refrigerate the specimen or place it on ice during collection.

Urine 17-ketogenic steroids

This test determines urine levels of 17-ketogenic steroids (17-KGS), which consist of the 17-OHCS, such as cortisol and its metabolites, and other adrenocortical steroids, such as pregnanetriol, that can be oxidized in the laboratory to 17-KS.

For accurate diagnosis of specific disease, 17-KGS must be compared with results of other tests, including plasma corticotropin, plasma cortisol, corticotropin stimulation, single-dose metyrapone, and dexamethasone suppression.

What it all means

The following are reference values for 17-KGS:
- *men:* 5 to 23 mg/24 hours (SI, 17 to 80 µmol/day)
- *women:* 3 to 15 mg/24 hours (SI, 10 to 52 µmol/day)
- *children:* less than 2 to 6 mg/24 hours (SI, 6 to 17 µmol/day).

The lowdown on levels

Elevated 17-KGS levels reflect hyperadrenalism, as in Cushing's syndrome; adrenal carcinoma or adenoma; and some cases of adrenogenital syndrome such as congenital adrenal hyperplasia. Levels also rise with severe physical or emotional stress.

Low levels may reflect hypoadrenalism, as in Addison's disease as well as panhypopituitarism, cretinism, and general wasting. (See *Urine 17-KGS test interference*, page 192.)

What needs to be done

- Check the patient's history for drugs that may affect 17-KGS levels.
- The patient should avoid excessive physical exercise and stressful situations during the collection period.
- Collect a 24-hour urine specimen in a bottle containing a preservative to keep the specimen at a pH of 4.0 to 4.5.
- Refrigerate the specimen or keep it on ice during the collection period.

Warning!

Urine 17-KS test interference

- Meprobamate, phenothiazines, spironolactone, aldactone, corticotropin, dexamethasone, and antibiotics may elevate levels.
- Estrogens, penicillin, ethacrynic acid, and phenytoin may suppress levels.

The urine 17-KGS test evaluates adrenocortical function and aids diagnosis of Cushing's syndrome and Addison's disease.

Warning!

Urine 17-KGS test interference

- Corticotropin therapy and drugs, such as meprobamate, phenothiazines, spironolactone, penicillin, and hydralazine, may elevate results.
- Levels may be suppressed by estrogens, quinine, reserpine, thiazide diuretics, and long-term corticosteroid therapy.
- Nalidixic acid and dexamethasone may elevate or suppress levels.

Proteins and protein metabolites

Urine Bence Jones protein

Bence Jones proteins are abnormal light-chain immunoglobulins of low molecular weight that derive from the clone of a single plasma cell (monoclonal). This globulin appears in the urine of 50% to 80% of patients with multiple myeloma and in most patients with Waldenström's macroglobulinemia.

What it all means

Urine should contain no Bence Jones proteins. The presence of these proteins in urine suggests multiple myeloma or Waldenström's macroglobulinemia. Very low levels in the absence of other symptoms may result from benign monoclonal gammopathy. (See *Bence Jones protein test interference*.)

In patients with clinical signs of multiple melanoma, the urine Bence Jones protein test can confirm the diagnosis.

Warning!

Bence Jones protein test interference

- False-positive results may occur in connective tissue disease, renal insufficiency, and certain cancers.
- Contamination of the specimen with menstrual blood, prostatic secretions, or semen may alter results.

What needs to be done

- Teach the patient how to collect a clean-catch urine specimen.
- Collect an early morning urine specimen of at least 50 ml.
- If transport to the laboratory is delayed, refrigerate the specimen.

Urine creatinine

The urine creatinine test measures urine levels of creatinine, the chief metabolite of creatine. Produced in amounts proportional to total body muscle mass, creatinine is removed from the plasma primarily by glomerular filtration and is excreted in the urine.

Because creatinine isn't recycled in the body, it has a relatively high, constant clearance rate, making it an efficient indicator of renal function.

> Because creatinine excretion levels are relatively constant, urine creatinine testing can evaluate the accuracy of a 24-hour urine collection.

What it all means

The normal range for urine creatinine levels in men is 1 to 1.9 g/24 hours (SI, 8.8 to 17.6 mmol/day); in women, 0.8 to 1.7 g/24 hours (SI, 7 to 15.8 mmol/day).

Decreased levels...renal impairment

Decreased urine creatinine levels may result from impaired renal perfusion (associated with shock, for example) or from renal disease caused by urinary tract obstruction. Chronic bilateral pyelonephritis, acute or chronic glomerulonephritis, and polycystic kidney disease may also depress creatinine levels.

Increased levels...not a problem

Increased urine creatinine levels generally have little diagnostic significance. (See *Urine creatinine test interference*.)

What needs to be done

- Check the patient's history for drugs that may affect creatinine levels.
- Tell the patient not to eat an excessive amount of meat and to avoid strenuous physical exercise during the collection period.
- Collect a 24-hour urine specimen in a refrigerated specimen bottle without a preservative.
- Refrigerate the specimen or keep it on ice during the collection period.

Warning!

Urine creatinine test interference

Drugs that may affect urine creatinine levels include corticosteroids, gentamicin, tetracyclines, diuretics, and amphotericin B.

Creatinine clearance

Creatinine is formed and excreted in constant amounts by an irreversible reaction, and it functions solely as the main end product of creatine. Creatinine production is proportional to total muscle mass and is relatively unaffected by normal physical activity, diet, or urine volume.

The rate of clearance is expressed in terms of the volume of blood (in milliliters) that can be cleared of creatinine in 1 minute. Creatinine levels become abnormal when more than 50% of the total nephron units have been damaged.

What it all means

At age 20, creatinine clearance normally ranges from 85 to 125 ml/ minute (SI, 1.41 to 2.08 ml/s/1.73 m^2) for men and from 75 to 115 ml/minute (SI, 1.21 to 1.91ml/s/1.73 m^2) for women.

Creatinine levels are proportional to total muscle mass and aren't affected by other variables. So, testing creatinine clearance can assess renal function and monitor progression of renal insufficiency.

When creatinine isn't clearing out

Low creatinine clearance may result from reduced renal blood flow, which is associated with shock or renal artery obstruction; acute tubular necrosis; acute or chronic glomerulonephritis; advanced bilateral chronic pyelonephritis; advanced bilateral renal lesions, such as in polycystic kidney disease, cancer, or renal tuberculosis; or nephrosclerosis. Heart failure and severe dehydration may also cause creatinine clearance to fall below normal. (See *Creatinine clearance test interference*.)

What needs to be done

• Check the patient's history for drugs that may affect creatinine clearance.
• Tell the patient that this test requires a timed urine specimen and at least one blood sample. Be sure to explain how the urine will be collected.
• Tell the patient to avoid strenuous exercise and to not eat an excessive amount of meat during the testing period.
• Collect a timed urine specimen at 2, 6, 12, or 24 hours in a bottle containing a preservative to prevent degradation of the creatinine.
• Perform a venipuncture anytime during the collection period, and collect the sample in a 7-ml tube without additives.
• Refrigerate the specimen or keep it on ice during the collection period.

Warning!

Creatinine clearance test interference

• A high-protein diet before the test or strenuous physical exercise during the collection period may alter results.
• Drugs that may affect creatinine clearance include amphotericin B, thiazide diuretics, furosemide, and aminoglycosides.

Urine uric acid

Urine uric acid testing supplements serum uric acid testing to identify disorders that alter production or excretion of uric acid. Derived from dietary purines in organ meats and from endogenous nucleoproteins, uric acid (as urate) is found normally in the blood and in other tissues in amounts totaling about 1 g. Its primary site of formation is the liver, although the intestinal mucosa is also involved in urate production.

As the chief end product of purine catabolism, urate passes from the liver through the bloodstream to the kidneys, where roughly 50% is excreted daily in the urine.

Testing urine uric acid is a good way to detect enzyme deficiencies and metabolic disturbances.

What it all means

Normal urine uric acid values vary with diet but generally range from 250 to 750 mg/24 hours (SI, 1.5 to 4.5 mmol/day). (See *Urine uric acid test intererence.*)

Acid elevation

Elevated urine uric acid levels may result from chronic myeloid leukemia, polycythemia vera, multiple myeloma, early remission in pernicious anemia, as well as lymphosarcoma and lymphatic leukemia during radiation therapy. High levels also result from tubular reabsorption defects, such as Fanconi's syndrome and hepatolenticular degeneration (Wilson's disease).

Acid depression

Low urine uric acid levels occur in gout and in severe renal damage, as occurs in chronic glomerulonephritis, diabetic glomerulosclerosis, and collagen disorders.

Warning!

Urine uric acid test interference

- A diet high or low in purine may alter results.
- Allopurinol increases uric acid excretion.
- Pyrazinamide and diuretics, such as furosemide and ethacrynic acid, decrease levels.
- Low doses of salicylates, phenylbutazone, and probenecid lower uric acid levels; high doses cause above-normal levels.

What needs to be done

• Check the patient's history for drugs that may influence uric acid levels.
• Collect a 24-hour urine specimen.

Pigments

Urine hemoglobin

Contained in red blood cells (RBCs), hemoglobin combines with oxygen and carbon dioxide to allow RBCs to transport these gases between the lungs and the tissues.

RBC destruction

Aging RBCs are constantly being destroyed by normal mechanisms within the reticuloendothelial system (the system of those cells that are able to ingest particles). However, when RBC destruction occurs within the circulation instead, as in intravascular hemolysis, free hemoglobin enters the plasma and binds with haptoglobin. If the plasma level of hemoglobin exceeds that of haptoglobin, the excess hemoglobin is excreted in the urine. This condition is known as hemoglobinuria.

Testing for urine blood pigments can be performed at the patient's bedside. (See *Bedside testing for urine blood pigments*.)

> Urine hemoglobin measurement aids diagnosis of hemolytic anemias, infection, or severe intravascular hemolysis from a transfusion reaction.

What it all means

Hemoglobin shouldn't be present in urine. Hemoglobinuria may result from severe intravascular hemolysis resulting from a blood transfusion reaction, burns, or a crushing injury; from acquired hemolytic anemias caused by chemical or drug intoxication or malaria; or from the hemolytic anemia known as paroxysmal nocturnal hemoglobinuria. Hemoglobinuria may also result from congenital hemolytic anemias, as in hemoglobinopathies or enzyme defects and, less commonly, from cystitis, ureteral calculi, or urethritis. Hemoglobinuria and hematuria occur in renal tumor, tuberculosis, or in renal epithelial damage, such as in acute glomerulonephritis or pyelonephritis. (See *Urine hemoglobin test interference*.)

Peak technique

Bedside testing for urine blood pigments

To test a patient's urine for blood pigments at the bedside, use one of the following methods.

Dipstick, Multistix, or Chemstrips
- Collect a urine specimen.
- Dip the stick into the specimen and withdraw it.
- After 30 seconds, compare the stick to the color chart. Blue indicates a positive reaction; the intensity of color indicates pigment concentration.

Occult solution
- Collect a urine specimen.
- After placing one drop of urine on the filter paper, close the package and turn it over. Open the opposite side and place two drops of solution on the filter paper.
- After 30 seconds, inspect the filter paper. Blue indicates a positive reaction; the intensity of color indicates pigment concentration.

Because these methods detect only blood pigments, immunochemical studies are necessary to differentiate hemoglobin from other blood pigments such as myoglobin.

Warning!

Urine hemoglobin test interference

- Large doses of vitamin C or drugs that contain vitamin C as a preservative, such as certain antibiotics, can inhibit reagent activity.
- Nephrotoxic drugs or anticoagulants may cause a positive result for hemoglobinuria or hematuria.
- Lysis of red blood cells in stale or alkaline urine and specimen contamination with menstrual blood alter test results.
- Bacterial peroxidases in highly infected specimens may alter results.

What needs to be done
- Check the patient's history for drugs that may affect free hemoglobin levels.
- If the patient is a female who is menstruating, reschedule the test.
- Collect a random urine specimen.

Urine myoglobin

Myoglobin is a red pigment found in the cytoplasm of cardiac and skeletal muscle cells. The urine myoglobin test measures the level of this pigment in the urine.

The oxygen reservoir

Myoglobin probably serves as a reservoir of oxygen, facilitating its movement within muscle. When muscle cells are extensively damaged, myoglobin is released into the blood, quickly cleared by renal glomerular filtration, and eliminated in the urine.

Warning!

Urine myoglobin test interference

- If performed with reagent strips, recent ingestion of large vitamin C amounts can inhibit the reaction.
- Urine contamination with iodine may alter results.
- Dilute urine can reduce test sensitivity.

> Myoglobin helps muscle cells receive oxygen. Myoglobin testing aids diagnosis of muscle disease or damage.

What it all means

Myoglobin shouldn't appear in the urine. Myoglobinuria occurs in acute or chronic muscular disease, alcoholic polymyopathy, familial myoglobinuria, and extensive myocardial infarction. It also results from severe trauma to the skeletal muscles, such as in a crushing injury, extreme hyperthermia, or severe burns. Transient myoglobinuria, known as "march" myoglobinuria, may follow strenuous or prolonged exercise but disappears after rest. (See *Urine myoglobin test interference.*)

What needs to be done

- Collect a random urine specimen and send it to the laboratory.

Urine bilirubin

The urine bilirubin screening test detects abnormally high urine levels of direct, or conjugated, bilirubin. Detectable amounts of bilirubin in the urine may indicate liver disease caused by infection, biliary disease, or hepatotoxicity. The analysis can be performed at the bedside, using a bilirubin reagent strip, or in the laboratory.

> The urine bilirubin test helps identify the cause of jaundice.

What it all means

Normally, bilirubin isn't found in urine in a routine screening test. High levels of direct bilirubin in urine may be evident from the specimen's appearance, which is dark with a yellow foam.

Three-way diagnosis

To diagnose jaundice, however, the presence or absence of direct bilirubin in urine must be correlated with serum test results and

Warning!

Urine bilirubin test interference

- Phenazopyridine and phenothiazine derivatives can cause false-positive results.
- Dipstrip testing, such as with Chemstrip or N-Multistix, is affected by large amounts of ascorbic acid and nitrite.

with urine and fecal urobilinogen levels. (See *Urine bilirubin test interference.*)

What needs to be done

- Collect a random, freshly voided urine specimen. Bilirubin disintegrates after 30 minutes of exposure to room temperature or light. For bedside analysis, use one of the following procedures:
  – *Dipstrip* — Dip the reagent strip into the specimen, and remove it immediately. After 20 seconds, compare the strip color with the color standards.
  – *Ictotest* — Place five drops of urine on the asbestos-cellulose test mat. If bilirubin is present, it will be absorbed into the mat. Next, put a reagent tablet on the wet area of the mat and place two drops of water on the tablet. If bilirubin is present, a blue to purple coloration will develop on the mat. Pink or red indicates that no bilirubin is present — a negative test.
- Send the specimen to the laboratory as appropriate.

Urine urobilinogen

The urine urobilinogen test measures urine levels of urobilinogen, the colorless, water-soluble product that results from the reduction of bilirubin by intestinal bacteria. Up to 50% of intestinal urobilinogen returns to the liver, where some of it is resecreted into bile and, eventually, into the intestine through enterohepatic circulation. Small amounts of the reabsorbed urobilinogen also enter general circulation for ultimate excretion in the urine, a condition called urobilinogenuria.

Eliminated in large amounts in the feces and in small amounts in the urine, urobilinogen reflects bile pigment metabolism.

> Urobilinogen measurement aids diagnosis of extrahepatic obstruction, such as a bile duct blockage and hepatic disorder.

Peak technique

Using a random specimen to test for urobilinogen

Quantitative tests for urinary urobilinogen excretion can be performed with reagent strips, such as Bili-Labstix or N-Multistix (dip-and-read tests).

To perform such tests, collect a clean-catch urine specimen in a clean, dry container—preferably in the afternoon, when urine uro-bilinogen levels peak—and test the specimen immediately. A fresh urine specimen is essential for reliable results because urobilinogen is unstable when exposed to room temperature and light.

Dip the strip into the urine and, as you remove it, start timing the re-action. Carefully remove excess urine by tapping the edge of the strip against the container or a clean, dry surface to prevent color changes along the edge of the test area. When using N-Multistix (or a similar product for multiple testing), hold the strip in a horizontal position to prevent mixing chemicals from adjacent reagent areas. Place the strip near the color block on the bottle and carefully compare the colors. Read the results at 45 seconds. The color results correspond to the number of Ehrlich units per deciliter of urine, as shown below.

Normally, a random specimen contains small amounts of urobilino-gen. This test can't determine the absence of urobilinogen in the speci-men being tested.

Color	Value
Yellow-green to yellow (normal)	0.1 to 1 Ehrlich unit
Yellow-orange (positive)	2 Ehrlich units
Medium yellow-orange (positive)	4 Ehrlich units
Light brown-orange (positive)	8 Ehrlich units
Brown-orange (positive)	12 Ehrlich units

Check out the cool color coding!

What it all means

Normally, urine urobilinogen values in women range from 0.1 to 1.1 mg/2 hours (SI, 0.2 to 1.9 µmol/2 hours); in men, from 0.3 to 2.1 mg/2 hours (SI, 0.5 to 3.6 µmol/2 hours). Absence of urine urobilinogen may result from complete obstructive jaundice or from treatment with broad-spectrum antibiotics, which destroy the intestinal flora. Low urine urobilinogen levels may result from congenital enzymatic jaundice or from treatment with drugs that acidify urine, such as ammonium chloride or ascorbic acid.

Elevated levels may indicate hemolytic jaundice, hepatitis, or cirrhosis. (See *Urine urobilinogen test interference.*)

What needs to be done

• Check the patient's history for drugs that may affect urine urobilinogen levels.
• The patient need not restrict food or fluids, except for bananas, which he should avoid for 48 hours before the test.
• Depending on the laboratory's request, collect a random urine specimen or a 2-hour specimen, usually during the afternoon — ideally between 1 p.m. and 3 p.m. — when urobilinogen levels peak. (See *Using a random specimen to test for urobilinogen.*)
• Send the specimen to the laboratory immediately. This test must be performed within 30 minutes of collection because urobilinogen quickly oxidizes to an orange compound called urobilin.

Warning!

Urine urobilinogen test interference

• Bananas eaten up to 48 hours before the test may raise levels.
• Drugs that affect the accuracy of test results include para-aminosalicylic acid, phenazopyridine, procaine, phenothiazines, mandelate, and sulfonamides.
• Highly alkaline urine, which may be caused by acetazolamide or sodium bicarbonate, may elevate levels.

Sugars, ketones, and mucopolysaccharides

Urine glucose

The glucose urine test, which involves the use of commercial, plastic-coated reagent strips (Clinistix, Diastix, or Tes-Tape) is a specific, qualitative test for glycosuria, which is routinely associated with diabetes mellitus.

Glucose spillover

Normally, nearly all glucose passes into the glomerular filtrate and is reabsorbed by the proximal renal tubule. However, if the blood glucose level exceeds the reabsorption capacity of the tubule, glucose spills into the urine.

What it all means

Glucose shouldn't be present in urine. Glycosuria occurs in diabetes mellitus, adrenal and thyroid disorders, hepatic and central nervous system diseases, Fanconi's syndrome and other conditions involving low renal threshold, toxic renal tubular disease, heavy metal poisoning, glomerulonephritis, nephrosis, pregnancy, and total parenteral nutrition (TPN). It also occurs when administering large amounts of glucose or niacin, prolonged use of phenothiazines, and use of certain other drugs, such as asparaginase, corticosteroids, carbamazepine, ammonium chloride, thiazide diuretics, dextrothyroxine, and lithium carbonate. (See *Urine glucose test interference.*)

The urine glucose test is an effective screen for diabetes.

What needs to be done

• Have the patient void, then give him a drink of water. After 30 to 45 minutes, collect a second-voided urine specimen, using one of the following procedures:

– *Clinistix test* — Dip the test area of the reagent strip in the specimen for 2 seconds. Remove excess urine by tapping the strip against a clean surface or the side of the container and begin timing. Hold the strip in the air and "read" the color exactly 10 seconds after taking the strip out of the urine by comparing it with the reference color blocks on the container label. Ignore color changes that develop after 10 seconds.

– *Diastix test* — Dip the reagent strip in the specimen for 2 seconds. Remove excess urine by tapping the strip against the container and begin timing. Hold the strip in the air and compare the color to the color chart *exactly 30 seconds* after taking the strip out of the urine. Ignore color changes that develop after 30 seconds.

– *Tes-Tape* — Withdraw about 1½" (4 cm) of the reagent tape from the dispenser; dip ¼" (0.6 cm) in the specimen for 2 seconds. Remove excess urine by tapping the strip against the side of the container and begin timing. Hold the tape in the air and compare the color of the darkest part of the tape to the color chart *exactly 60 seconds* after taking the strip out of the urine. If the tape indicates 0.5% or higher, wait an additional 60 seconds to make the final color comparison.

Warning!

Urine glucose test interference

• Medications, such as tetracycline, levodopa, ascorbic acid, phenazopyridine, methyldopa, and salicylates, may cause false-negative results.
• Diluted, stale urine or bacterial contamination of the specimen may alter results.

Urine ketones

Ketones are products of fat metabolism not normally found in the urine. However, ketones may be found with excessive fat metabolism, which occurs when the body can't metabolize carbohydrates, carbohydrate intake is inadequate, metabolic demand increases, or excessive carbohydrates are lost. In the urine ketone test, the action of urine on a commercially prepared product (Acetest tablet, Ketostix, or Keto-Diastix) measures the urine level of ketone bodies (ketones).

> The urine ketone test helps identify diabetic ketoacidosis and carbohydrate deprivation.

Checking the ketone bodies

Each product measures a specific ketone body. For example, Acetest measures acetone, and Ketostix measures acetoacetic acid. The urine determinations reflect serum concentration.

What it all means

Ketones shouldn't be present in urine. Ketonuria is present in uncontrolled diabetes mellitus and starvation; it also occurs as a metabolic complication of TPN. (See *Urine ketone test interference*.)

What needs to be done

• Have the patient void; then give him a drink of water. About 30 minutes later, collect a second-voided urine specimen, and use one of the following procedures to test the specimen:
– *Acetest* — Lay the tablet on a piece of white paper and place one drop of urine on the tablet. After 30 seconds, compare the tablet color (white, lavender, or purple) with the color chart. (If the patient is taking levodopa or phenazopyridine or has recently received sulfobromophthalein, Acetest tablets must be used because reagent strips will give inaccurate results.)
– *Ketostix* — Dip the reagent stick into the specimen and remove it immediately. After 15 seconds, compare the stick color (buff or purple) with the color chart.
– *Keto-Diastix* — Dip the reagent strip into the specimen and remove it immediately. Tap the edge of the strip against the container or a clean, dry surface to remove excess urine. Hold the strip horizontally to prevent mixing the chemicals from the two areas. Interpret each area of the strip separately. After exactly 15 seconds, compare the color of the ketone section (buff or purple) with the appropriate color chart; after 30 seconds, compare the color of the glucose section. Ignore color changes that occur after the specified waiting periods.

Warning!

Urine ketone test interference

• Levodopa, phenazopyridine, and sulfobromophthalein produce false-positive test results when either Ketostix or Keto-Diastix is used.
• Bacterial contamination of the specimen causes false-negative results.

Minerals

Urine sodium and chloride

The urine sodium and chloride test determines urine levels of sodium, the major extracellular cation, and chloride, the major extracellular anion.

Sodium and chloride — in tandem

Sodium and chloride help maintain osmotic pressure and water and acid-base balance. After these ions are absorbed by the intestinal tract, they're regulated by the kidneys and rise and fall in tandem. The kidneys conserve constant serum levels of sodium and chloride — even at the risk of dehydration or edema — or excrete excessive amounts.

What it all means

Although levels of sodium and chloride in the urine vary greatly with dietary salt intake and perspiration, the normal range for urine sodium excretion is 30 to 280 mEq/24 hours (SI, 30 to 280 mmol/day); for urine chloride excretion, 110 to 250 mEq/24 hours; and for urine sodium-chloride excretion, 5 to 20 g/24 hours (SI, 110 to 250 mmol/day).

Out of sync levels...

Usually, urine sodium and chloride levels are parallel, rising and falling in tandem. Elevated urine sodium levels may reflect increased salt intake, adrenal failure, salicylate toxicity, diabetic acidosis, salt-losing nephritis, or water-deficient dehydration. Decreased urine sodium levels suggest decreased salt intake, primary aldosteronism, acute renal failure, or heart failure.

...elevated levels...

Elevated urine chloride levels may result from water-deficient dehydration, salicylate toxicity, diabetic acidosis, adrenocortical insufficiency (Addison's disease), or salt-losing renal disease.

...and decreased levels

Decreased levels may result from excessive diaphoresis, heart failure, or hypochloremic metabolic alkalosis caused by prolonged vomiting or gastric suctioning. (See *Urine sodium and chloride test interference.*)

> Testing for sodium and chloride can help monitor the effects of a low-salt diet. These minerals help maintain fluid and electrolyte balance.

What needs to be done
• Check the patient's medication history for drugs that may influence test results.
• Collect a 24-hour urine specimen, and send it to the laboratory on completion.

Urine potassium

This quantitative test measures urine levels of potassium, a major intracellular cation (positively charged ion) that helps regulate acid-base balance and neuromuscular function. The kidneys regulate potassium balance through potassium excretion in the urine.

What it all means
Normal potassium excretion is 25 to 125 mEq/24 hours (SI, 125 to 125 mmol/day), with an average potassium concentration of 25 to 100 mEq/L.

Potassium puzzle

In a patient with hypokalemia and normal kidney function, potassium concentration will be less than 10 mEq/L (SI, 10 mmol/L), indicating that potassium loss is most likely the result of a GI disorder such as malabsorption syndrome.

In a patient with hypokalemia lasting more than 3 days, urine potassium levels above 10 mEq/L (SI, 10 mmol/L) indicate renal losses that may result from such disorders as aldosteronism, renal tubular acidosis, or chronic renal failure. However, extrarenal disorders, such as dehydration, starvation, Cushing's disease, and salicylate intoxication, may also elevate urine potassium levels. (See *Urine potassium test interference*, page 206.)

What needs to be done
• Check the patient's history for drugs that may alter test results.
• Collect a 24-hour urine specimen.
• Refrigerate the specimen or place it on ice during the collection period.

Urine magnesium

The urine magnesium test measures the urine level of magnesium, an important cation absorbed in the intestinal tract and excreted in urine. Measurement of urine magnesium was rarely used in the

Warning!

Urine sodium and chloride test interference

• Ammonium chloride and potassium chloride elevate urine chloride levels.
• Sodium bicarbonate and thiazide diuretics raise urine sodium levels; steroids suppress them.

Testing urine potassium determines whether hypokalemia stems from renal or extrarenal disorders.

Warning!

Urine potassium test interference

- Excess dietary potassium raises levels.
- Potassium-wasting medications, such as ammonium chloride, thiazide diuretics, and acetazolamide, raise levels.
- Excessive vomiting or stomach suctioning produces false results.

past, but it's becoming more widely used because magnesium deficiency is detectable earlier in urine than in serum.

Magnesium facts

Magnesium is found primarily in the bones and in intracellular fluid; a small amount is present in extracellular fluid. This element activates many enzyme systems, helps transport sodium and potassium across cell membranes, affects nucleic acid and protein metabolism, and influences intracellular calcium levels through its effect on parathyroid hormone secretion.

What it all means

Normal urinary excretion of magnesium is 3 to 5 mEq/24 hours (SI, 3 to 5 mmol/day).

The lowdown on levels

Low urine magnesium levels may result from malabsorption, acute or chronic diarrhea, diabetic acidosis, dehydration, pancreatitis, advanced renal failure, primary aldosteronism, or decreased dietary intake of magnesium.

Elevated urine magnesium levels may result from early chronic renal disease, adrenocortical insufficiency (Addison's disease), chronic alcoholism, or chronic ingestion of magnesium-containing antacids. (See *Urine magnesium test interference*.)

What needs to be done

- Note if the patient is receiving magnesium-containing antacids, ethacrynic acid, thiazide diuretics, or aldosterone.
- Collect a 24-hour urine specimen, and send it to the laboratory upon completion.

Urine magnesium testing rules out magnesium deficiency in patients with CNS irritation.

Urine calcium and phosphates

This test measures the urine levels of calcium and phosphates, elements essential for the formation and resorption of bone. Urine calcium and phosphate levels generally parallel serum levels.

Normally absorbed in the upper intestine and excreted in stool and urine, calcium and phosphates help maintain tissue and fluid pH, electrolyte balance in cells and extracellular fluids, and permeability of cell membranes. Calcium promotes enzymatic processes, aids blood coagulation, and lowers neuromuscular irritability; phosphates aid carbohydrate metabolism.

What it all means

Normal values depend on dietary intake. Males excrete less than 275 mg of calcium/24 hours (SI, less than 6.8 mmol/day); females, less than 250 mg/24 hours (SI, less than 6.2 mmol/day). Normal excretion of phosphates is 0.9 to 1.3 g/24 hours (SI, 29 to 42 mmol/day). (See *Disorders that affect urine calcium and phosphate levels*, page 208, and *Urine calcium and phosphate test interference*, page 208.)

What needs to be done

- Note the patient's recent use of thiazide diuretics, sodium phosphate, or glucocorticoids.
- Tell the patient that he needs to be as active as possible before the test.
- As ordered, provide the Albright-Reifenstein diet, which contains about 130 mg of calcium/24 hours, for 3 days before the test, or provide a copy of the diet for the patient to follow at home.
- Collect a 24-hour urine specimen.
- Send the specimen to the laboratory on completion.

Warning!

Urine magnesium test interference

- Increased calcium intake reduces levels.
- Ethacrynic acid, thiazide diuretics, aldosterone, or excessive amounts of magnesium-containing antacids elevate levels.
- Spironolactone lowers levels.

Urine calcium and phosphates testing evaluates calcium and phosphate metabolism and excretion.

Advice from the experts

Disorders that affect urine calcium and phosphate levels

The following disorders can cause changes in urine calcium or phosphate levels.

Disorder	Urine calcium level	Urine phosphate level
Hyperparathyroidism	Elevated	Elevated
Vitamin D intoxication	Elevated	Suppressed
Metastatic carcinoma	Elevated	Normal
Sarcoidosis	Elevated	Suppressed
Multiple myeloma	Elevated or normal	Elevated or normal
Hypoparathyroidism	Suppressed	Suppressed
Nephrosis	Suppressed	Suppressed or normal
Acute nephritis	Suppressed	Suppressed
Renal insufficiency	Suppressed	Suppressed

Warning!

Urine calcium and phosphate test interference

- Thiazide diuretics decrease calcium excretion.
- Prolonged inactivity and use of corticosteroids, sodium phosphate, or calcitonin increase excretion.
- Vitamin D increases phosphate absorption and excretion.
- Parathyroid hormone increases urinary phosphate excretion and decreases urinary calcium excretion.

Quick quiz

1.   Your patient's urine specific gravity measures 1.001. Based on this finding, your patient may have which disorder?
    A.   Diabetes insipidus
    B.   Heart failure
    C.   Acute glomerulonephritis

Answer: A. Low specific gravity (less than 1.005) is characteristic of diabetes insipidus.

2. Before obtaining a specimen for urine amylase testing, the patient should refrain from taking:

    A.   furosemide.

    B.   bumetanide.

    C.   hydrochlorothiazide.

Answer: C. Thiazide diuretics such as hydrochlorothiazide should be withheld for 24 hours before obtaining a specimen for urine amylase testing. Thiazide diuretics may raise urine amylase levels.

3. When teaching the patient about urine aldosterone testing, you should include which instruction?

    A.   Avoid alcohol for 24 hours before the test.

    B.   Avoid sodium-rich foods during the collection period.

    C.   Restrict fluids for 8 hours before the test.

Answer: B. Before urine aldosterone testing, you should instruct the patient to avoid sodium-rich foods, strenuous exercise, and stressful situations during the collection period.

4. Your pregnant patient's total urine estrogens measure 6,000 μg/24 hours (SI, 6,000 μg/day). This result is normal for which trimester?

    A.   First

    B.   Second

    C.   Third

Answer: C. Total urine estrogen levels range from 0 to 800 μg/24 hours (SI, 0 to 800 μg/day) in the first trimester; 800 to 5,000μg/24 hours (SI, 800 to 5,000 μg/day) in the second trimester; and 5,000 to 50,000 μg/24 hours (SI, 5,000 to 50,000 μg/day) in the third trimester.

5. A patient complains of bone pain and fatigue. The doctor orders a urine Bence Jones protein test. Why?

    A.   To confirm multiple myeloma

    B.   To confirm acute leukemia

    C.   To rule out myocardial damage

Answer: A. Urine testing for Bence Jones protein confirms multiple myeloma in patients with classic signs and symptoms, such as bone pain and persistent anemia and fatigue.

Scoring

☆☆☆ If you answered all five questions correctly, great! "Ur-in" top form!

☆☆ If you answered three or four questions correctly, super! You're 17-KS above the rest!

☆ If you answered fewer than three correctly, chin up! A little more practice and you'll be Queen of the Bilirubin Ball.

6

Other specimen tests

Just the facts

In this chapter, you'll learn:

♦ about other specimen tests

♦ what patient care is associated with these tests

♦ what factors can interfere with test results

♦ what test results may indicate.

A look at other specimen tests

Other specimen tests include pleural fluid analysis, gastric acid stimulation, peritoneal fluid analysis, fecal occult blood, fecal lipids, stool for ova and parasite, stool for rotavirus antigen, amniotic fluid analysis, Papanicolaou test, semen analysis, cerebrospinal fluid analysis, pericardial fluid analysis, and sweat test. Each test is unique and requires its own procedure to collect the specimen. Explain the procedure to the patient in simple terms to allay his anxiety.

Pleural fluid analysis can help determine the cause of pleural damage, pulmonary compression, and respiratory distress.

Respiratory system

Pleural fluid analysis

In pleural fluid aspiration, also known as thoracentesis, the thoracic wall is punctured to obtain a specimen of pleural fluid for analysis or to relieve pulmonary compression and resultant respiratory distress. Locating the fluid before thoracentesis reduces the risk of puncturing the lung, liver, or spleen.

What it all means

The pleural cavity should contain less than 20 ml of serous fluid. Pleural effusion results from the abnormal formation or reabsorption of pleural fluid. Certain characteristics classify pleural fluid as either a transudate or an exudate.

Abnormal findings

Pleural fluid may contain blood, chyle, or pus and necrotic tissue. A high percentage of neutrophils suggests septic inflammation. Pleural fluid glucose levels that are 30 to 40 mg/dl (SI, 1.5 to 2 mmol/L) lower than blood glucose levels may indicate cancer, bacterial infection, nonseptic inflammation, or metastasis. Increased amylase levels occur with pleural effusions associated with pancreatitis. (See *Characteristics of pulmonary transudate and exudate* and *Pleural fluid analysis interference*, page 214.)

Memory jogger

To remember the difference between transudate and exudate, focus on the prefixes: *trans-* means "across," as in the transcontinental railroad, and *ex-* means "out of," as in exhale.

Advice from the experts

Characteristics of pulmonary transudate and exudate

The following characteristics help classify pleural fluid as either a transudate or an exudate.

Characteristic	Transudate	Exudate
Appearance	Clear	Cloudy, turbid
Specific gravity	< 1.016	> 1.016
Clot (fibrinogen)	Absent	Present
Protein	< 3 g/dl (SI, < 30 g/L)	> 3 g/dl (SI, > 30 g/L)
White blood cells	Few lymphocytes	Many lymphocytes; may be purulent
Red blood cells	Few	Variable
Glucose level	Equal to serum level	May be less than serum level
Lactate dehydrogenase	Low	High

Peak technique

Positioning the patient for thoracentesis

To prepare the patient for thoracentesis, place him in one of the three positions shown below: sitting on the edge of the bed with his arms on an overbed table, sitting up in bed with his arms on an overbed table, or lying partially on the side, partially on the back with his arms over his head. These positions serve to widen the intercostal spaces and permit easy access to the pleural cavity. Using pillows (as shown) will make the patient more comfortable.

Sitting on edge of bed

Pillow

Sitting up in bed

Pillows

Lying partially on unaffected side with head of bed raised 30 to 45 degrees

Pillow

Rolled-up towel

What needs to be done

• Check the patient's history for bleeding disorders or anticoagulant therapy.
• Explain that a chest X-ray or ultrasound study may precede the test.
• Explain the procedure to the patient.
• Instruct the patient not to cough, breathe deeply, or move during the test to minimize the risk of lung injury.
• Record the patient's baseline vital signs.
• Shave the area around the needle insertion site, if necessary, and position the patient properly. (See *Positioning the patient for thoracentesis.*)

Doctor does A...

• The doctor disinfects the skin, drapes the area, injects a local anesthetic, and inserts the thoracentesis needle above the rib. When the needle reaches the pocket of fluid, he attaches the 50-ml syringe and the stopcock and opens the clamps on the tubing to aspirate fluid into the container.

Recognizing complications of thoracentesis

You can identify the following complications of thoracentesis by watching for characteristic signs and symptoms:
• pneumothorax—apprehension, increased restlessness, cyanosis, sudden breathlessness, tachycardia, chest pain
• tension pneumothorax—dyspnea, chest pain, tachycardia, hypotension, absent or diminished breath sounds on the affected side
• subcutaneous emphysema—local tissue swelling, crackling on palpation of site
• infection—fever, rapid pulse rate, pain
• mediastinal shift—labored breathing, cardiac arrhythmias, pulmonary edema.

Warning!

Pleural fluid analysis interference

Antimicrobial therapy before aspiration of fluid for culture may decrease the number of bacteria, making isolation of the infecting organism difficult.

...while you do B, C, and D

• During aspiration, check the patient for signs of respiratory distress.
• After the needle is withdrawn, apply slight pressure and a small adhesive bandage to the puncture site.
• Reposition the patient on the affected side or as ordered. Tell him to remain on this side for at least 1 hour to seal the puncture site. Elevate the head of the bed to facilitate breathing.

Waiting and watchful

• Monitor vital signs every 30 minutes for 2 hours, then every 4 hours until they're stable.
• Watch for signs and symptoms of complications. (See *Recognizing complications of thoracentesis.*)

Gastrointestinal system

Gastric acid stimulation

The gastric acid stimulation test measures gastric acid secretion for 1 hour after subcutaneous injection of pentagastrin or a similar drug that stimulates gastric acid output. It's usually performed if the basal secretion test suggests abnormal gastric secretion.

The gastric acid stimulation test helps diagnose duodenal ulcers, Zollinger-Ellison syndrome, pernicious anemia, and gastric carcinoma.

What it all means

Normally, gastric secretion following stimulation ranges from 18 to 28 mEq/hour (SI, 18 to 28 mmol/hour) for males and from 11 to 21 mEq/hour (SI, 11 to 21 mmol/hour) for females. (See *Gastric acid stimulation test interference.*)

Abnormal findings

Increased gastric secretion may indicate duodenal ulcer; markedly elevated secretion suggests Zollinger-Ellison syndrome. Decreased secretion may indicate gastric carcinoma; achlorhydria may indicate pernicious anemia.

What needs to be done

• Tell the patient that the test requires passing a nasogastric (NG) tube and injecting pentagastrin subcutaneously and takes 1 hour.
• Instruct the patient to refrain from eating, drinking, and smoking after midnight before the test and to report adverse effects, such as abdominal pain, nausea, dizziness, and numbness of extremities, immediately.
• After basal gastric secretions have been collected, keep the NG tube in place. Pentagastrin is then injected subcutaneously. Wait 15 minutes and then collect a specimen every 15 minutes for 1 hour.

Read and record

• Record the color and odor of each specimen, and note presence of food, mucus, bile, or blood. Label all specimens "Stimulated contents," and number them 1 through 4. If the NG tube will be left in place, clamp it or attach it to low intermittent suction, as ordered.
• Watch for adverse effects after removal of the NG tube.

Gastric acid stimulation test interference

Gastric acid levels are elevated by cholinergics, adrenergic blockers, and reserpine and depressed by antacids, anticholinergics, hydrogen blockers, and proton pump inhibitors.

Peritoneal fluid analysis determines the cause of ascites and helps detect abdominal trauma.

Peritoneal fluid analysis

Peritoneal fluid analysis assesses a sample of peritoneal fluid obtained by paracentesis, a procedure that entails inserting a trocar and cannula through the abdominal wall. For this procedure, the patient receives a local anesthetic.

What it all means

Peritoneal fluid is normally odorless and clear to pale yellow. (See *Normal peritoneal fluid profile*, page 216, and *Peritoneal fluid analysis interference*, page 216.)

Advice from the experts

Normal peritoneal fluid profile

The table below shows normal findings in peritoneal fluid analysis. Any deviation in these results can help pinpoint disorders or injury to the peritoneum.

Element	Normal findings
Gross appearance	Sterile, odorless, clear to pale yellow color; scant amount (< 50 ml)
Red blood cells	None
White blood cells	< 300/µl (SI, < 300 × 10^9/L)
Protein	0.3 to 4.1 g/dl (SI, 3 to 41 g/L)
Glucose	70 to 100 mg/dl (SI, 3.5 to 5 mmol/L)
Amylase	138 to 404 amylase U/L (SI, 138 to 404 U/L)
Ammonia	< 50 µg/dl (SI, < 29 µmol/L)
Alkaline phosphatase	30 to 110 U/L (SI, 30 to 110 U/L)
Cytology	No malignant cells present
Bacteria	None
Fungi	None

Warning!

Peritoneal fluid analysis interference

Injury to underlying structures during paracentesis may contaminate the sample with bile, blood, urine, or feces.

Judging by looks

Milk-colored peritoneal fluid may result from a malignant tumor, lymphoma, tuberculosis, a parasitic infection, an adhesion, or hepatic cirrhosis. Cloudy or turbid fluid may indicate peritonitis. Bloody fluid may result from a benign or malignant tumor, hemorrhagic pancreatitis, perforated intestine, duodenal ulcer, neoplasm, tuberculosis, or intra-abdominal trauma.

The lowdown on levels

A white blood cell count over 300/µl (SI, 300 × 10^9/L), with more than 25% neutrophils, occurs with spontaneous bacterial peritonitis and cirrhosis. A high percentage of lymphocytes suggests tuberculous peritonitis or chylous ascites. Numerous mesothelial cells indicate tuberculous peritonitis.

Protein levels rise in cancer and tuberculous peritonitis. Peritoneal fluid glucose levels fall in tuberculous peritonitis and peritoneal carcinomatosis.

Amylase levels rise in pancreatic trauma, pancreatic pseudocyst, or acute pancreatitis and may also rise in intestinal necrosis or strangulation. Peritoneal alkaline phosphatase levels rise to more than twice the normal serum levels in a ruptured or strangulated small intestine. Peritoneal ammonia levels also exceed twice the normal serum levels in ruptured or strangulated large and small intestines and in a ruptured ulcer or appendix.

Cytologic examination accurately detects malignant cells. Microbiological examination can reveal bacteria and fungi.

What needs to be done

• Tell the patient this test requires a peritoneal fluid sample and may take up to 45 minutes to perform. Explain that he'll receive a local anesthetic to ease discomfort. Instruct him to urinate just before the test to help prevent accidental bladder injury.
• Position the patient on a bed or in a chair, as ordered, with his feet flat on the floor and his back well supported. If he can't tolerate being out of bed, place him in high Fowler's position.
• Shave the puncture site, prepare the skin, and drape the area.

Aspiration station

• A local anesthetic is injected and the needle or trocar and cannula are inserted, usually 1″ to 2″ (2.5 to 5 cm) below the umbilicus. If a trocar and cannula are used, a small incision is made to facilitate insertion. When the needle pierces the peritoneum, it "gives" with an audible sound. The trocar is removed, and a sample of fluid is aspirated with a 50-ml Luer-lock syringe. The fluid is then aspirated (no more than 1,500 ml).

Pressure dressing

• If fluid aspiration is difficult, reposition the patient as ordered. After aspiration, the trocar or needle is removed, and a pressure dressing is applied.
• Check the dressing frequently and reinforce or apply a pressure dressing if needed. Wear gloves during dressing changes.

On the lookout

• Monitor vital signs, and have the patient maintain bed rest until his vital signs are stable. Monitor his urine output for at least 24 hours and watch for hematuria.

- Weigh the patient and measure abdominal girth; compare these with baseline measurements.
- If a large amount of fluid was aspirated, watch for signs of shock.
- Watch for increasing pain and abdominal tenderness, which may indicate a perforated intestine—or puncture of the inferior epigastric artery—hematoma of the anterior cecal wall, or rupture of the iliac vein or bladder.
- Observe the patient with severe hepatic disease for signs of hepatic coma.
- Administer I.V. infusions and albumin as ordered. Check electrolyte (especially sodium) and serum protein levels.

Fecal occult blood

Fecal occult blood, invisible because of its minute quantity, can be detected by microscopic analysis or by chemical tests for hemoglobin, such as the guaiac test.

Detection tests

Because small amounts of blood (2 to 2.5 ml/day) normally appear in the feces, tests for occult blood are designed to detect quantities larger than this. The most commonly used screening test is the Hemoccult test, which uses guaiac.

What it all means

Less than 2.5 ml of blood should be present, causing the indicator to turn green. (See *Fecal occult blood test interference.*)

Abnormal findings

A positive test, in which the indicator turns blue, indicates GI bleeding, which may result from many disorders. This test is particularly important for early diagnosis of colorectal cancer because 80% of people with this type of cancer demonstrate positive results. Further tests are necessary to define the site and extent of bleeding.

What needs to be done

Inform the patient that this test requires collection of three stool specimens. (Occasionally, only a random specimen is collected.) (See *Collecting a stool specimen at home.*)

- Instruct the patient to maintain a high-fiber diet and to refrain from eating red meat, poultry, fish, turnips, and horserad-

Testing for fecal occult blood detects GI bleeding and aids early diagnosis of colorectal cancer.

Listen up!

Collecting a stool specimen at home

When teaching the patient how to collect a stool specimen, tell him to:
• collect it in a clean container with a tight-fitting lid
• wrap the container in a brown paper bag
• keep it in the refrigerator (separate from food items) until it can be transported.

Warning!

Fecal occult blood test interference

• Iron preparations, bromides, rauwolfia derivatives, indomethacin, colchicine, phenylbutazone, steroids, or ascorbic acid (vitamin C) affects results.
• Ingestion of 2 to 5 ml of blood (for example, from bleeding gums) can cause abnormal results.
• Active bleeding from hemorrhoids may cause false-positive results.

ish for 48 to 72 hours before the test and throughout the collection period.

• As ordered, the patient should withhold iron preparations, bromides, iodides, rauwolfia derivatives, indomethacin, colchicine, salicylates, phenylbutazone, steroids, and ascorbic acid for 48 hours before the test and during the collection period. If these drugs must be continued, note this on the laboratory request.

• Wearing gloves, collect three stool specimens or a random specimen, as ordered. Be sure to obtain specimens from two different areas of each stool.

• For the Hemoccult slide test, open the flap on the slide packet and use a wooden applicator to apply a thin smear of the stool specimen to the guaiac-impregnated filter paper exposed in box A. Or, after performing a digital rectal examination, wipe the examination finger on a square of the filter paper. Apply a second smear from another part of the specimen to the filter paper exposed in box B because some parts of the specimen may not contain blood.

Don't be blue

• Allow the specimen to dry for 3 to 5 minutes. Open the flap at the rear of the slide package and place 2 drops of Hemoccult developing solution on the paper over each smear. A blue reaction will appear in 30 to 60 seconds if the test is positive. Record the results and discard the slide package.

Fecal lipids

Lipids excreted in feces include monoglycerides, diglycerides, triglycerides, phospholipids, glycolipids, soaps (fatty acids and fatty acid salts), sterols, and cholesterol esters.

The fecal lipid test can confirm steatorrhea, or excess fat in the stool.

Lipid origins

These lipids are derived from sloughed intestinal bacterial cells and epithelial cells, unabsorbed dietary lipids, and GI secretions. Normally, dietary lipids emulsified by bile are almost completely absorbed in the small intestine, provided that biliary and pancreatic secretions are adequate. However, excessive excretion of fecal lipids (steatorrhea) occurs in various malabsorption syndromes.

Both qualitative and quantitative tests can detect excessive excretion of lipids; however, only the quantitative test can confirm steatorrhea.

What it all means

Fecal lipids normally make up less than 20% of excreted solids, with excretion of less than 7 g/24 hours (SI, 7 g/d). Both digestive and absorptive disorders cause steatorrhea. (See *Fecal lipids test interference.*)

What needs to be done

- Inform the patient to abstain from alcohol and to maintain a high-fat diet (100 g/day) for 3 days before the test and during the collection period.
- Collect a 72-hour stool specimen.
- Don't use a waxed collection container because the wax may become incorporated in the stool and interfere with test results.
- Refrigerate the collection container between defecations.
- Inform the patient to resume his usual diet and medications withheld, as ordered.

Warning!

Fecal lipids test interference

Azathioprine, bisacodyl, cholestyramine, kanamycin, neomycin, colchicine, aluminum hydroxide, calcium carbonate, alcohol, potassium chloride, and mineral oil may cause inaccurate results.

Stool examination for ova and parasites

Examination of a stool specimen can detect several types of intestinal parasites. Some of these parasites live in nonpathogenic symbiosis; others cause intestinal disease. In the United States, the most common parasites include the roundworm *Ascaris lumbricoides* and the hookworm *Necator americanus;* the tapeworms *Diphyllobothrium latum, Taenia saginata* and, rarely, *Taenia solium;* the amoeba *Entamoeba histolytica;* and the flagellate *Giardia lamblia.* Detection of pinworm requires a different collection method. (See *Collection procedure for pinworm.*)

Get off of my back! Stool examination for ova and parasites can confirm or rule out intestinal parasitic infection.

What it all means

No parasites or ova should appear in stool.

Peak technique

Collection procedure for pinworm

The ova of the pinworm *Enterobius vermicularis* seldom appear in feces because the female migrates to the anus and deposits her ova there. To collect them, place a piece of cellophane tape, sticky side out, on the end of a tongue blade, and press it firmly on the anal area. Then transfer the tape, sticky side down, to a slide (kits with tape and a slide or a sticky paddle are available). Because the female usually deposits her ova at night, collect the specimen early in the morning, before the patient bathes or defecates. Pinworm infection shouldn't be ruled out until five consecutive negative specimens have been obtained.

Warning!

Stool ova and parasite test interference

• Radiographic contrast media within 5 to 10 days before specimen collection alters results.
• Collection of too few specimens may cause false-negative results.
• Excessive heat or excessive cold can destroy parasites.

Parasitic presence

The presence of *E. histolytica* confirms amebiasis; *G. lamblia* confirms giardiasis. Because injury to the host is difficult to detect — even when helminth ova or larvae appear — the number of worms is usually correlated with the patient's clinical symptoms to distinguish between helminth infestation and helminth diseases. Eosinophilia may also indicate parasitic infection. (See *Stool ova and parasite test interference.*)

What needs to be done

• Check the patient's history for use of antiparasitic drugs within 2 weeks of the test.
• If the patient has diarrhea, record recent dietary and travel history.
• Instruct the patient to avoid treatments with castor or mineral oil, bismuth, magnesium or antidiarrheal compounds, barium enemas, and antibiotics for 7 to 10 days before the test.
• Collect a stool specimen directly in the container or in a clean, dry bedpan; then, using a tongue blade, transfer it into a properly labeled container. Remember to wear gloves throughout collection and handling of the specimen.

Contamination cautions

• Don't contaminate the stool specimen with urine.
• Don't collect stool from a toilet bowl because water is toxic to trophozoites and may contain organisms that interfere with test results.

Immediate action

• Send the specimen to the laboratory immediately. If a liquid or soft stool specimen can't be examined within 30 minutes of passage, place some of it in a preservative; if a formed stool specimen can't be examined immediately, refrigerate it or place it in preservative.

• If the entire stool can't be sent to the laboratory, include macroscopic worms or worm segments as well as bloody and mucoid portions of the specimen.

Stool examination for rotavirus antigen

Rotavirus (previously referred to as orbivirus, reovirus-like agent, duovirus, and gastroenteritis virus) is the most frequent cause of infectious diarrhea in infants and young children.

Virus detection

Human rotaviruses don't replicate efficiently in the usual laboratory cell cultures. Therefore, detection of the typical virus particles in stool specimens by electron microscopy has been replaced by sensitive, specific enzyme immunoassays that can provide results within minutes or a few hours (depending on the assay) after the specimen is received in the laboratory.

The rotavirus stool examination diagnoses rotavirus gastroenteritis.

What it all means

The detection of rotavirus by enzyme immunoassay is evidence of current infection with the organism. (See *Stool rotavirus antigen test interference.*)

What needs to be done

• A stool specimen (1 g in a screw-capped tube or vial) is preferred for detecting rotaviruses. If a microbiologic transport swab is used, it must be heavily stained with feces to be diagnostically productive for rotavirus.

• Avoid using collection containers with preservatives, metal ions, detergents, or serum, which may interfere with the assay.

• Store stool specimens for up to 24 hours at 35.6° to 46.4° F (2° to 8° C). If a longer period of storage or shipment is necessary, freeze the specimens at –4° F (–20° C) or colder.

• Don't store the specimen in a self-defrosting freezer.

• Remember to use gloves when handling all specimens.

Warning!

Stool rotavirus antigen test interference

Repeated freezing and thawing causes the specimen to deteriorate and yields misleading results.

Reproductive system

Amniotic fluid analysis

Amniocentesis is the transabdominal needle aspiration of 10 to 20 ml of amniotic fluid for laboratory analysis. Amniotic fluid reflects important metabolic changes in the fetus, the placenta, and the mother. Amniocentesis can be performed only when the amniotic fluid level reaches 150 ml, usually after the 16th week of pregnancy. It's indicated when a pregnant woman is over age 35; has a family history of genetic, chromosomal, or neural tube defects; or has had a previous miscarriage. Rare complications from this test include spontaneous abortion, trauma to the fetus or placenta, bleeding, premature labor, infection, and Rh sensitization from fetal bleeding into the maternal circulation.

> Amniotic fluid analysis detects fetal abnormalities, assesses fetal health, and can determine fetal age and maturity!

What it all means

Amniotic fluid should be clear but may contain white flecks of vernix caseosa when the fetus is near term. (See *Amniotic fluid analysis findings*, page 224.)

Enzyme time

Laboratory analysis can identify at least 25 different enzymes—usually in low concentrations—in amniotic fluid. The enzymes have few known clinical implications, although elevated acetylcholinesterase levels may occur with neural tube defects, exomphalos, and other serious malformations.

X marks the spot

When the mother carries an X-linked disorder, determining the fetus's sex is important. A male fetus has a 50% chance of being affected; a female fetus won't be affected but has a 50% chance of being a carrier.

Chorionic villi sampling can detect fetal abnormalities up to 10 weeks sooner than amniocentesis. (See *Chorionic villi sampling*, page 225, and *Amniotic fluid analysis interference*, page 226.)

What needs to be done

• Explain the procedure to the patient.
• Instruct the patient to urinate just before the test to minimize the risk of puncturing the bladder. Have her fold her hands behind

Advice from the experts

Amniotic fluid analysis findings

Amniotic fluid analysis can provide important information about the condition of the mother, fetus, and placenta. The table shows normal findings and abnormal findings and their implications.

Test component	Normal findings	Fetal implications of abnormal findings
Color	Clear, with white flecks of vernix caseosa in a mature fetus	Blood of maternal origin is usually harmless. "Port wine" fluid may indicate abruptio placentae. Fetal blood may indicate damage to the fetal, placental, or umbilical cord vessels.
Bilirubin	Absent at term	High levels indicate hemolytic disease of the newborn.
Meconium	Absent (except in breach presentation)	Presence indicates fetal hypotension or distress.
Creatinine	More than 2 mg/dl (SI, 177 µmol/L) in a mature fetus	Decrease may indicate fetus less than 37 weeks.
Lecithin-sphingomyelin ratio	More than 2	Less than 2 indicates pulmonary immaturity.
Phosphatidylglycerol	Present	Absence indicates pulmonary immaturity.
Glucose	Less than 45 mg/dl (SI, 2.3 mmol/L)	Excessive increases at term or near term indicate hypertrophied fetal pancreas.
Alpha-fetoprotein	Variable, depending on gestation age and laboratory technique	Inappropriate increases indicate neural tube defects, such as spina bifida or anencephaly, impending fetal death, congenital nephrosis, or contamination of fetal blood.
Bacteria	Absent	Presence indicates chorioamnionitis.
Chromosome	Normal karyotype	Abnormal karyotype indicates fetal chromosome disorders.
Acetylcholinesterase	Absent	Presence may indicate neural tube defects, exomphalos, or other serious malformations.

her head to prevent her from accidentally touching the sterile field.

• After determining fetal and placental position, usually through palpation and ultrasonography, the doctor locates a pool of amni-

Chorionic villi sampling

Chorionic villi sampling (CVS) is a prenatal test for quick detection of fetal chromosomal and biochemical disorders that's performed during the first trimester of pregnancy. Preliminary results may be available within hours; complete results within a few days. In contrast, amniocentesis can't be performed before the 16th week of pregnancy, and the results aren't available for at least 2 weeks. Thus, CVS can detect fetal abnormalities up to 10 weeks sooner than amniocentesis.

Chorionic villi are fingerlike projections that surround the embryonic membrane and eventually give rise to the placenta. Cells obtained from sample are of fetal, rather than maternal, origin and thus can be analyzed for fetal abnormalities. Samples are best obtained between the 8th and 10th weeks of pregnancy.

Procedure

To collect a chorionic villi sample, place the patient in the lithotomy position. The doctor checks the placement of the uterus bimanually, inserts a Graves' speculum, and swabs the cervix with an antiseptic solution. If necessary, he may use a tenaculum to straighten an acutely flexed uterus, permitting cannula insertion. Guided by ultrasound and possibly endoscopy, he directs the catheter through the cannula to the villi. He applies suction to the catheter to remove about 30 mg of tissue from the villi. Then he withdraws the sample, places it in a Petri dish, and examines it with a microscope. Part of the specimen is then cultured for further testing.

Complications

Possible complications are similar to those for amniocentesis: a small risk of spontaneous abortion, cramps, infection, and bleeding. Studies have found limb malformations in neonates whose mothers underwent CVS.

Symphysis

Bladder

Catheter

Rectum

Ultrasound scanner

Placenta
Yolk sac
Chorion

Uterus

Amnion

otic fluid. After preparing the skin with an antiseptic and alcohol, he injects 1 ml of 1% lidocaine with a 25G needle, first intradermally and then subcutaneously. Then he inserts the 20G to 22G spinal needle with a style into the amniotic cavity and withdraws the stylet. After attaching a 10-ml syringe to the needle, he aspirates the fluid and places it in an amber or foil-covered test tube. Approximately 20 to 30 ml of fluid is drawn when cells from amniotic fluid are needed for culturing. After the needle is withdrawn, an adhesive bandage is placed over the needle insertion site.

During the test

- Monitor fetal heart rate and maternal vital signs every 15 minutes for at least 30 minutes.
- If the patient feels faint or nauseated or perspires profusely, position her on the left side to counteract uterine pressure on the vena cava.

After the test

- Before the patient is discharged, instruct her to notify the doctor immediately if she experiences abdominal pain or cramping, chills, fever, vaginal bleeding or leakage of serous vaginal fluid, or fetal hyperactivity or unusual fetal lethargy.
- Send the specimen to the laboratory immediately.

Warning!

Amniotic fluid analysis interference

- Blood or meconium in the fluid adversely affects the lecithin-spingomyelin ratio.
- Maternal blood in the fluid may lower creatinine levels.
- Fetal blood in the fluid specimen invalidates alpha-fetoprotein results.

Papanicolaou test

The Papanicolaou (Pap) test is a cytologic test of the cervix. To perform this test, a doctor or a specially trained nurse scrapes cells from the patient's cervix and spreads them on a slide. The slide is immersed in a fixative and sent to the laboratory for cytologic analysis.

Versatility is a virtue! The Pap test can detect malignant cells, assess inflammatory tissue changes, assess response to chemotherapy and radiation therapy, and detect viral, fungal, and parasitic invasion.

What it all means

No malignant cells or abnormalities are present in a normal specimen. (See *Pap test interference*.)

Grading the Pap

A Pap smear may be graded in different ways, so check your laboratory's reporting format. In the Bethesda system—the current standardized method—potentially premalignant squamous lesions fall into three categories: atypical squamous cells of undetermined significance, low-grade squamous intraepithelial lesions, and high-grade squamous intraepithelial lesions. The low-grade category includes mild dysplasia and the changes of the human papillomavirus. The high-grade category includes moderate to severe dysplasia and carcinoma in situ.

To confirm a suggestive or positive cytology report, the test may be repeated, followed by a biopsy, or both. (See *ThinPrep for greater accuracy*.)

Now I get it!

ThinPrep for greater accuracy

A new tool for analyzing cervical cells, ThinPrep is collected in the same manner as a Papanicolaou (Pap) test using a cytobrush and plastic spatula. Specimens are deposited in a bottle provided with a fixative and sent to a specialized laboratory. A filter is then inserted into the bottle and excess mucus, blood, and inflammatory cells are filtered out by centrifuge. Remaining cells are then placed on a slide in a uniform, thin layer and read as a Pap test. This causes fewer slides to be classified as unreadable, significantly reducing the incidence of false negatives and the need for repeat tests.

Warning!

Pap test interference

Exclusive use of a specimen collected from the vaginal fornix and collection during menstruation may alter results.

What needs to be done

- Instruct the patient to avoid intercourse for 24 hours, douching for 48 hours, and vaginal creams or medications for 1 week.
- Just before the test, instruct the patient to empty her bladder. During the procedure, she may experience slight discomfort but no pain from the speculum; however, she may feel some pain when the cervix is scraped. Explain that the procedure takes only 5 to 10 minutes to perform.
- Instruct the patient to disrobe from the waist down and to drape herself. Ask her to lie on the examining table and to place her heels in the stirrups. Tell her to slide her buttocks to the edge of the table.

The examiner's role

- The examiner puts on gloves and inserts an unlubricated speculum into the vagina. To make insertion easier, he may moisten the speculum with warm water.
- The examiner collects secretions from the cervix and material from the endocervical canal. Then he spreads the specimen on the slide, according to laboratory policy, and immediately immerses the slide in a fixative or sprays it with fixative held 9″ to 12″ (23 to 30.5 cm) from the slide.

Actions after collection

- Label the specimen appropriately. A bimanual examination may follow removal of the speculum.
- If cervical bleeding occurs, give the patient a sanitary napkin.

> The Pap test shouldn't be scheduled during your menstrual period. The best time to test is midcycle.

- Examine the consistency of the specimen. It should be just thick enough that it isn't transparent. A specimen that's too thin will dry and leave too few cells for adequate screening; if it's too thick, the stain won't penetrate.
- If vaginal or vulval lesions are present, scrapings taken directly from the lesion are preferred.
- In a patient whose uterus is involuting or atrophying from age, use a small pipette, if necessary, to aspirate cells from the squamocolumnar junction and the cervical canal. Use two slides to reduce air-drying artifact.

Semen analysis

Inexpensive, technically simple, and reasonably definitive, semen analysis is usually the first test performed on a male to evaluate fertility.

Volume, motility, morphology

The procedure for analyzing semen for infertility usually includes measuring the volume of seminal fluid, assessing the sperm count, and examining the specimen under a microscope. Sperm are counted in much the same way that red and white blood cells and platelets are counted on an anticoagulated blood sample. Staining and microscopic examination of a drop of semen permits the sperms' motility and morphology to be evaluated.

Some laboratories offer specialized semen tests such as screening for antibodies to spermatozoa.

What it all means

Semen volume normally ranges from 0.7 to 6.5 ml. Liquefied semen is generally highly viscid, translucent, and gray-white, with a musty or acrid odor. After liquefaction, specimens of normal viscosity can be poured in drops. Normally, semen is slightly alkaline, with a pH of 7.3 to 7.9. Other normal characteristics of semen include immediate coagulation and liquefaction within 20 minutes. Normal sperm count ranges from 20 to 150 million/ml (SI, 20 to 150×10^6/ml); at least 40% of spermatozoa have normal morphology, and at least 20% of spermatozoa show progressive motility within 4 hours of collection.

Abnormal findings

Abnormal semen isn't synonymous with infertility. Although a normal sperm count is more than 20 million/ml (SI, 20×10^6/ml), many males with sperm counts below 1 million/ml (SI, 1×10^6/ml) have fathered normal children. Only males who can't deliver any

Semen analysis can evaluate male fertility, determine the effectiveness of vasectomy and, in rare cases, rule out paternity on grounds of complete sterility.

viable spermatozoa in their ejaculate during sexual intercourse are absolutely sterile. Nevertheless, subnormal sperm counts, decreased sperm motility, and abnormal morphology are usually associated with decreased fertility. (See *Semen analysis test interference.*)

What needs to be done

• Preparation for semen analysis varies with the test purpose. The steps below refer to fertility evaluation. (For instructions on collecting a semen specimen from a rape victim, see *Obtaining semen from a rape victim.*)

Fertility evaluation

• In most cases, it's helpful to provide written instructions for specimen collection.
• Explain to the patient that the most desirable specimen requires masturbation, ideally in a doctor's office or a laboratory, and that

Warning!

Semen analysis test interference

• The most common cause of an abnormal postcoital test is poor timing within the menstrual cycle.
• Prior cervical conization or cryotherapy as well as some drugs, such as clomiphene citrate, may adversely affect cervical mucus and yield abnormal postcoital test results.

Obtaining semen from a rape victim

When collecting a semen specimen from a rape victim, follow these guidelines:
• Inform the patient that the doctor will try to obtain a semen specimen from her vagina. Encourage her to express her fears and anxieties, and listen sympathetically. Prepare her for speculum insertion. If she's scheduled for vaginal lavage, tell her to expect a cold sensation when saline solution is instilled to wash out the specimen.
• Just before the test, instruct her to urinate, but warn her not to wipe the vulva afterward, because this may remove semen. During the test, she should breathe deeply and slowly through her mouth.
• Handle the patient's clothes as little as possible. If her clothes are moist, put them in a paper bag—not a plastic bag, which causes seminal stains and secretions to mold. Label the bag properly and send it to the laboratory immediately.
• Be aware that the doctor obtains a specimen from the vagina by direct aspiration, saline lavage, or a direct smear of vaginal contents, using a Papanicolaou stick or, less desirably, a cotton-tipped applicator. Dried smears are usually collected from the skin by gently washing with gauze moistened with physiologic saline solution. Before a postcoital examination, the examiner wipes excess mucus from the external cervix and collects the specimen by direct aspiration of the cervical canal.

Legal precautions
Prepare direct smears on glass microscopic slides after labeling the frosted end. Immediately place the slides in Coplin jars containing 95% ethanol. Use extreme caution in securing, labeling, and delivering specimens to be used for medicolegal purposes. If your facility uses routing slips for such specimens, fill them out carefully, and place them in the permanent medicolegal file.

the semen should be collected in a clean, plastic specimen container. Instruct him to follow the doctor's orders regarding the period of continence before the test.

• If he prefers to collect the specimen at home, he should deliver the specimen to the laboratory within 1 hour after collection. Warn him not to expose it to extreme temperatures or direct sunlight, which can also increase its temperature. Ideally, it should remain at body temperature until liquefaction is complete (about 20 minutes). If the weather is cold, instruct him to keep the specimen container in a coat pocket to protect it from the cold.

• Alternatives to collection by masturbation include coitus interruptus or the use of a condom or special sheath. For collection by coitus interruptus, instruct the patient to withdraw immediately before ejaculation and to deposit the ejaculate in a suitable specimen container.

• For collection by condom, tell the patient to wash the condom with soap and water, rinse it thoroughly, and allow it to dry completely. (Powders or lubricants applied to the condom may be spermicidal.) Special sheaths that don't contain spermicides are also available for semen collection. After collection, instruct the patient to tie the condom, place it in a glass jar, and deliver it to the laboratory promptly.

Miscellaneous specimen tests

Cerebrospinal fluid analysis

Cerebrospinal fluid (CSF), a clear substance that circulates in the subarachnoid space, has many vital functions. It protects the brain and spinal cord from injury and transports products of neurosecretion, cellular biosynthesis, and cellular metabolism through the central nervous system.

Obtaining by puncture

For qualitative analysis, CSF is most commonly obtained by lumbar puncture, usually between the third and fourth lumbar vertebrae; in rare instances, it's obtained by cisternal or ventricular puncture. Specimens of CSF for laboratory analysis are commonly obtained during other neurologic tests such as myelography.

CSF analysis measures CSF pressure and circulation; helps diagnose meningitis, brain hemorrhages, tumors, and abscesses; and can be used in the diagnosis of Alzheimer's disease.

What it all means

Normally, the doctor records CSF pressure and checks the appearance of the specimen. Three tubes are routinely collected and sent to the laboratory for analysis of protein, glucose, red blood cell and white blood cell (WBC) counts as well as for serologic testing, such as the Venereal Disease Research Laboratory test for neurosyphilis. A separate specimen is also sent to the laboratory for culture and sensitivity testing. Electrolyte analysis and Gram stain may be ordered as supplementary tests. CSF electrolyte levels are of special interest in patients with abnormal serum electrolyte levels or CSF infection and in those receiving hyperosmolar agents. (For the implications of abnormal CSF analysis findings, see *Interpreting CSF findings*, page 232, and *CSF analysis interference*, page 233.)

What needs to be done

- Tell the patient this test usually takes at least 15 minutes.
- Inform him that a headache is the most common adverse effect of lumbar puncture, but reassure him that his cooperation during the test helps minimize this reaction.

Assume the position

- Position the patient on his side at the edge of the bed with his knees drawn up to his abdomen and his chin tucked against his chest (fetal position). Provide pillows to support the spine on a horizontal plane. This position allows easy access to the lumbar subarachnoid space.

Puncture, pain...

- After the skin is prepared for injection, the area is draped. Instruct the patient to remain still and breathe normally; movement and hyperventilation can alter pressure readings or cause injury.
- The anesthetic is injected, and the spinal needle is inserted in the midline between the spinous vertebral processes, usually between the third and fourth lumbar vertebrae. When the stylet is removed from the needle, CSF drips from it if the needle is properly positioned. A stopcock and manometer are attached to the needle to measure initial (opening) CSF pressure.

...and postpunctural procedures

- After the specimen is collected, label the containers in the order in which they were filled and record the doctor's specific instructions for the laboratory. A final pressure reading is taken, and the needle is removed. Clean the puncture site with a local antiseptic, such as povidone-iodine solution, and apply a small adhesive bandage. Send the form and labeled specimens to the laboratory immediately.

Advice from the experts

Interpreting CSF findings

Obtaining a cerebrospinal fluid (CSF) specimen and interpreting the results helps diagnose various conditions. The table below shows normal CSF findings as well as abnormal findings and their implications.

Test	Normal	Abnormal	Implications
Pressure	50 to 180 mm H_2O	Increase	Increased intracranial pressure
		Decrease	Spinal subarachnoid obstruction above puncture site
Appearance	Clear, colorless	Cloudy	Infection
		Xanthochromic or bloody	Subarachnoid, intracerebral, or intraventricular hemorrhage; spinal cord obstruction; traumatic lumbar puncture
		Brown, orange	Elevated protein levels, yellow or red blood cell (RBC) breakdown
Protein	15 to 50 mg/dl (SI, 0.15 to 0.5 q/L)	Marked increase	Tumors, trauma, hemorrhage, diabetes mellitus, polyneuritis, blood in CSF
		Marked decrease	Rapid CSF production
Gamma globulin	3% to 12% of total protein	Increase	Demyelinating disease, neurosyphilis, Guillain-Barré syndrome
Glucose	50 to 80 mg/dl (SI, 2.8 to 4.4 mmol/L)	Increase	Systemic hyperglycemia
		Decrease	Systemic hypoglycemia, bacterial or fungal infection, meningitis, mumps, postsubarachnoid hemorrhage
Cell count	0 to 5 WBCs; no RBCs	Increase	Active disease: meningitis, acute infection, onset of chronic illness, tumor, abscess, infarction, demyelinating disease
	No RBCs	RBCs	Hemorrhage or traumatic lumbar puncture
VDRL test for syphilis and other serologic tests	Nonreactive	Positive	Neurosyphilis
Chloride	118 to 130 mEq/L (SI, 118 to 130 mmol/L)	Decrease	Infected meninges
Gram stain	No organisms	Gram-positive or gram-negative organisms	Bacterial meningitis

Resting reminders

• In most cases, you'll be instructed to keep the patient lying flat for 8 hours after lumbar puncture, but some doctors allow a 30-degree elevation. Encourage him to drink fluids.

Red alert

• Check the puncture site for redness, swelling, and drainage every hour for the first 4 hours, then every 4 hours for the first 24 hours. Watch for complications such as a reaction to the anesthetic, meningitis, bleeding into the spinal canal, and cerebellar tonsillar herniation and medullary compression. Observe closely for signs of an adverse reaction, such as elevated pulse rate, pallor, or clammy skin. Alert the doctor immediately to significant changes.

• Infection at the puncture site contraindicates removal of CSF; in a patient with increased intracranial pressure, CSF should be removed with extreme caution because the rapid reduction in pressure that follows withdrawal of fluid can cause cerebellar tonsillar herniation and medullary compression.

In case of elevation

• If CSF pressure is elevated, assess neurologic status every 15 minutes for 4 hours. If the patient is stable, assess every hour for 2 hours, then every 4 hours or according to the pretest schedule.

Warning!

CSF analysis interference

• Patient position and activity can alter cerebrospinal fluid (CSF) pressure.

• Crying, coughing, or straining may increase pressure.

• Delay between collection time and laboratory testing may alter results.

Pericardial fluid analysis

Pericardial fluid analysis involves the needle aspiration—pericardiocentesis—and analysis of pericardial fluid. Both therapeutic and diagnostic, it's most useful as an emergency measure to relieve cardiac tamponade. It can also provide a fluid sample to confirm and identify the cause of pericardial effusion (excess pericardial fluid).

Possible complications

Pericardiocentesis should be performed cautiously because of the risk of potentially fatal complications, such as laceration of a coronary artery or the myocardium; other possible complications include ventricular fibrillation or vasovagal arrest, pleural infection, and accidental puncture of the lung, liver, or stomach. To minimize the risk of complications, echocardiography should precede pericardiocentesis to determine the effusion site. Generally, surgical drainage and biopsy are safer than pericardiocentesis.

What it all means

The pericardium normally contains 10 to 50 ml of sterile fluid. Pericardial fluid is clear and straw colored, without evidence of

Pericardial fluid analysis helps identify the cause of pericardial effusion and helps determine appropriate therapy.

pathogens, blood, or malignant cells. The WBC count in the fluid is usually less than 1,000/µl (SI, 1 x 10⁹ L). Its glucose concentration should approximate the glucose levels in whole blood.

Transudates and exudates

Pericardial effusions are typically classified as transudates or exudates. *Transudates* are protein-poor effusions that usually arise from mechanical factors altering fluid formation or resorption, such as increased hydrostatic pressure, decreased plasma oncotic pressure, or obstruction of the pericardial lymphatic drainage system by a tumor.

Most *exudates* result from inflammation and contain large amounts of protein. Inflammation damages the capillary membrane, allowing protein molecules to leak into the pericardial fluid. Both effusion types occur in pericarditis, neoplasms, acute myocardial infarction, tuberculosis, rheumatoid disease, and systemic lupus erythematosus. (See *Pericardial fluid analysis interference*.)

What needs to be done

- Check the patient's history for current use of antimicrobial drugs. Let him know that it takes 10 to 20 minutes. Inform him that he need not restrict food or fluids.
- Explain the procedure to the patient. Inform him that an I.V. line will be started and he'll receive I.V. sedation as ordered.
- Place the patient in a supine position with the thorax elevated 60 degrees and tell him to remain still during the procedure. After the skin is prepared, a local anesthetic is administered at the insertion site.

How it's done

- With the three-way stopcock open, a 50-ml syringe is attached to one end and the cardiac needle to the other. The patient is connected to monitor, which is set to read lead V. (Make sure resuscitation equipment is nearby.) The needle is inserted through the chest wall into the pericardial sac, maintaining gentle aspiration until fluid appears in the syringe. The needle is angled 35 to 45 degrees toward the tip of the right scapula between the left costal margin and the xiphoid process.
- When the needle is properly positioned, a Kelly clamp is attached at the skin surface so the needle won't advance further. During asiration, fluid specimen tubes are labeled and numbered. When the needle is withdrawn, pressure is applied to the site *immediately* with sterile gauze pads for 3 to 5 minutes. Then a bandage is applied. (See *Aspirating pericardial fluid*.)
- Watch for grossly bloody aspirate—a sign of inadvertent puncture of a cardiac chamber.

By the end of this test, I'll be filled with pericardial fluid.

Peak technique

Aspirating pericardial fluid

In pericardiocentesis, a needle and syringe assembly is inserted through the chest wall into the pericardial sac (as illustrated below). Electrocardiographic (ECG) monitoring, with a leadwire attached to the needle and electrodes placed on the limbs (right arm [RA], right leg [RL], left arm [LA], and left leg [LL]), helps ensure proper needle placement and avoids damage to the heart.

Warning!

Pericardial fluid analysis interference

Antimicrobial therapy can prevent isolation of the causative organism.

On alert

• Check vital signs and heart sounds every 15 minutes until stable, then every half hour for 2 hours, every hour for 4 hours, and every 4 hours thereafter.
• Be alert for respiratory or cardiac distress. Watch especially for signs of cardiac tamponade.

Collection technique

• Clean the top of the culture and sensitivity tube with povidone-iodine solution to reduce the risk of extrinsic contamination.
• If bacterial culture and sensitivity tests are scheduled, record on the laboratory request any antimicrobial drugs the patient is receiving. If anaerobic organisms are suspected, consult the laboratory about proper collection technique to avoid exposing the aspirate to air.
• Send all specimens to the laboratory immediately.

Sweat test

The sweat test quantitatively measures electrolyte concentrations — primarily sodium and chloride — in sweat, usually through pilocarpine iontophoresis (pilocarpine is a sweat inducer). This test is used almost exclusively in children.

The sweat test confirms cystic fibrosis.

What it all means

Normal sodium values in sweat range from 10 to 30 mEq/L (SI, 10 to 30 mmol/L). Normal chloride values range from 10 to 35 mEq/L (SI, 10 to 35 mmol/L).

Abnormal findings

Abnormal sodium values range from 50 to 130 mEq/L (SI, 50 to 130 mmol/L). Abnormal chloride values range from 50 to 110 mEq/L (SI, 50 to 110 mmol/L). Sodium and chloride concentrations of 50 to 60 mEq/L (SI, 50 to 60 mmol/L) strongly suggest cystic fibrosis. Concentrations above 60 mEq/L (SI, above 60 mmol/L) with typical clinical features confirm the diagnosis. Only a few conditions other than cystic fibrosis cause elevated sweat electrolyte levels — most notably, untreated adrenal insufficiency as well as type I glycogen storage disease, vasopressin-resistant diabetes insipidus, meconium ileus, and renal failure. However, only cystic fibrosis raises sweat electrolyte levels above 80 mEq/L (SI, above 80 mmol/L).

In females, sweat electrolyte levels fluctuate cyclically: Chloride concentrations usually peak 5 to 10 days before onset of menses, and most women retain fluid before menses. Males also show fluctuations (up to 70 mEq/L [SI, 70 mmol/L]). (See *Sweat test interference.*)

What needs to be done

• Tell the patient the test takes 20 to 45 minutes. Explain that he may feel a slight tickling sensation but won't feel pain. Stay with the child during the test to help minimize anxiety.
• With distilled water, wash the test area; then dry it. The flexor surface of the right forearm is commonly used; if the patient's arm is too small to secure electrodes, the right thigh is used.
• Place a gauze pad saturated with premeasured pilocarpine solution on the positive electrode; place a gauze pad saturated with normal saline solution on the negative electrode. Apply both electrodes to the area to be tested and secure them with straps.

Electro-precautions

• Leadwires to the analyzer are given a current of 4 mA in 15 to 20 seconds. This process (iontophoresis) is continued at 15- to 20-

second intervals for 5 minutes. After iontophoresis, remove both electrodes. Discard the pads, clean the patient's skin with distilled water, and then dry it. (Always perform iontophoresis on the right arm or right thigh).

Halt!

• Stop the test immediately if the patient complains of a burning sensation, which usually indicates that the positive electrode is exposed or positioned improperly. Adjust the electrode and then continue the test.

Sweat collection

• Using forceps, place a dry gauze pad or filter paper (previously weighed on a gram scale) on the area where the pilocarpine was used. Cover the pad or filter paper with a slightly larger piece of plastic and seal the edges of the plastic with waterproof adhesive tape. Leave the gauze pad or filter paper in place for about 45 minutes. Make sure that at least 100 mg of sweat is collected in 45 minutes. (Droplets on the plastic usually indicate induction of an adequate amount of sweat.)

• Remove the pad or filter paper with the forceps, place it immediately in the weighing bottle, and insert the stopper in the bottle. Send the bottle to the laboratory immediately. The difference between the first and second weights indicate the weight of the sweat specimen collected.

After collection

• Wash the tested area with soap and water and dry it thoroughly.
• If the area looks red, reassure the patient that this is normal and that the redness will disappear within a few hours.
• Tell the patient he may resume his usual activities.

Warning!

Sweat test interference

• Dehydration and edema, especially in the collection area, may alter results.
• Pure salt depletion (common during hot weather) may cause false-normal test results.

Quick quiz

1.   Which of the following are adverse effects of gastric acid stimulation testing?
    A.   Tachycardia, cyanosis, and chest pain
    B.   Abdominal pain, nausea, and dizziness
    C.   Fever, tachycardia, and sudden breathlessness

Answer: B. Adverse effects of gastric acid stimulation testing include abdominal pain, nausea, dizziness, and numbness of the extremities. Report these findings to the doctor immediately.

2. When preparing the patient for fecal occult blood testing, instruct him to refrain from consuming which of the following for 48 to 72 hours before testing?
- A.   Horseradish, turnips, fish, and red meat
- B.   Alcohol, high-fiber foods, and high-sodium foods
- C.   High-fat foods, alcohol, and foods containing vanilla

Answer: A. The patient should maintain a high-fiber diet and refrain from eating red meat, poultry, fish, turnips, and horseradish for 48 to 72 hours before the fecal occult blood test and throughout the collection period.

3. Amniocentesis can be performed only when the amniotic fluid level reaches 150 ml. This typically occurs after which week of gestation?
- A.   12th week
- B.   16th week
- C.   24th week

Answer: B. Amniocentesis can be performed only when the amniotic fluid level reaches 150 ml, usually after week 16 of pregnancy.

4. Which factor may alter Pap test results?
- A.   Douching within 72 hours of the test
- B.   Collecting the specimen immediately after menstruation
- C.   Having intercourse within 24 hours of the test

Answer: C. Douching within 48 hours or having intercourse within 24 hours of a Pap test can wash away cellular deposits, altering results.

Scoring

☆☆☆   If you answered all four questions correctly, superb! You're one heck of a specimen!

☆☆   If you answered three questions correctly, terrific! You're testing your way to perfection!

☆   If you answered fewer than three questions correctly, don't worry! Your specimen-collecting skills will be perfect in no time!

7

Cultures

Just the facts

In this chapter, you'll learn:

♦ about cultures
♦ what patient care is associated with cultures
♦ what factors can interfere with these tests
♦ what culture results may indicate.

A look at cultures

Cultures are performed to isolate organisms and determine the cause of infection. Each culture requires its own specimen collection technique. Explain the procedure to the patient to ensure proper collection and avoid inadvertent specimen contamination.

Urine cultures

Although urine in the kidneys and bladder is normally sterile, a small number of bacteria are usually present in the urethra and, consequently, may pass into the urine. A single negative culture doesn't always rule out infection, as in chronic, low-grade pyelonephritis.

Colony count

Significant results of urine culture are possible only after quantitative examination. To distinguish between true bacteriuria and contamination, it's necessary to know the number of organisms in a milliliter of urine, estimated by a culture technique known as a "colony count." In addition, a quick centrifugation test can determine where a urinary tract infection (UTI) originates. (See *Quick centrifugation test*, page 240.)

A urine culture diagnoses UTI and monitors microorganism colonization after urinary catheter insertion.

Collecting a clean-catch midstream specimen

To teach a patient how to collect a clean-catch midstream urine specimen, tell him to:
• clean the periurethral area with soap and water
• wipe the area three times, each time with a fresh 2″ × 2″ gauze pad soaked in povidone-iodine solution or with the wipes provided in a commercial kit
• begin voiding after cleaning
• then, without stopping the urine stream, move the collection container into the stream, collecting 30 to 50 ml at the midstream portion of voiding
• finish voiding into toilet, bedpan, or urinal
• wash his hands.

Quick centrifugation test

The quick centrifugation test can determine whether the source of a urinary tract infection (UTI) is in the lower tract (bladder) or the upper tract (kidneys). The test involves urine centrifugation in a test tube, followed by staining of the sediment with fluorescein. If at least one-fourth of the bacteria fluoresce when viewed under a fluorescent microscope, an upper tract UTI is present; lack of fluorescence means a lower tract UTI.

Clean-voided midstream collection is the method of choice for obtaining a urine specimen.

What it all means

Culture results of sterile urine are normally reported as "no growth," which usually indicates the absence of UTI.

Overpopulation problem

Bacterial counts of 100,000 or more organisms of a single microbe species per milliliter indicate probable UTI. Counts under 100,000/ml may be significant, depending on the patient's age, sex, history, and other individual factors. All growths from catheterized urine or suprapubic aspirations are considered significant and are investigated by using susceptibility tests to identify the causative organism. Isolation of more than two species of organisms or of vaginal or skin organisms usually suggests contamination and requires a repeat culture. Urine cultures also identify pathogenic fungi. (See *Urine culture test interference.*)

What needs to be done

• Check the patient's history for current use of antimicrobial drugs. Explain to the patient that this test requires the collection of a clean-catch midstream specimen. (See *Collecting a clean-catch midstream specimen.*)
• If appropriate, explain catheterization or suprapubic aspiration to the patient.
• Put on gloves and collect a urine specimen. Collect at least 3 ml of urine; don't fill the specimen cup more than halfway.

- Record current antimicrobial therapy and fluid- or drug-induced diuresis on the laboratory request.
- Seal the cup with a sterile lid and send it to the laboratory at once.
- If transport is delayed for more than 30 minutes, store the specimen at 39.2° F (4° C) or place it on ice, unless a urine transport tube containing preservative is used.

Stool culture

Normally, feces contain many species of bacterial flora and several potentially pathogenic organisms. Identifying these organisms is vital to treatment to prevent possibly fatal complications (especially in a debilitated patient), and to confine these severe infectious diseases. A sensitivity test may follow pathogen isolation.

Stool culture may also detect viruses, such as enterovirus, which can cause aseptic meningitis.

What it all means

More than 95% of normal fecal flora consist of anaerobes, including non-spore-forming bacilli, clostridia, and anaerobic streptococci. The remainder consist of aerobes, including gram-negative bacilli (predominantly *Escherichia coli* and other Enterobacteriaceae, plus small amounts of *Pseudomonas*), gram-positive cocci (mostly enterococci), and a few yeasts.

Abnormal findings

Isolation of some pathogens indicates bacterial infection or other disorders. (See *Pathogens of the GI tract*, page 242.)

If a stool culture shows no unusual growth, detection of viruses by immunoassay or electron microscopy may diagnose nonbacterial gastroenteritis. (See *Stool culture test interference*, page 242.)

What needs to be done

- Check the patient's history for dietary patterns, recent antimicrobial therapy, and recent travel that might suggest an endemic infection or infestation.
- Collect the specimen before antimicrobial therapy is started.
- Explain to the patient that this test may require the collection of a stool specimen on 3 consecutive days.
- Collect a stool specimen directly in the container. If the patient isn't ambulatory, collect it in a clean, dry bedpan. Using a tongue blade, transfer the specimen to the container. If the specimen is

Warning!

Urine culture test interference

Fluid- or drug-induced diuresis and antimicrobial therapy may alter test results.

A stool culture identifies pathogenic organisms causing GI disease, detects viruses, and identifies carrier states.

Advice from the experts

Pathogens of the GI tract

The presence of the following pathogens in a stool culture may indicate certain disorders:
- *Aeromonas hydrophila:* gastroenteritis, which causes diarrhea, especially in children
- *Bacillus cereus:* food poisoning, acute gastroenteritis (rare)
- *Campylobacter jejuni:* gastroenteritis
- *Clostridium botulinum:* food poisoning and infant botulism (a possible cause of sudden infant death syndrome)
- Toxin-producing *Clostridium difficile:* pseudomembranous enterocolitis
- *Clostridium perfringens:* food poisoning
- Enterotoxigenic *Escherichia coli:* gastroenteritis (resembles cholera or shigellosis)
- *Salmonella:* gastroenteritis, typhoid fever, nontyphoidal salmonellosis, paratyphoid fever, enteric fever
- *Shigella:* shigellosis, bacillary dysentery
- *Staphylococcus aureus:* food poisoning, suppression of normal bowel flora from antimicrobial therapy
- *Vibrio cholerae:* cholera
- *V. parahaemolyticus:* food poisoning, especially seafood
- *Yersinia enterocolitica:* gastroenteritis, enterocolitis (resembles appendicitis), mesenteric lymphadenitis, ileitis.

Warning!

Stool culture test interference

Antimicrobial therapy may decrease bacterial growth in the specimen.

collected by rectal swab, insert the swab past the anal sphincter, rotate it gently, and withdraw it. Then place the swab in the appropriate container.
- Use gloves when handling the specimen; put the specimen container in a leakproof bag.
- Check with the laboratory for the collection procedure for a virus test.
- Send the specimen to the laboratory immediately; be sure to include mucoid and bloody portions and always represent the first, middle, and last portion of the feces passed. If a specimen can't be transported to the laboratory within 1 hour, refrigerate it or place it in transport media.
- Indicate the suspected cause of the patient's GI disorder and current antimicrobial therapy on the laboratory request.

Throat culture

A throat culture requires swabbing the throat, streaking a culture plate, and allowing the organisms to grow for isolation and identification of pathogens. A Gram-stained smear may provide preliminary identification, which may guide clinical management and determine the need for further tests. Culture results must be interpreted in light of clinical status, recent antimicrobial therapy, and the amount of normal flora.

What it all means

Throat flora normally include nonhemolytic and alpha-hemolytic streptococci, *Neisseria* species, staphylococci, diptheroids, some *Haemophilus* species, pneumococci, yeasts, enteric gram-negative organisms, spirochetes, *Veillonella* species, and *Micrococcus* species.

Abnormal findings

Possible pathogens cultured include group A beta-hemolytic streptococci (*Streptococcus pyogenes*), which can cause scarlet fever or pharyngitis; *Candida albicans*, which can cause thrush; *Corynebacterium diphtheriae*, which can cause diphtheria; and *Bordetella pertussis*, which can cause whooping cough. Other cultured bacteria include *Legionella* species, *Mycoplasma pneumoniae*, *Staphylococcus aureus*, *Streptococcus pneumoniae*, and *H. influenzae*. It's also used to screen for carriers of *N. meningitidis*. Fungi include *Histoplasma capsulatum*, *Coccidioides immitis*, and *Blastomyces dermatitidis*. Viruses include adenovirus, enterovirus, herpesvirus, rhinovirus, influenza virus, and parainfluenza virus. (See *Throat culture test interference*, page 244.)

Throat cultures isolate and identify pathogens, particularly group A beta-hemolytic streptococci, and screen asymptomatic carriers of pathogens, especially *Neisseria meningitidis*.

What needs to be done

• Check for a recent history of antimicrobial therapy, and obtain the throat specimen before beginning antimicrobial therapy.
• Explain to the patient that this test helps identify the microorganisms and takes about 30 seconds. Tell him he may gag during swabbing.
• Use gloves when performing the procedure and handling specimens.
• Have the patient tilt his head back and close his eyes. With the throat well illuminated, check for inflamed areas, using a tongue blade.

Swab the deck

• Swab the tonsillar areas from side to side; include inflamed or purulent sites. *Don't* touch the tongue, cheeks, or teeth with the swab.
• Immediately place the swab in the culture tube. If a commercial sterile collection and transport system is used, crush the ampule and force the swab into the medium to keep it moist.

Special delivery

• Note recent antimicrobial therapy on the laboratory request. Also indicate the suspected organism.
• Send the specimen to the laboratory immediately; keep the container upright during transport. Don't refrigerate specimens.

Warning!

Throat culture test interference

Failure to report recent or current antimicrobial therapy may alter test results.

Nasopharyngeal culture

Direct microscopic inspection of a Gram-stained smear of the nasopharyngeal specimen provides preliminary identification of organisms, which may guide clinical management and determine the need for additional testing. Streaking a culture plate with the swab allowing any organisms present to grow permits isolation and identification of pathogens. Cultured pathogens may require susceptibility testing to determine the appropriate antimicrobial agent.

What it all means

Flora commonly found in the nasopharynx include nonhemolytic streptococci, alpha-hemolytic streptococci, *Neisseria* species (except *N. meningitidis* and *N. gonorrhoeae*), *Staphylococcus epidermidis* and, occasionally, *S. aureus*. (See *Nasopharyngeal culture test interference.*)

Abnormal findings

Pathogens may include group A beta-hemolytic streptococci; occasionally groups B, C, and G beta-hemolytic streptococci; *B. pertussis; C. diphtheriae; S. aureus;* large numbers of pneumococci; *H. influenzae; Myxovirus influenzae;* paramyxoviruses; *C. albicans; Mycoplasma* species; *Mycobacterium tuberculosis; B. pertussis;* and *N. meningitidis.* Viruses can be isolated, especially carriers of influenza virus A and B.

A nasopharyngeal culture can identify pathogens that can cause upper respiratory tract symptoms.

Peak technique

Obtaining a nasopharyngeal specimen

When the swab passes into the nasopharynx, gently but quickly rotate it to collect a specimen. Then remove the swab, taking care not to injure the nasal mucous membrane.

Warning!

Nasopharyngeal culture test interference

Recent antimicrobial therapy decreases bacterial growth.

What needs to be done

• Inform the patient of how and where the specimen will be obtained and that he may experience slight discomfort and may gag.
• Put on gloves. Moisten the swab with sterile water or saline. Ask the patient to cough before you begin collecting the specimen, and then position the patient with his head tilted back.
• Using a penlight and a tongue blade, inspect the nasopharyngeal area. Next, without touching the sides of the patient's nostril or his tongue, gently pass the swab through the nostril and into the nasopharynx, keeping the swab near the septum and floor of the nose. (See *Obtaining a nasopharyngeal specimen*.)
• If *B. pertussis* is suspected, Dacron or calcium alginate minitipped swabs should be used for collection.

Lab notes

• If the specimen is for isolation of a virus, verify the laboratory's recommended collection and refrigeration techniques.
• Note recent antimicrobial therapy or chemotherapy on the laboratory request.
• Tell the laboratory if *Corynebacterium diphtheriae* or *B. pertussis* is suspected; these organisms need special growth media.
• Keep the container upright.

Sputum culture

Bacteriologic examination of sputum—material raised from the lungs and bronchi during deep coughing—is an important aid in managing lung disease.

The usual method of specimen collection is expectoration. Other methods include tracheal suctioning and bronchoscopy. A Gram stain of expectorated sputum must be examined to ensure that it's representative of secretions from the lower respirato-

A sputum culture isolates and identifies the cause of a pulmonary infection.

ry tract rather than contaminated by oral flora. Careful examination of an acid-fast sputum smear may provide presumptive evidence of a mycobacterial infection, such as tuberculosis.

What it all means

Flora commonly found in the respiratory tract include alpha-hemolytic streptococci, *Neisseria* species, diptheroids, some *Haemophilus* species, pneumococci, staphylococci, and yeasts such as *Candida*. However, the presence of normal flora doesn't rule out infection. A culture isolate must be interpreted in light of the patient's overall clinical condition.

On-site organisms

Pathogenic organisms most often found in sputum include *Streptococcus pneumoniae*, *Mycobacterium tuberculosis*, *Klebsiella pneumoniae* (and other Enterobacteriaceae), *H. influenzae*, *Staphylococcus aureus*, and *Pseudomonas aeruginosa*. Other pathogens, such as *Pneumocystis carinii*, *Legionella* species, *Mycoplasma pneumoniae*, and respiratory viruses, may exist in the sputum and can cause lung disease, but they usually require serologic or histologic diagnosis rather than diagnosis by sputum culture. (See *Sputum culture test interference*.)

What needs to be done

• Explain to the patient that this test requires sputum, not saliva. Instruct him to brush his teeth and gargle with water immediately before obtaining the specimen and teach him how to expectorate.
• *For expectoration:* Put on gloves and a mask. Instruct the patient to cough deeply and expectorate into the container. If the cough is nonproductive, use chest physiotherapy or nebulization to induce sputum, as ordered. Using aseptic technique, close the container securely and place it in a leakproof bag before sending it to the laboratory.
• *For tracheal suctioning:* Administer oxygen to the patient, as necessary. Using sterile gloves, lubricate the catheter with normal saline solution and pass the catheter through the nostril, without suction. (The patient will cough when the catheter passes through the larynx.) Advance the catheter into the trachea. Apply suction for no longer than 15 seconds to obtain the specimen. Stop suction and gently remove the catheter. Discard the catheter and gloves. Then detach the in-line sputum trap from the suction apparatus and cap the opening. If the patient becomes hypoxic or cyanotic, remove the catheter immediately and administer oxygen. (See *Using an in-line trap.*)

Warning!

Sputum culture test interference

• Failure to report current or recent antimicrobial therapy may alter results.
• Sputum collected over an extended period may cause pathogens to deteriorate or become overgrown by commensals (one of two or more organisms that live in an intimate, nonparasitic relationship).

Peak technique

Using an in-line trap

Put on sterile gloves. Push the suction tubing onto the male adapter of the in-line trap.

Insert the suction catheter into the rubber tubing of the trap. Then suction the patient.

After suctioning, disconnect the in-line trap from the suction tubing and catheter.

To seal the container, connect the rubber tubing to the female adapter of the trap.

• *For bronchoscopy:* After a local anesthetic is sprayed into the patient's throat or the patient gargles with a local anesthetic, the bronchoscope is inserted through the pharynx and trachea into the bronchus. Secretions are then collected with a bronchial brush or aspirated through the inner channel of the scope, using an irrigating solution, such as normal saline solution, if necessary. After the specimen is obtained, the bronchoscope is removed.

• After bronchoscopy, observe the patient carefully for signs of hypoxemia, laryngospasm, bronchospasm, pneumothorax, perforation of the trachea or bronchus (subcutaneous crepitus), or trauma to respiratory structures. Check for difficulty breathing or swallowing. *Don't* give liquids until the gag reflex returns. In a patient with asthma or chronic bronchitis, watch for aggravated bronchospasms.

• Include on the laboratory request the nature and origin of the specimen, the date and time of collection, the initial diagnosis, and any current antimicrobial therapy.

• Send the specimen to the laboratory immediately.

Blood culture

A blood culture involves inoculating a culture medium with a blood sample and incubating it for isolation and identification of the causative pathogens in bacteremia (bacterial invasion of the bloodstream) and septicemia (systemic spread of such infection). Blood cultures can identify about 67% of pathogens within 24 hours and up to 90% within 72 hours. Blood cultures are ideally performed on 2 consecutive days.

Time factor

Bacteremia may be transient, intermittent, or continuous. The timing of specimen collection for blood cultures varies; it usually depends on the type of suspected bacteremia — either intermittent or continuous — and on whether drug therapy needs to be started regardless of test results.

> A blood culture confirms bacteremia and identifies the causative organism in bacteremia and septicemia.

What it all means

Blood normally has no pathogenic organisms.

Common pathogens

Common blood pathogens include *Neisseria meningitidis*, *Streptococcus pneumoniae* and other *Streptococcus* species, *Haemophilus influenzae*, *Staphylococcus aureus*, *Pseudomonas aeruginosa*, *Brucella*, and organisms classified as Bacteroidaceae and Enterobacteriaceae.

Immunodeficiency issues

Debilitated or immunocompromised patients may have isolates of *Candida albicans*. In patients with human immunodeficiency virus infection, *Mycobacterium tuberculosis* and *M. avium* complex may be isolated as well as other *Mycobacterium* species on a less frequent basis. (See *Blood culture test interference.*)

What needs to be done

• Inform the patient of the number of samples required and that some discomfort may be felt from the needle punctures and the pressure of the tourniquet. Let him know that dietary restrictions aren't necessary before the test.
• Put on gloves. After cleaning the venipuncture site with an alcohol swab, clean it again with a povidone-iodine swab, starting at the site and working outward in a circular motion. Wait at least 1 minute for the skin to dry, and then remove the residual iodine with an alcohol swab. Apply the tourniquet.

Venipuncture procedures

• Clean the diaphragm tops of the culture bottles with alcohol or iodine, and change the needle on the syringe. If broth is being used, add blood to each bottle until a 1:5 or 1:10 dilution is achieved. If a special resin is being used, add blood to the resin in the bottles and invert gently to mix.
• Perform a venipuncture and draw 10 to 20 ml of blood for an adult or 2 to 6 ml for a child. Draw the blood directly into a special collection-processing tube if the lysis-centrifugation technique (Isolator) is being used. Whenever possible, blood cultures should be collected before administering antimicrobial agents.
• Note current or recent antimicrobial therapy on the laboratory request slip.
• If a hematoma develops at the venipuncture site, apply warm soaks.
• Send each sample to the laboratory immediately after collection.

Warning!

Blood culture test interference

Previous or current antimicrobial therapy may give false-negative results.

Wound culture

A wound culture consists of microscopic analysis of a specimen from a lesion to confirm infection.

Aerobic and anaerobic

Wound cultures may be aerobic (for detection of organisms that usually require oxygen to grow and typically appear in a superficial wound) or anaerobic (for organisms that need little or no oxygen and appear in areas of poor tissue perfusion, such as postoperative wounds, ulcers, or compound fractures).

Indications for wound culture include fever as well as inflammation and drainage in damaged tissue.

What it all means

A clean wound has no pathogenic organism. (See *Wound culture test interference*, page 250.)

Abnormal findings

The most common aerobic pathogens in wounds are *Staphylococcus aureus*, group A beta-hemolytic streptococci, *Proteus* species, *Escherichia coli* and other Enterobacteriaceae, and some *Pseudomonas* species; the most common anaerobic pathogens are some *Clostridium*, *Bacteroides*, *Peptococcus*, and *Streptococcus* species.

Memory jogger

To remember the difference between aerobic and anaerobic, think of jogging. When you jog, an aerobic activity, your body requires oxygen — aerobic means oxygen is required. Anaerobic means without oxygen.

Peak technique

Anaerobic specimen collector

Some anaerobes die when they're exposed to the slightest bit of oxygen. To facilitate anaerobic collection and culturing, tubes filled with carbon dioxide (CO_2) or nitrogen are used for oxygen-free transport.

The anaerobic specimen collector shown here consists of a rubber-stoppered tube filled with CO_2, a small inner tube, and a swab attached to a plastic plunger. The drawing on the left shows the tube before specimen collection. The small inner tube containing the swab is held in place by the rubber stopper.

After specimen collection (right), the swab is quickly replaced in the inner tube and the plunger depressed. This separates the inner tube from the stopper, forcing it into the larger tube and exposing the specimen to the CO_2-rich environment. Keep the tube upright.

Warning!

Wound culture test interference

Failure to report recent or current antimicrobial therapy

Before   After

Wound cultures, which may be aerobic or anaerobic, can identify an infectious microbe in a wound.

What needs to be done

• Using gloves, prepare a sterile field and clean the area around the wound with antiseptic solution.

Culture differences

• *For aerobic culture:* Express the wound and swab as much exudate as possible, or insert the swab deep into the wound and gently rotate. Obtain exudate from the entire wound, using more

than one swab. Immediately place the swab in the aerobic culture tube.
• *For anaerobic culture:* Insert the swab deep into the wound, gently rotate it, and immediately place it in the anaerobic culture tube; or insert the needle into the wound, aspirate 1 to 5 ml of exudate, and immediately inject the exudate into the anaerobic culture tube. (See *Anaerobic specimen collector.*)

Completing the culture

• Dress the wound as ordered.
• Record on the laboratory request recent antimicrobial therapy, the source of the specimen, and the suspected organism.
• If the needle is covered with a rubber stopper, the aspirate may be sent to the laboratory in the syringe.
• Send the specimen to the laboratory within 15 minutes to prevent growth or deterioration of microbes.

Quick Quiz

1. What is the *least* amount of urine required to perform a urine culture?

    A.   30 ml
    B.   10 ml
    C.   3 ml

Answer: C. When collecting a urine specimen for urine culture, at least 3 ml of urine is required; don't fill the specimen cup more than halfway.

2. How should you position the patient when collecting a nasopharyngeal specimen?

    A.   With his head tilted toward one side
    B.   With his head tilted forward
    C.   With his head tilted back

Answer: C. Ask the patient to cough before you begin collecting the specimen; then position him with his head tilted back.

3. What is the usual method for collecting a sputum culture?

    A.   Tracheal suctioning
    B.   Expectoration
    C.   Bronchoscopy

Answer: B. The usual method for sputum specimen collection is expectoration; other methods include tracheal suctioning and bronchoscopy.

4.   Which of the following is an aerobic pathogen commonly found in wounds?

    A.   *Clostridium*
    B.   *Bacteroides*
    C.   *Staphylococcus aureus*

Answer: C. The most common aerobic pathogens in wounds are *S. aureus*, group A beta-hemolytic streptococci, *Proteus* species, *Escherichia coli* and other Enterobacteriaceae, and some *Pseudomonas* species.

Scoring

⭐⭐⭐ If you answered all four questions correctly, wow! You represent the *highest* of cultures!

⭐⭐ If you answered three questions correctly, great! You'll have a cult following in no time!

⭐ If you answered less than three correctly, don't fret. You'll be cruising through cultures before you know it.

8

Biopsy

Just the facts

In this chapter, you'll learn:

♦ about biopsies and how they're performed
♦ what patient care is associated with these tests
♦ what factors can interfere with these tests
♦ what biopsy results may indicate.

A look at biopsy

Typically, a biopsy is performed to confirm cancer when other tests point to that diagnosis. In a biopsy, tissue samples are examined microscopically. The sample may be obtained during surgery, from a local excision or needle aspiration, or with special instruments (such as tissue punches or curettes). Common biopsy sites include the lung, breast, prostate gland, cervix, and skin.

Because of the possible cancer diagnosis, expect the patient to be anxious. Explain the procedure in terms he can understand, and provide emotional support to ease his anxiety.

Respiratory system

Lung biopsy

In a lung biopsy, a specimen of pulmonary tissue is excised for examination, using either the closed or open technique. The closed technique, performed under local anesthesia, includes both needle and transbronchial biopsies. The open technique, performed under general anesthesia in the operating room, includes both limited and standard thoracotomies.

Easy access

Needle biopsy is appropriate when the lesion is readily accessible. This procedure provides a much smaller specimen than the open technique. Transbronchial biopsy, the removal of multiple tissue specimens through a fiber-optic bronchoscope, is appropriate for some lung abnormalities or when the patient's condition won't tolerate an open biopsy.

What it all means

Examination of lung tissue specimens can reveal squamous cell or oat cell carcinoma and adenocarcinoma.

What needs to be done

• Describe the test to the patient and tell him that the test takes 30 to 60 minutes. Instruct him to fast after midnight before the procedure.
• Make sure the patient has signed a consent form. Check his history for hypersensitivity to the local anesthetic.

You... are...getting...very...sleepy

• Administer a mild sedative, as ordered, 30 minutes before the biopsy to help the patient relax.
• After the biopsy site is selected, lead markers are placed on the patient's skin, and X-rays are ordered to verify the markers' correct placement.
• Place the patient in a sitting position, with arms folded on a table in front of him; instruct him to remain as still as possible and to refrain from coughing.
• During biopsy, observe for signs of respiratory distress—shortness of breath, elevated pulse rate, and cyanosis (late sign); if such signs develop, report them immediately.

Damage control

• The skin over the biopsy site is prepared, and the area is draped. To prevent damage to intercostal nerves and vessels, a local anesthetic is injected with a 25G needle just above the lower rib.
• Using a 22G needle, the examiner anesthetizes the intercostal muscles and parietal pleura, makes a small incision (2 to 3 mm) with a scalpel, and introduces the needle through the incision, chest wall, and pleura, into the tumor or pulmonary tissue.

Lung biopsy helps confirm lung lesions and diseases.

Needle biopsy provides a smaller specimen than open biopsy.

- When the needle is in the tumor or pulmonary tissue, the specimen is obtained and the needle is withdrawn.
- Pressure is exerted on the biopsy site to stop the bleeding, and a small bandage is applied.

Distress signals

- Check vital signs every 15 minutes for 1 hour, every hour for 4 hours, and then every 4 hours for 24 hours. Watch for bleeding, shortness of breath, increased pulse, diminished breath sounds on the biopsy side and, eventually, cyanosis. Make sure the chest X-ray is repeated immediately after the biopsy.

Pleural biopsy

Pleural biopsy is the removal of pleural tissue, by needle biopsy or open biopsy, for examination. Performed under local anesthesia, pleural biopsy usually follows thoracentesis — aspiration of pleural fluid — which is performed when the cause of the effusion is unknown. However, it can be performed separately.

Open pleural biopsy, performed in the absence of pleural effusion, permits direct visualization of the pleura and the underlying lung. It's performed in the operating room.

What it all means

Microscopic examination of the tissue specimen can reveal malignant disease, tuberculosis, or viral, fungal, parasitic, or collagen vascular disease. Primary tumors of the pleura are commonly fibrous and epithelial.

What needs to be done

- Explain the procedure to the patient and tell him that it typically takes 30 to 45 minutes. Let him know that blood studies will be necessary before the biopsy and that chest X-rays will be taken before and after the biopsy.
- Make sure the patient has signed a consent form. Check the patient history for hypersensitivity to the local anesthetic. Just before the procedure, record vital signs.
- Seat the patient on the side of the bed, with his feet resting on a stool and his arms supported by the overbed table or his upper body. If he can't sit up, place him in a side-lying position with the side to be biopsied facing up.
- Tell him to remain still during the procedure. Prepare the skin and drape the area.
- The local anesthetic is then administered.

Pleural biopsy helps differentiate between nonmalignant and malignant disease. It also helps diagnose viral, fungal, parasitic, and collagen vascular disease.

Long John Silverman

- If your patient is having a Vim-Silverman needle biopsy, the needle is inserted through the appropriate intercostal space into the biopsy site, with the outer tip distal to the pleura and the central portion pushed in deeper and held in place. The outer case is inserted about ⅜″ (1 cm), the entire assembly is rotated 360 degrees, and the needle and tissue specimen are withdrawn.

Cope-ing with a needle biopsy

- When the biopsy is performed using a Cope's needle, a trocar is introduced through the appropriate intercostal space into the biopsy site. The sharp obturator is then removed, and a hooked stylet is inserted through the trocar. The opened notch is directed against the pleura, along the intercostal space, and is slowly withdrawn. While the outer tube is held stationary, the inner tube is twisted to cut off the tissue specimen and the assembly is withdrawn. (See *Scoping out a Cope's needle.*)

Peak technique

Scoping out a Cope's needle

Used to obtain a pleural biopsy specimen, a Cope's needle consists of three parts: a sharp obturator (A) and a cannula (B), which when fitted together are called a trocar, and a blunt-ended, hooked stylet (C). The trocar is used to gain access to the pleural cavity. Then the obturator is removed, leaving the cannula in place. The stylet is passed through the cannula to excise a tissue specimen, as shown below.

Specimen treatment

- The specimen is immediately put in a special solution in a labeled specimen bottle. Then the skin around the biopsy site is cleaned, and an adhesive bandage is applied.

Close attention

- After the biopsy, check the patient's vital signs every 15 minutes for 1 hour and then every hour for 4 hours or until his condition is stable. Make sure the chest X-ray is repeated immediately after the biopsy. Instruct the patient to lie on his unaffected side to promote healing of the biopsy site.
- Watch for signs of respiratory distress (shortness of breath), shoulder pain, and such other complications as pneumothorax (immediate) and pneumonia (delayed).
- Send the specimen to the laboratory immediately.
- Pleural biopsy is contraindicated in patients with severe bleeding disorders.

Reproductive system

Breast biopsy

Breast biopsy is necessary to confirm or rule out cancer. Needle biopsy or fine-needle biopsy can provide a core of tissue or a fluid aspirate, but needle biopsy should be restricted to fluid-filled cysts and advanced malignant lesions. Both methods have limited diagnostic value because of the small and perhaps unrepresentative specimens they provide. Open biopsy provides a complete tissue specimen, which can be sectioned to allow more accurate evaluation. All three techniques require only a local anesthetic and commonly are performed on outpatients.

Stereotactic biopsy is available in some medical centers. (See *Making breast biopsy more accurate*, page 258.)

Breast tissue analysis commonly includes an estrogen and progesterone receptor assay to help select therapy if the mass is malignant.

What it all means

Breast tissue normally consists of cellular and noncellular connective tissue, fat lobules, and various lactiferous ducts. It's normally pink, more fatty than fibrous, and shows no abnormal development of cells or tissue elements.

Breast biopsy helps differentiate benign and malignant tumors but may be inconclusive.

Making breast biopsy more accurate

Numerous medical centers in the United States now offer the Advanced Breast Biopsy Instrument procedure, a technique that improves the accuracy of breast biopsies. Using computers linked to radiographs, the procedure causes less pain and carries a lower risk of deformity than conventional biopsies. It requires only local anesthesia and can be completed in about 1 hour.

To be exact...
In the past, doctors had to rely on two-dimensional radiographs to locate calcium deposits for biopsy, and they couldn't be sure they were cutting into the correct area. With the Advanced Breast Biopsy Instrument procedure, the computer pinpoints the exact location of the area to be biopsied. Using computer coordinates, a probing tube is inserted into the breast to remove a tissue specimen as the patient lies facedown on a raised operating table. A rotating camera under the table takes radiographs of the breast from every angle. The doctor then matches up the coordinates to make sure the specimen comes from the correct area.

Test results usually take less than 2 days. According to surgeons who have used it, the method is 100% accurate, pinpointing the exact three-dimensional location of calcium deposits.

Abnormal breast tissue may exhibit a wide range of malignant or benign pathology.

Tumor evaluation

The receptor assays evaluate tumors for estrogen and progesterone protein and assign a positive or negative value to the estrogen and progesterone receptors. This positive or negative value assists in the prognosis and treatment of breast cancer.

What needs to be done

• Before the test, obtain a complete medical history.
• Explain how the test is done and that it permits a microscopic examination of a breast tissue specimen. Tell the patient the biopsy will take 15 to 30 minutes. If she's to receive a general anesthetic, advise her to fast from midnight before the test until after the biopsy. Explain that pretest studies, such as blood tests, urine tests, and chest radiographs may be required.
• Make sure the patient has signed a consent form. Check her history for hypersensitivity to anesthetics. Offer her emotional support, and assure her that breast masses don't always indicate cancer.

I know you're scared, but breast masses don't always indicate cancer.

What's your type?

- The procedure varies with the type of biopsy your patient requires. She may require a needle biopsy or an open biopsy.

Needle biopsy

- Instruct your patient to undress to the waist.
- After guiding her to a sitting or recumbent position with her hands at her sides, tell her to remain still.
- The doctor then prepares the biopsy site, administers a local anesthetic, and introduces the syringe (luer-lock syringe for aspiration, Vim-Silverman needle for tissue specimen) into the lesion.
- Fluid aspirated from the breast is expelled into a properly labeled, heparinized tube; the tissue specimen is placed in a labeled specimen bottle containing normal saline solution or formalin.
- Send both specimens to the laboratory immediately. (With fine-needle aspiration, a slide is made and viewed immediately under a microscope.)
- Because breast fluid aspiration isn't diagnostically accurate, some doctors aspirate fluid only from cysts. If such fluid is clear yellow and the mass disappears, the aspiration is both diagnostic and therapeutic, and the aspirate is discarded. If aspiration yields no fluid or if the lesion recurs two or three times, an open biopsy is then considered appropriate.
- After the procedure, pressure is exerted on the biopsy site and, after bleeding has stopped, an adhesive bandage is applied.

Open biopsy

- Incisional biopsy generally provides an adequate specimen for analysis. After administering a general or local anesthetic, the doctor makes an incision in the breast to expose the mass. He may then incise a portion of tissue or excise the entire mass. If the mass is smaller than ¾" (1.9 cm) in diameter and appears benign, it's usually excised. If it's larger or appears malignant, a specimen is usually incised before the mass is excised.
- The specimen is placed in a properly labeled specimen bottle containing 10% formalin solution. Tissue that appears malignant is sent for frozen section and receptor assays. Receptor assay specimens must not be placed in the formalin solution. Specimens must be sent to the laboratory immediately.
- After the procedure, the wound is sutured and an adhesive bandage is applied.

Aftercare

- If the patient has received a local anesthetic during needle or open biopsy, check her vital signs and provide medication for pain, as ordered. Watch for and report bleeding, tenderness, or redness at the biopsy site.

• If the patient received a general anesthetic, check vital signs every 30 minutes for the first 4 hours, every hour for the next 4 hours, and then every 4 hours. Give an analgesic as ordered. Watch for and report bleeding, tenderness, or redness at the biopsy site.

• An ice bag at the biopsy site may provide comfort. Instruct the patient to wear a support bra at all times until healing is complete.

• Provide emotional support to the patient who is awaiting diagnosis.

Prostate gland biopsy

Prostate gland biopsy is the needle excision of a prostate tissue specimen for examination. A perineal, transrectal, or transurethral approach may be used; the transrectal approach is usually used for high prostatic lesions. Indications include potentially malignant prostatic hypertrophy and prostatic nodules.

What it all means

The prostate gland normally consists of a thin, fibrous capsule surrounding the stroma, which is made up of elastic and connective tissues and smooth-muscle fibers. The epithelial glands, found in these tissues and muscle fibers, drain into the chief excreting ducts. Microscopic tissue examination can confirm cancer.

What needs to be done

• Before the biopsy, describe the procedure to the patient and explain that it takes less than 30 minutes.

• Make sure the patient has signed a consent form. Check his history for hypersensitivity to the anesthetic or to other drugs. For a transrectal approach, prepare the bowel by administering enemas until the return is clear. As ordered, give an antibacterial to minimize the risk of infection. Just before the biopsy, check vital signs and give a sedative, as ordered.

• The doctor may choose the perineal, transurethral, or transrectal approach. An alternative method to the transrectal approach is the automated cone biopsy.

> Prostate biopsy can help confirm prostate cancer or determine the cause of prostatic hyperplasia.

Perineal approach

- Place the patient in the proper position (left lateral, knee-chest, or lithotomy), and clean the perineal skin.
- After giving the local anesthetic, the doctor makes a 2-mm incision into the perineum. He immobilizes the prostate by inserting a finger into the rectum and inserts the needle into a prostate lobe. He rotates the needle gently, pulls it out about 5 mm, and reinserts it at another angle, repeating the procedure in several areas.
- Specimens are placed immediately in a labeled specimen bottle containing 10% formalin solution. Pressure is exerted on the puncture site, which is then bandaged.

Transurethral approach

- Position the patient on a special table. Place his legs in stirrups and drape him to maintain privacy.
- The doctor passes an endoscopic instrument through the urethra, permitting direct viewing of the prostate and passage of a cutting loop. The loop is rotated to chip away pieces of tissue and is then withdrawn.
- The specimen is placed immediately in a labeled specimen bottle containing 10% formalin solution.

Transrectal approach

- Place the patient in a left lateral position.
- The doctor attaches a curved needle guide to the finger palpating the rectum and pushes the biopsy needle along the guide, into the prostate. As the needle enters the prostate, the patient may experience pain. The doctor rotates the needle to cut off the tissue and then withdraws it.
- The specimen is placed immediately in a bottle containing 10% formalin solution.

Automated cone biopsy

- Position the patient on a special table. Place his legs in stirrups and drape him to maintain privacy.
- The doctor uses a spring-powered device with an inner trocar needle to cut through prostatic tissue. This technique is quick and reportedly painless.
- The specimen is placed immediately in a labeled specimen bottle containing 10% formalin solution.

Aftercare

- Check vital signs immediately after the procedure, every 2 hours for 4 hours, and then every 4 hours.
- Observe the biopsy site for a hematoma and signs of infection, such as redness, swelling, and pain.
- Watch for urine retention, urinary frequency, and hematuria.

Cervical punch biopsy

Cervical punch biopsy is the excision by sharp forceps of a cervical tissue specimen for microscopic examination. Generally, multiple biopsies are done to obtain specimens from different areas.

What it all means

Cervical tissue should have no dysplasia or abnormal cell growth. Microscopic examination of a cervical tissue specimen identifies abnormal cells and differentiates the tissue as intraepithelial neoplasia or invasive cancer.

Cone biopsy

If cervical biopsy doesn't show the cause of an abnormal Papanicolaou test or if the specimen shows advanced dysplasia (abnormal tissue changes) or carcinoma in situ (malignant cell changes in the epithelial tissue that don't extend beyond the basement membrane), a cone biopsy is done in the operating room under general anesthesia. A cone biopsy collects a larger tissue specimen and allows more accurate evaluation of dysplasia.

What needs to be done

• Explain the procedure to the patient. Tell her that the biopsy takes about 15 minutes and provides a cervical tissue specimen for microscopic study.
• Make sure the patient has signed a consent form, and instruct her to void just before the biopsy. If she's an outpatient, she should have someone accompany her home after the biopsy.
• Biopsy sites are selected by direct visualization of the cervix with a colposcope (the most accurate method) or by Schiller's test, which stains normal squamous epithelium a dark mahogany but fails to color abnormal tissue.

Direct visualization

• Place the patient in the lithotomy position, and tell her to relax as the unlubricated speculum is inserted.
• For direct visualization, the doctor inserts the colposcope through the speculum, locates the biopsy site, and cleans the cervix with a swab soaked in 3% acetic acid solution. He then inserts the biopsy forceps through the speculum or the colposcope and removes tissue from any lesion or from selected sites, starting from the posterior lip to avoid obscuring other sites with blood.
• The doctor immediately places each specimen in 10% formalin solution in a labeled bottle.

Cervical punch biopsy is used to evaluate suspicious cervical lesions and to diagnose cervical cancer.

Listen up!

Recovering from cervical punch biopsy

After a cervical punch biopsy, encourage the outpatient to rest briefly before leaving the office. To help her recover from the procedure, provide the following teaching:
• Avoid strenuous exercise for 8 to 24 hours.
• If a tampon was inserted after the biopsy, leave it in place for 8 to 24 hours, as ordered.
• Know that some bleeding may occur, but report bleeding that's heavier than menstrual bleeding.
• Avoid using additional tampons, according to the doctor's directions, because tampons can irritate the cervix and provoke bleeding.
• If you had cryotherapy or laser treatment during the procedure, avoid douching and refrain from intercourse for up to 2 weeks, or as directed.
• Be aware that a foul-smelling, gray-green vaginal discharge is normal for several days after the biopsy and may persist for 3 weeks.

• To control bleeding after biopsy, the doctor swabs the cervix with 5% silver nitrate solution (cautery or sutures may be used instead). If bleeding persists, the doctor may insert a tampon.

Schiller's test

• With this test, the doctor inserts an applicator stick saturated with iodine solution through the speculum. This stains the cervix to identify lesions for biopsy.

Make your request

• Record the patient's and doctor's names and the biopsy sites on the laboratory request and send the specimens immediately.
• Instruct the patient in aftercare. (See *Recovering from cervical punch biopsy.*)

Two's company! Make sure someone accompanies the outpatient home after the biopsy.

Other organ-specific biopsies

Bone marrow aspiration and biopsy

Bone marrow, the soft tissue contained in the medullary canals of long bone and the interstices of cancellous bone, may be removed by aspiration or needle biopsy under local anesthesia. In aspiration biopsy, a fluid specimen in which pustulae of marrow are suspended is removed. In needle biopsy, a core of marrow — cells, not fluid—is removed. These methods are commonly used concurrently to obtain the best possible marrow specimens.

What it all means

Yellow marrow contains fat cells and connective tissue; red marrow contains hematopoietic cells, fat cells, and connective tissue. Special stains that detect hematologic disorders produce these normal findings: the iron stain, which measures hemosiderin (storage iron), has a +2 level; the Sudan black B (SBB) stain, which shows granulocytes, is negative; and the periodic acid–Schiff (PAS) stain, which detects glycogen reactions, is negative.

Abnormal findings

Histologic examination of a bone marrow specimen can help detect myelofibrosis, granulomas, lymphomas, or cancer. Hematologic analysis, including the differential count and the myeloid-erythroid ratio, can implicate a wide range of disorders. (See *Normal bone marrow values*.)

In an iron stain, decreased hemosiderin levels may indicate a true iron deficiency. Increased levels may accompany other anemias or blood disorders. A positive SBB stain can distinguish acute myelogenous leukemia from acute lymphoblastic leukemia (negative SBB), or it may indicate granulation in myeloblasts. A positive PAS stain may mean acute or chronic lymphocytic leukemia, amyloidosis, thalassemia, lymphoma, infectious mononucleosis, iron deficiency anemia, or sideroblastic anemia.

What needs to be done

• Explain the procedure to the patient. A mild sedative will be given 1 hour before the test, if ordered. Tell the patient the test usually takes only 5 to 10 minutes and that more than one bone marrow specimen may be required. Let him know a blood sample will be collected before the biopsy for laboratory testing

History and consent

• Make sure the patient has signed a consent form. Check his history for hypersensitivity to the local anesthetic. After checking with the doctor, tell the patient which bone—sternum, anterior or posterior iliac crest, vertebral spinous process, rib, or tibia—will be used as the biopsy site. (See *Common bone marrow aspiration and biopsy sites*, page 266.) A child requires additional steps. (See *Preparing a child for bone marrow biopsy*, page 266.)
• A bone marrow specimen can be collected by bone marrow aspiration or needle biopsy. For both procedures position the patient and instruct him to remain as still as possible.

Bone marrow aspiration and biopsy helps diagnose hematologic disorders and metastatic tumors. It also can determine the cause of infection and monitor the effectiveness of chemotherapy.

Normal bone marrow values

Cell type	Normal adult mean values
Normoblasts, total	25.6%
Pronormoblasts	0.2% to 1.3%
Basophilic	0.5% to 2.4%
Polychromatic	17.9% to 29.2%
Orthochromatic	0.4% to 4.6%
Neutrophils, total	56.5%
Myeloblasts	0.2% to 1.5%
Promyelocytes	2.1% to 4.1%
Myelocytes	8.2% to 15.7%
Metamyelocytes	9.6% to 24.6%
Bands	9.5% to 15.3%
Segmented	6% to 12%
Eosinophils	3.1%
Basophils	0.01%
Lymphocytes	16.2%
Plasma cells	1.3%
Megakaryocytes	0.1%
Myeloid-erythroid ratio	2.3%

- During the biopsy, talk to the patient quietly, describe what's being done, and answer questions.

Aspiration biopsy

- The doctor prepares the biopsy site and injects a local anesthetic. He then inserts the needle through the skin, the subcutaneous tissue, and the cortex of the bone. The doctor removes the stylet from the needle and attaches a 10- to 20-ml syringe. He aspirates 0.2 to 0.5 ml of marrow and withdraws the needle.
- Pressure is applied to the site for 5 minutes while the marrow slides are being prepared. If the patient has thrombocytopenia, pressure is applied for 10 to 15 minutes.
- The biopsy site is cleaned again, and a sterile adhesive bandage is applied.

Bone marrow biopsy is contraindicated in patients with severe bleeding disorders.

Common bone marrow aspiration and biopsy sites

These illustrations show commonly used sites for bone marrow aspiration and biopsy.

Usually, the *posterior superior iliac spine* is preferred for bone marrow aspiration because no vital organs or vessels are located nearby.

The *sternum* involves the greatest risk. However, it's commonly used for marrow aspiration because it's near the surface, the cortical bone is thin, and the marrow cavity contains numerous cells and relatively little fat or supporting bone.

The *spinous process* is the preferred site if multiple punctures are necessary, marrow is absent at other sites, or the patient objects to sternal puncture.

The *tibia* is the site of choice for infants under age 1.

Listen up!

Preparing a child for bone marrow biopsy

To prepare a child for bone marrow biopsy, give him his own biopsy kit: a syringe without a needle, cotton balls, and adhesive bandages. Act out the procedure by using a doll or stuffed animal as a model. This will help you gain the child's confidence and answer questions he may have. Be sure to describe the kinds of pressure and discomfort he'll feel during the procedure.

Show and tell

Before the biopsy, show the child the equipment on the tray and explain what it's for in simple terms. Encourage the parents to get involved by helping you hold the child still and reassuring him. Tell the child that he'll feel some pain when the clinician aspirates the bone marrow and that it's okay to cry or yell if he wants to. Reassure him that the pain will go away quickly.

• If the doctor doesn't obtain an adequate marrow specimen on the first attempt, he may reposition the needle or remove and reinsert it in another site within the anesthetized area. If the second attempt fails, a needle biopsy may be necessary.

Needle biopsy

• With a needle biopsy, the site is prepared and the skin is marked at the site with an indelible pencil or marking pen.
• The doctor then injects a local anesthetic intradermally, subcutaneously, and at the surface of the bone.
• He inserts the biopsy needle into the periosteum and sets the needle guard as indicated.
• He advances the needle until the outer needle passes through the cortex of the bone, and then inserts the inner needle into the outer needle and removes the stylet.
• Alternately rotating the inner needle clockwise and counterclockwise, the doctor directs the needle into the marrow cavity and removes a tissue plug. He withdraws the needle assembly and places the marrow in a labeled bottle containing a special fixative.
• After the biopsy site is cleaned, a sterile adhesive bandage or a pressure dressing is applied.

Aftercare

• Check the biopsy site for bleeding and inflammation.
• Observe the patient for signs of hemorrhage and infection, such as rapid pulse rate, low blood pressure, and fever.
• Send the specimen or slides to the laboratory immediately.

Thyroid biopsy

Thyroid biopsy—excision of a thyroid tissue specimen for microscopic examination—is indicated for patients with thyroid enlargement or nodules (even if serum triiodothyronine [T_3] and serum thyroxine [T_4] levels are normal), breathing and swallowing difficulties, vocal cord paralysis, weight loss, hemoptysis, or a full sensation in the neck. It's commonly performed when noninvasive tests, such as thyroid ultrasonography, are abnormal or inconclusive.

Needle versus open biopsy

A thyroid tissue specimen may be obtained with a hollow needle under local anesthesia or during open biopsy under general anesthesia. Fine-needle aspiration with a microscopic examination can aid diagnosis and replace an open biopsy. Open biopsy, performed in the operating room, is more complex and provides more direct

Thyroid biopsy differentiates various thyroid diseases.

information; the surgeon obtains a tissue specimen from the exposed thyroid and sends it to the laboratory for rapid analysis. Open biopsy also permits immediate excision of suspicious thyroid tissue. Coagulation studies should precede thyroid biopsy.

What it all means

Examination of normal tissue shows fibrous networks dividing the gland into pseudolobules that consist of follicles and capillaries. Cuboidal epithelium lines the follicle walls and contains the protein thyroglobulin, which stores T_3 and T_4. Malignant tumors appear as well-encapsulated, solitary nodules of uniform but abnormal structure. Papillary carcinoma is the most common type of thyroid cancer. Follicular carcinoma, a less common form, strongly resembles normal cells.

Benign distinctions

Such benign conditions as nontoxic nodular goiter demonstrate hypertrophy, hyperplasia, and hypervascularity. Distinct histologic patterns characterize subacute granulomatous thyroiditis, Hashimoto's disease, and hyperthyroidism.

Missed malignancy

Because many malignant thyroid tumors are multicentric and small, a negative report doesn't necessarily rule out cancer.

Thyroid biopsy should be used cautiously in patients with coagulation defects.

What needs to be done

• Explain the procedure to the patient. If he'll receive a general anesthetic, explain that he needs to restrict food and fluids. Inform him that test results are typically available in 1 day.
• Make sure the patient has signed a consent form. Check for hypersensitivity to anesthetics or analgesics.
• For needle biopsy, place the patient in the supine position with a pillow under his shoulder blades.
• Prepare the skin over the biopsy site. As the doctor prepares to inject the local anesthetic, warn the patient not to swallow.
• After the anesthetic is injected, the carotid artery is palpated and the biopsy needle is inserted parallel to and about 1″ (2.5 cm) from the thyroid cartilage to prevent damage to the deep structures and the larynx. When the specimen is obtained, the needle is removed and the specimen is immediately placed in formalin.

When the biopsy is over

• Apply pressure to the biopsy site to stop bleeding. If bleeding continues for more than a few minutes, press on the site for up to 15 minutes more. Apply an adhesive bandage.

- To make the patient more comfortable, place him in semi-Fowler's position. Tell him that to avoid strain on the biopsy site he should put both hands behind his neck when he sits up.
- Observe for difficulty breathing. Check the back of the neck and the patient's pillow for bleeding every hour for 8 hours. Report bleeding immediately.
- Keep the biopsy site clean and dry.

Lymph node biopsy

Lymph node biopsy is the surgical excision of an active lymph node or needle aspiration of a nodal specimen for histologic examination. Both techniques usually use local anesthesia and sample superficial nodes in the cervical, supraclavicular, axillary, or inguinal region. Excision, the preferred technique, provides a larger specimen.

What it all means

Microscopic examination of the tissue specimen distinguishes malignant from nonmalignant causes of lymph node enlargement. Hodgkin's disease, a lymphoma affecting the entire lymph system, is the leading cancer in adolescents and young adults. Lymph node malignancy may also result from metastatic cancer.

What needs to be done

- Describe the procedure to the patient. For excisional biopsy, instruct him to restrict food from midnight and to drink only clear liquids. For a needle biopsy, explain that the procedure takes 15 to 30 minutes and analysis takes 1 day.
- Make sure the patient has signed a consent form. Check his history for hypersensitivity to the anesthetic. Just before the biopsy, record baseline vital signs.

Excisional biopsy

- For excisional biopsy, prepare the skin over the biopsy site, and drape the area for privacy.
- The doctor administers the anesthetic. He then makes an incision, removes an entire node, and places it in a properly labeled bottle containing normal saline solution.
- After the biopsy, he sutures the wound and applies a sterile dressing.

Needle biopsy

- For needle biopsy, the doctor prepares the site and administers a local anesthetic.

Lymph node biopsy can distinguish between benign and malignant tumors and stage metastatic cancer.

• He grasps the node between thumb and forefinger, inserts the needle directly into the node, and obtains a small core specimen.
• He then removes the needle and places the specimen in a properly labeled bottle containing normal saline solution.
• Pressure is exerted on the biopsy site to control bleeding, and an adhesive bandage is applied.

Aftercare

• Check vital signs and watch for bleeding, tenderness, and redness at the biopsy site.
• Tell the patient that he may resume his usual diet.

Skin biopsy

Skin biopsy is the removal of a small piece of tissue, under local anesthesia, from a lesion suspected of being malignant.

Three techniques

A specimen may be secured by one of three techniques: shave, punch, or excision. A shave biopsy cuts the lesion above the skin line and leaves the lower layers of dermis intact, permitting further biopsy at the site. A punch biopsy removes an oval core from the center of a lesion. An excisional biopsy, the procedure of choice, removes the entire lesion. It's indicated for rapidly expanding lesions; sclerotic, bullous, or atrophic lesions; and examination of a lesion's border and surrounding normal skin.

What it all means

Normal skin consists of squamous epithelium (epidermis) and fibrous connective tissue (dermis). Microscopic examination of the tissue specimen may reveal a benign or malignant lesion.

Growths may be benign...

Benign growths include cysts, seborrheic keratoses, warts, keloids, pigmented nevi, dermatofibromas, and multiple neurofibromas.

...or malignant.

Malignant skin cancers include basal cell carcinoma, squamous cell carcinoma, and malignant melanoma. Basal cell carcinoma occurs on hair-bearing skin, the most common location being the face, including the nose and its folds. Squamous cell carcinoma most commonly appears on the lips, mouth, and genitalia. Malignant melanoma, the most deadly skin cancer, can spread throughout the body by way of the lymphatic system and the blood vessels.

Skin biopsy can differentiate among skin cancers and benign growths. It's also useful for diagnosing chronic bacterial or fungal skin infections.

What needs to be done

• Describe the procedure to the patient. Tell him the biopsy should take about 15 minutes.
• Make sure the patient has signed a consent form. Check his history for hypersensitivity to the local anesthetic.
• Position the patient comfortably and clean the biopsy site before the doctor administers a local anesthetic.

Shave biopsy

• During a shave biopsy, the doctor cuts off the protruding growth at the skin line with a #15 scalpel and immediately places the tissue in a specimen bottle containing 10% formalin solution.
• Pressure is applied to the area to stop the bleeding.

Punch biopsy

• With a punch biopsy, the doctor pulls taut the skin surrounding the lesion, firmly introduces the punch into the lesion, and rotates to obtain a tissue specimen. He then lifts the plug with forceps or a needle and severs as deeply into the fat layer as possible.
• The specimen is placed in specimen bottle containing 10% formalin solution or, if indicated, in a sterile container.
• The doctor then closes the wound.

Excisional biopsy

• For excisional biopsy, the doctor uses a #15 scalpel to excise the lesion completely.
• He removes the tissue specimen and immediately places it in a specimen bottle containing 10% formalin solution.
• Pressure is applied to the site to stop the bleeding.
• The doctor typically closes the wound using 4-0 sutures.

Finishing up

• Check the biopsy site for bleeding.
• Administer pain medication as needed and ordered.
• Advise the patient with sutures to keep the area as clean and dry as possible. Instruct him to leave adhesive strips in place for 14 to 21 days or until they fall off.
• Send the specimen to the laboratory immediately.

Quick quiz

1. During lung biopsy, monitor your patient for complications such as:
- A.   respiratory distress.
- B.   shoulder pain.
- C.   abdominal pain.

Answer: A. During lung biopsy, monitor for signs of respiratory distress, such as shortness of breath, elevated pulse rate, and cyanosis.

2. During a needle biopsy of the thyroid, the patient is placed in:
- A.   the supine position.
- B.   the supine position with the neck extended.
- C.   the supine position with a pillow under the shoulder blades.

Answer: C. The supine position with a pillow under the shoulder blades pushes the trachea and thyroid forward and allows neck veins to fall backward.

3. The preferred procedure for skin biopsy is:
- A.   shave biopsy.
- B.   punch biopsy.
- C.   excisional biopsy.

Answer: C. Excisional biopsy is the procedure of choice because it removes the entire lesion.

Scoring

☆☆☆   If you answered all three questions correctly, congratulations! You've just been inducted to the Biopsy Hall of Fame!

☆☆   If you answered two questions correctly, way to go! You've been elected MVB!

☆   If you answered just one question correctly, don't worry! You'll be winning the biopsy game in no time!

9

Endoscopy

Just the facts

In this chapter, you'll learn:

♦ about endoscopic procedures and how they're performed

♦ what patient care is associated with these tests

♦ what factors can interfere with these tests

♦ what endoscopic results may indicate.

A look at endoscopy

Endoscopy, which allows direct visualization using a fiber-optic scope, helps diagnose abnormalities of the GI tract, lungs, and reproductive system. When explaining the procedure to your patient, be sure to use terms he can understand. Ask him if he has any allergies, and tell him he'll receive a sedative beforehand to help him relax.

Gastrointestinal system

Colonoscopy

Colonoscopy is the visual examination of the lining of the large intestine using a flexible fiber-optic endoscope. This test is indicated for patients with a history of constipation and diarrhea, persistent rectal bleeding, or lower abdominal pain when results of proctosigmoidoscopy and a barium enema test prove negative or inconclusive.

Although usually a safe procedure, colonoscopy can cause perforation of the large intestine, exces-

Colonoscopy is versatile! It can diagnose inflammatory and ulcerative bowel disease, locate the origin of lower GI bleeding, and diagnose colonic strictures, polyps, and lesions.

sive bleeding, and retroperitoneal emphysema. The test may be performed on an inpatient or an outpatient basis.

Colonoscopy is contraindicated in near-term pregnancy, a recent history of acute MI or abdominal surgery, ischemic bowel disease, acute diverticulitis, peritonitis, fulminant granulomatous colitis, fulminant ulcerative colitis, and a perforated viscus.

What it all means

The normal mucosa of the large intestine beyond the sigmoid colon appears light pink-orange and is marked by semilunar folds and deep tubular pits. Blood vessels are visible beneath the intestinal mucosa, which glistens from mucus secretions.

Abnormal findings

Colonoscopy, along with microscopic test results, may reveal proctitis, granulomatous and ulcerative colitis, Crohn's disease, and malignant or benign lesions. Colonoscopy alone can detect diverticular disease or the site of lower GI bleeding. (See *Colonoscopy interference*.)

What needs to be done

• Explain to the patient that this test permits examination of the lining of the large intestine by inserting a flexible instrument through his anus. Instruct him to maintain a clear liquid diet for 24 to 48 hours before the test and to take nothing by mouth after midnight the night before the procedure. (See *Following a clear liquid diet*.)
• Tell the patient the procedure usually takes 30 to 60 minutes and that he must arrange for transportation home because he shouldn't drive for 12 hours afterward.

Quick cleaning

• Inform the patient that the large intestine must be thoroughly cleaned to be clearly visible. Give him a laxative, such as 10 oz (296 ml) of magnesium citrate, 3 tbs (45 ml) of castor oil, or a gallon of GoLYTELY solution in the evening. Chill the solution to make it more palatable. If you're using GoLYTELY, instruct the patient to drink the preparation quickly, drinking 8 oz (236.6 ml) every 10 minutes until the entire gallon is consumed. This laxative produces watery diarrhea in 30 to 60 minutes and clears the bowel in 4 to 5 hours.
• If fecal results still aren't clear, the patient will receive a laxative, suppository, or tap-water enema. Don't administer a soap-suds enema because this irritates the mucosa and stimulates mucous secretions that may hinder the examination.

Warning!

Colonoscopy interference

The following factors may interfere with test results by inhibiting visual examination or colonoscope passage:
• barium retained in the intestine from previous diagnostic studies
• blood from acute colonic hemorrhage
• sigmoid colon fixation from inflammatory bowel disease, surgery, or radiation therapy.

Listen up!

Following a clear liquid diet

You'll need to teach your patient about following a clear liquid diet before certain intestinal tests. The diet consists of transparent foods that are liquid or that will liquefy at room temperature. This diet reduces stool volume in the bowels, letting the doctor see the inside of the bowels more easily.

Listed below are the only foods and beverages your patient should eat or drink when following a clear liquid diet:

- water
- ice chips
- clear tea (no milk or lemon)
- strained, clear fruit juices, such as apple, grape, and cranberry (no pulp)
- decaffeinated coffee (may vary with facility)
- clear carbonated beverages
- plain fruit gelatin (no fruit added)
- chicken or beef broth (fat-free only)
- chicken or beef bouillon
- frozen ice pops (no fruit or pulp)
- clear, fruit-flavored drink mixes.

Sedate and consent

- Tell the patient he may receive a sedative to help him relax.
- Make sure the patient or responsible family member has signed a consent form. Check the patient's vital signs 30 minutes before the test; if they're stable, give the sedative as ordered.

Baselines and other basic

- Obtain baseline vital signs, and monitor vital signs throughout the procedure. Attach the patient to a continuous electrocardiogram monitor and pulse oximeter.
- Place the patient on his left side, with his knees flexed, and drape him. Instruct him to breathe deeply and slowly through his mouth as the doctor inserts his gloved, lubricated index finger into the anus and rectum and palpates the mucosa. After a water-soluble lubricant has been applied to the patient's anus and to the tip of the colonoscope, tell the patient the colonoscope is about to be inserted.

After drinking all these liquids to prepare for colonoscopy, I may never be thirsty again!

Scoping out the situation

- After the colonoscope is inserted through the patient's anus, a small amount of air is blown in to locate the bowel lumen. The scope is advanced through the rectum into the sigmoid colon under direct vision. When the instrument reaches the descending sigmoid junction, assist the patient to a supine position to aid the scope's advance, if necessary. After the scope has passed the splenic flexure, it's advanced through the transverse colon and hepatic flexure, into the ascending colon and cecum.
- The doctor may pass biopsy forceps or a cytology brush through a channel in the colonoscope to obtain specimens for microscopic examination; he may use a special instrument to remove polyps. If the doctor removes a tissue specimen, immediately place it in a specimen bottle containing 10% formalin; immediately place cytology smears in a Coplin jar containing 95% ethyl alcohol.
- If the doctor obtains a tissue or cell specimen, send it to the appropriate laboratory immediately.

A safe watch

- Observe the patient closely for signs of bowel perforation, including malaise, rectal bleeding, abdominal pain and distention, fever, and mucopurulent drainage. Notify the doctor immediately if such signs develop.
- Check vital signs until they're stable.
- Watch closely for adverse effects of the sedative, such as respiratory depression, hypotension, excessive diaphoresis, bradycardia, and confusion. Have emergency resuscitation equipment available and a narcotic antagonist such as naloxone for I.V. use, if necessary. Monitor level of consciousness.

Get on the horn! After colonoscopy, immediately report rectal bleeding, abdominal pain, and other signs of bowel perforation.

Resuming and recovering

- Provide a safe environment until the patient has recovered from sedation; then tell him he may resume his usual diet.
- Tell the patient he may pass large amounts of flatus resulting from the air blown into the colon during the procedure. Provide privacy to minimize embarrassment.
- If a polyp has been removed, inform the patient that there may be some blood in his stool and that he should report excessive bleeding immediately.
- Outpatients may be discharged when fully awake. Make sure the patient has transportation home.
- Advise the patient to avoid alcohol for 24 hours after being sedated.

Endoscopic ultrasound

Endoscopic ultrasound (EUS) combines ultrasonography with endoscopy to visualize the GI wall and adjacent structures. Incorporation of the ultrasound probe at the distal end of the ultrasonic endoscope allows ultrasound imaging that provides a detailed picture.

Check me out! Endoscopic ultrasound is used to stage certain GI tract cancers and evaluate bile duct abnormalities.

What it all means

EUS usually reveals normal anatomy with no evidence of tumor.

Abnormal EGD EUS findings

If endoscopic ultrasonography is used in combination with an esophagogastroduodenoscopy (EGD), results may reveal acute or chronic ulcers, benign or malignant tumors, or inflammatory disease, including gastritis, esophagitis, and duodenitis. They may also show diverticula, varices, Mallory-Weiss syndrome, esophageal and pyloric stenosis, and esophageal hiatal hernia.

Abnormal colonoscopy EUS findings

When combined with colonoscopy, EUS findings may indicate ulcerative colitis, Crohn's disease, diverticular disease, or malignant or benign lesions of the colon. It may also isolate the site of lower GI bleeding.

Abnormal sigmoidoscopy EUS findings

EUS findings when combined with sigmoidoscopy may reveal benign or malignant tumors. (See *EUS interference.*)

What needs to be done

- Explain the procedure to the patient and tell him the test generally takes 30 to 90 minutes. Check his history for allergies, medications, and information pertinent to his current complaint. Instruct him to fast for 6 to 8 hours before the test. If he's undergoing colonscopy or sigmoidoscopy, tell him he may have to take a laxative the evening before the procedure.
- Inform the patient that he may receive an I.V. sedative to help him relax before the endoscope is inserted. If the patient is an outpatient, advise him to arrange for someone to drive him home. Make sure he or a responsible family member has signed the consent form.
- Obtain baseline vital signs, and leave the blood pressure cuff in place for monitoring throughout the procedure, according to your facility's policy. Throughout the procedure, observe the patient's

Warning!

EUS interference

The following factors may inhibit visual examination or endoscope passage:
- esophageal stricture
- barium retained in the intestine from previous diagnostic studies
- blood from acute colonic hemorrhage
- sigmoid colon fixation from inflammatory bowel disease, surgery, or radiation therapy.

skin color and temperature. Monitor his level of consciousness and pain tolerance, and observe for abdominal distention.

Esophageal approach

• With an EGD EUS, tell the patient to hold his breath while his mouth and throat are sprayed with a local anesthetic.
• Let him know that the anesthetic spray will cause him to lose some control of his secretions. Encourage him to let saliva drain from the side of his mouth to decrease the risk of aspiration.

Scope advancement

• After placing the patient in a left lateral position, ask him to bend his head forward and to open his mouth.
• The doctor inserts his finger into the mouth and guides the tip of the endoscope alongside his finger to the back of the throat. As the endoscope passes through the throat, the patient's head is slowly extended to aid scope advancement. The patient's chin must be kept at midline. The doctor then passes the endoscope along the esophagus under direct vision. When the endoscope is about 12″ (30 cm) into the esophagus, position the patient's head with his chin toward the table so saliva can drain from his mouth.
• When examination of the esophagus and the cardiac sphincter is complete, the doctor rotates the endoscope clockwise, with the tip angled upward, and advances it into the stomach. After examining the stomach lining the doctor advances the endoscope into the duodenum. Then he slowly withdraws the endoscope and reexamines suspicious areas of the gastric and esophageal lining.

A camera may be attached to the endoscope to photograph areas for later study, or a measuring tube may be passed through the endoscope to determine the size of a lesion.

Just passing through

• During the examination, the doctor may instill air into the GI tract to open the bowel lumen and flatten tissue folds or water to rinse material or fluids from the lens; he may apply suction to remove unnecessary insufflated air or secretions. The doctor may also pass biopsy forceps through the scope to obtain a tissue specimen or a cytology brush to obtain cells.
• Tissue specimens are immediately placed in a specimen bottle containing 10% formaldehyde solution; cell specimens are smeared on glass slides and placed in a Coplin jar containing 95% ethyl alcohol.

Keeping a close watch

• Observe the patient for possible perforation. Perforation in the cervical area of the esophagus produces pain on swallowing and with neck movement; thoracic perforation causes substernal or epigastric pain that increases with breathing or trunk movement; diaphragmatic perforation produces shoulder pain and dyspnea; gastric perforation causes abdominal or back pain, cyanosis, fever, or pleural effusion.

• Observe the patient for evidence of aspiration of gastric contents, which could precipitate aspiration pneumonia.

• For inpatients, check vital signs every 15 minutes for 4 hours, every hour for 4 hours, and then every 4 hours. Observe outpatients for a 30- to 60- minute recovery period, monitoring vital signs every 15 minutes. When fully awake, outpatients may be discharged if the gag reflex has returned.

• Provide a safe environment for the patient until he has recovered from the sedative. Keep his bed's side rails up.

• Withhold food and fluids until the gag reflex returns, which is usually within 1 hour. Test the gag reflex by touching the back of the throat with a tongue blade.

• Tell the patient he may burp some insufflated air and may have a sore throat for 3 to 4 days.

• Instruct the patient to watch for persistent difficulty swallowing and for pain, fever, black stools, or bloody vomitus. Tell him to notify the doctor immediately if any of these complications develop. Also, instruct him to avoid alcohol for 24 hours and driving for 12 hours.

Opposite-end approach

• If your patient requires a colonoscopic or sigmoidoscopic EUS, place him on his left side, with his knees flexed, and drape him. Instruct him to breathe deeply and slowly through his mouth as the doctor inserts his gloved, lubricated index finger into the anus and rectum and palpates the mucosa. After a water-soluble lubricant has been applied to the patient's anus and to the tip of the scope, tell the patient the scope is about to be inserted.

• After the doctor inserts the scope through the patient's anus, he blows a small amount of air into the bowel to locate the bowel lumen. He advances the scope through the rectum into the sigmoid colon. When the instrument reaches the descending sigmoid junction, assist the patient to a supine position to aid the scope's advance, if necessary. After the scope has passed the splenic flexure, the doctor advances it through the transverse colon and hepatic flexure, into the ascending colon and cecum, if a colonoscopy is being performed.

Specimen collection

• The doctor may pass biopsy forceps or a cytology brush through a channel in the endoscope to obtain specimens for microscopic examination; he may use a special instrument to re-

move polyps. If he removes a tissue specimen, immediately place it in a specimen bottle containing 10% formalin; immediately place cytology smears in a Coplin jar containing 95% ethyl alcohol.
• If the doctor obtains a tissue or cell specimen, send it to the appropriate laboratory immediately.

Check, check, and recheck

• For inpatients, check vital signs every 15 minutes for 4 hours, every hour for 4 hours, and then every 4 hours. Observe outpatients for a 30- to 60-minute recovery period, monitoring vital signs every 15 minutes. When fully awake, outpatients may be discharged. Because of sedation, outpatients shouldn't drive for 12 hours. Make sure these patients have transportation home.

Reproductive system

Colposcopy

In colposcopy, the cervix and vagina are visually examined by means of a colposcope — an instrument that contains a magnifying lens and a light. Colposcopy is primarily used to evaluate abnormal cytology or grossly suspicious lesions and to examine the cervix and vagina after a positive Papanicolaou (Pap) test. During the examination, a biopsy may be performed and photographs taken of suspicious lesions, using the colposcope and attachments. Biopsy risks include bleeding (especially during pregnancy) and infection.

What it all means

Surface contour of the cervical vessels should be smooth and pink; columnar epithelium should appear grapelike. Different tissue types should have definite borders.

Abnormal findings

Abnormal colposcopy findings include white epithelium or punctuation and mosaic patterns, which may indicate underlying cervical tissue abnormalities, indicating possible invasive cancer or precancerous tissue changes. Abnormal findings also include atypical vessels, which may indicate invasive cancer. Other abnormalities visible during colposcopy include inflammatory changes, atrophy, erosion, papilloma (benign epithelial tumor), and condyloma (wart-like growth). (See *Colposcopy interference.*)

Colposcopy helps confirm abnormal cervical tissue growth after a positive Pap test. It also helps evaluate vaginal and cervical lesions.

What needs to be done

• Explain the procedure to the patient. Tell her the procedure is safe and painless and takes 10 to 15 minutes. Advise her that a biopsy may be performed at the time of examination and may cause minimal but easily controlled bleeding and mild cramping.
• The doctor puts on gloves and, with the patient in the lithotomy position, inserts the speculum and, if indicated, performs a Pap test. Then he swabs the cervix with acetic acid solution to remove mucus. After examining the cervix and vagina, he performs a biopsy on areas that appear abnormal. Finally, he stops bleeding by applying pressure or hemostatic solutions or by cautery.

Brief abstinence

After a biopsy, instruct the patient to abstain from intercourse and avoid inserting anything in her vagina, including a tampon, until biopsy site healing is confirmed (approximately 10 days).

Warning!

Colposcopy interference

Failure to clean the cervix of foreign materials, such as creams and medications, may impair visualization.

Laparoscopy

Laparoscopy permits visualization of the peritoneal cavity by the insertion of a small fiber-optic telescope (laparoscope) through the anterior abdominal wall.

Laparoscopy has largely replaced laparotomy because it requires a smaller incision, is faster, and reduces the risk of postoperative adhesions. Nevertheless, laparotomy is usually preferred when extensive surgery is indicated. Potential laparoscopy risks include a punctured visceral organ, which can cause bleeding or spilling of intestinal contents into the peritoneum.

Laparoscopy can detect cysts, adhesions, fibroids, and infection. As a treatment, it can be used for adhesion destruction, tubal sterilization, and foreign body removal.

What it all means

Normal findings include mobile uterus and fallopian tubes of normal size and shape and with no adhesions. The ovaries are of normal size and shape; cysts and endometriosis are absent.

Abnormal findings

An ovarian cyst appears as a bubble on the surface of the ovary. The cyst may be clear, filled with follicular fluid or serous or mucous material, or red, blue, or brown, if filled with blood. Adhesions appear as sheets or strands of tissue that may be almost transparent or thick and fibrous. Endometriosis resembles small, blue powder burns on the peritoneum or the serous membrane of any pelvic or abdominal structure. Fibroids (fibrous, encapsulated connective tissue tumor) appear as lumps on the uterus; hydrosalpinx (distention of the fallopian tube caused by fluid), as an enlarged fallopian tube; ectopic pregnancy, as an enlarged or ruptured fallopian tube. In pelvic inflammatory disease, infection or abscess is evident. (See *Laraposcopy interference*.)

What needs to be done

• Explain the procedure to the patient. Instruct her to fast after midnight before the test or for at least 8 hours before surgery. Tell her the procedure generally takes 15 to 30 minutes.
• Inform the patient that she'll receive a local or general anesthetic, and tell her whether the procedure will require an outpatient visit or overnight hospitalization.

Don't know much about history?

• Make sure the patient or a responsible family member has signed a consent form. Check the patient history for hypersensitivity to the anesthetic. Make sure all laboratory work is completed and results reported before the test. Instruct the patient to empty her bladder just before the test.
• The patient is anesthetized and placed in the lithotomy position. The doctor catheterizes the bladder and then performs a bimanual examination of the pelvic area to detect abnormalities that may contraindicate the test and to ensure that the bladder is empty.
• The doctor makes an incision at the inferior rim of the umbilicus. He inserts a special needle into the peritoneal cavity and insufflates 2 to 3 L of carbon dioxide or nitrous oxide. Next, he removes the needle and inserts a trocar and sheath into the peritoneal cavity. After removing the trocar, he inserts the laparoscope through the sheath to examine the pelvis and abdomen.
• To evaluate tubal patency, the doctor infuses a dye through the cervix and observes the fimbria (the fringelike extremity of the fallopian tubes) for spillage.
• After the examination, he may perform minor surgical procedures such as ovarian biopsy. He may insert a second trocar at the pubic hairline to provide a channel for inserting other instruments.

Aftercare

• Monitor vital signs and urine output. Immediately report sudden changes; they may indicate complications.
• After administration of a general anesthetic, check for an allergic reaction and monitor electrolyte balance and hemoglobin level and hematocrit, as ordered. Help the patient ambulate after recovery as ordered.
• Tell the patient she may resume her normal diet as ordered.
• Instruct the patient to restrict activity for 2 to 7 days as ordered.

Warning!

Laparoscopy interference

Adhesions, marked obesity, or tissue or fluid that attaches to the lens may obstruct the field of vision.

Laparoscopy is commonly performed in place of laparotomy. It requires a smaller incision, which allows a faster recovery.

• Reassure the patient that some abdominal and shoulder pain is normal and should disappear within 24 to 36 hours. Provide analgesics as ordered.

Other endoscopies

Bronchoscopy

Bronchoscopy is the direct visualization of the larynx, trachea, and bronchi through a standard metal or fiberoptic bronchoscope, a slender flexible tube with mirrors and a light at its distal end. A brush, biopsy forceps, or a catheter may be passed through the bronchoscope to obtain specimens for cytologic examination.

A flexible fiber-optic bronchoscope is used most often because it's smaller, allows a better view of the smaller bronchial structures, and carries less risk of trauma than a rigid bronchoscope. However, a large, rigid bronchoscope must be used to remove foreign objects, excise endobronchial lesions, and control massive hemoptysis.

Possible complications of bronchoscopy include hypoxemia, cardiac arrhythmias, bleeding, infection, bronchospasm, and pneumothorax.

What it all means

The trachea normally consists of smooth muscle containing C-shaped rings of cartilage at regular intervals. The bronchi appear structurally similar to the trachea, with the right bronchus slightly larger and more vertical than the left. Smaller segmental bronchi branch off from the main bronchi.

Abnormalities

Abnormalities of the bronchial wall include inflammation, swelling, protruding cartilage, ulceration, tumors, and enlargement of the mucous gland orifices or submucosal lymph nodes.

Abnormalities that originate in the trachea include stenosis, compression, ectasia (dilation of tubular vessel), irregular bronchial branching, and abnormal separation into two branches resulting from a diverticulum.

Abnormal substances in the trachea or bronchi include blood, secretions, and foreign bodies.

Bronchoscopy allows visual examination and removal of a tumor or a foreign body in the tracheobronchial tree. It also helps diagnose cancer, tuberculosis, or other infections by obtaining a specimen for examination.

Small findings...big consequences

Results of tissue and cell studies may indicate interstitial pulmonary disease, lung cancer, tuberculosis, or other pulmonary infections. Lung cancers include squamous cell carcinoma, small-cell (oat cell) carcinoma, adenocarcinoma, and large-cell (undifferentiated) carcinoma. Bronchoscopy findings must be correlated with X-ray and microscopic findings as well as with the patient's signs and symptoms.

What needs to be done

• Describe the procedure to the patient, and explain that this test allows the doctor to examine the lower airways. Instruct the patient to fast for 6 to 12 hours before the test. Tell him that the room will be darkened and that the procedure takes 45 to 60 minutes. Advise him that test results are usually available in 1 day, except for a tuberculosis report, which may take up to 6 weeks.
• Tell the patient that a chest X-ray and blood studies, such as partial thromboplastin time, platelet count and, possibly, arterial blood gas analysis, will precede the bronchoscopy.

Expect the anesthetics

• Advise him that he may receive a sedative I.V. to help him relax.
• Make sure the patient or a responsible family member has signed the consent form. Check the patient history for hypersensitivity to the anesthetic, and obtain baseline vital signs. Administer the preoperative sedative as ordered. If the patient is wearing dentures, instruct him to remove them just before the test.

Ventilation station

• A patient with severe respiratory failure who can't breathe adequately by himself should be put on a ventilator before bronchoscopy.
• Place the patient in the supine position on a table or bed. Tell him to remain relaxed, with his arms at his sides, and to breathe through his nose. Provide supplemental oxygen by nasal cannula, if ordered. Make sure a handheld resuscitation bag with face mask is readily available.
• After the local anesthetic is sprayed into the patient's throat and takes effect, the doctor introduces the bronchoscope through the patient's mouth or nose. When the bronchoscope is just above the vocal cords, lidocaine is flushed through the inner channel of the scope to the vocal cords to anesthetize deeper areas. (See *Features of the bronchoscope.*)

Peak technique

Features of the bronchoscope

The bronchoscope, inserted through the nostril into the bronchi, has four channels (see inset): two light channels (A), which provide a light source; one visualizing channel (B) to see through; and one open channel (C), which accommodates biopsy forceps, a cytology brush, suction apparatus, a lavage device, anesthetic, or oxygen.

Side viewer for observer

Flexible bronchoscopic tube

Eyepiece

Open channel

Fiber-optic tube connected to light source

In-line sputum trap

Suction tubing

B
A
A
C

Detective work

• The doctor inspects the trachea and bronchi, observes the color of the mucosal lining, and notes masses or inflamed areas. Then he may use biopsy forceps to remove a tissue specimen from a suspect area, a bronchial brush to obtain cells from the surface of a lesion, or a suction apparatus to remove foreign bodies or mucous plugs. Lavage may be performed to diagnose the infectious causes of infiltrates or to remove thickened secretions. After the tissue, mucus, or secretion is collected, place the specimens in appropriate containers and label them properly.

Powers of observation

- Monitor vital signs. Notify the doctor immediately if the patient has an adverse reaction to the anesthetic or sedative. (See *Trouble signs*.)
- As ordered, place the conscious patient in semi-Fowler's position; place the unconscious patient on his side with the head of the bed slightly elevated to prevent aspiration.
- Provide an emesis basin, and instruct the patient to spit out saliva rather than swallow it. Observe sputum for blood, and notify the doctor immediately if excessive bleeding occurs.

Refrain, restrict, and reassure

- Tell the patient who has had a biopsy to refrain from clearing his throat and coughing, which could dislodge the clot at the biopsy site and cause hemorrhaging.
- Restrict food and fluids until the gag reflex returns (usually in 2 hours). Then let the patient resume his usual diet, beginning with sips of clear liquid or ice chips.
- Reassure the patient that hoarseness, loss of voice, and sore throat after this procedure are only temporary.
- Send the specimens to the laboratory immediately.

Arthroscopy

Most commonly used to examine the knee, arthroscopy is the visual examination of the interior of a joint with a specially designed fiber-optic endoscope. Unlike radiographic studies, arthroscopy permits concurrent surgery or biopsy using a technique called triangulation, in which instruments are passed through a separate cannula. Thus, arthroscopy provides a safe, convenient alternative to open surgery and separate biopsy.

Although arthroscopy is commonly performed under a local anesthetic, it may also be performed under a spinal or general anesthetic, particularly when surgery is anticipated. Arthroscopy complications include infection, hematoma, thrombophlebitis, and joint injury.

What it all means

The knee is a typical diarthrodial joint surrounded by muscles, ligaments, cartilage, and tendons and lined with synovial membrane. In children, the menisci (crescent-shaped cartilage) are smooth and opaque, with thick outer edges attached to the joint capsule

Trouble signs

Bronchoscopy can be a risky procedure. After your patient undergoes bronchoscopy, watch him carefully for the following complications:
- laryngeal edema or laryngospasm, such as laryngeal stridor and dyspnea
- hypoxemia
- pneumothorax (dyspnea, cyanosis, diminished breath sounds on the affected side)
- bronchospasm (dyspnea, wheezing) and bleeding (hemoptysis)
- tracheal or bronchial perforation (subcutaneous crepitus around the face and neck).

and inner edges lying snugly against the condylar (the rounded portion at the end of the bone) surfaces, unattached. Articular cartilage appears smooth and white; ligaments and tendons appear cablelike and silvery. The synovium (the membrane that lines the joint capsule) is smooth and marked by a fine vascular network. Degenerative changes begin during adolescence.

Abnormal findings

Arthroscopic examination can reveal a torn meniscus, chondromalacia (softening of the cartilage), dislocation, subluxation (partial or incomplete dislocation), fracture, degenerative articular cartilage, torn anterior cruciate or tibial collateral ligaments, Baker's cyst (cyst that contains synovial fluid) and ganglion cyst, synovitis, rheumatoid and degenerative arthritis, and foreign bodies associated with gout, pseudogout, and osteochondromatosis.

Depending on test findings, appropriate treatment or surgery can follow arthroscopy. If arthroscopic surgery can't be performed, arthrotomy (incision into the joint) is the procedure of choice. (See *Understanding knee arthroscopy findings*, page 288.)

What needs to be done

• Describe the procedure to the patient. Instruct him to fast after midnight before the procedure.

Razor sharp

• Make sure the patient or a responsible family member has signed a consent form. Check the patient history for hypersensitivity to the anesthetic. Just before the procedure, shave the area 5″ (12.7 cm) above and below the joint; then administer a sedative as ordered.

Technique time

• Arthroscopic techniques vary with the surgeon and the type of arthroscope used. In most cases, the doctor drains as much blood as possible from the leg by wrapping it in an elastic bandage and elevating it or he instills a mixture of lidocaine with epinephrine and sterile normal saline solution into the knee to distend the knee and help reduce bleeding. Then he anesthetizes the joint, makes a small incision, and passes a cannula through the incision and positions it in the joint cavity. Next, he inserts the arthroscope through the cannula and examines the knee structures. If necessary, he takes photographs for further study.

• When the examination is complete, the doctor performs a synovial biopsy or appropriate surgery. After the surgery, he removes

Arthroscopy can be a real saving grace. It can diagnose joint diseases and monitor their progression and therapy. Doctors also use the technique to perform joint surgery.

Now I get it!

Understanding knee arthroscopy findings

With the patient's knee flexed about 40 degrees, the arthroscope is introduced into the joint. The doctor moves the knee into various degrees of flexion, extension, and rotation to obtain different arthroscopic views of the joint space.

> Here, the articular surface of the patella shows evidence of chondromalacia.

> This view depicts a normal patellofemoral joint with smooth joint surfaces.

> This view reveals a tear in the anterior cruciate ligament.

> Arthroscopy should be avoided in patients with fibrous ankylosis when flexion is less than 50 degrees and in patients with local skin or wound infections.

the arthroscope, irrigates the joint, and applies an adhesive strip and compression bandage to the site.
• Watch for fever and swelling, increased pain, and localized inflammation at the incision site. If the patient reports discomfort, administer analgesics as ordered.
• Monitor the patient's circulation and sensation in his leg.

Crucial (and cruciate) instruction

- Instruct the patient to report fever, bleeding, drainage, or increased joint swelling or pain.
- If an immobilizer is ordered, teach the patient how to apply it.
- Tell the patient that showering is permitted after 48 hours, but a tub bath should be avoided until after the postoperative visit.
- Tell the patient that he may resume his usual diet.

Quick quiz

Advise the patient to elevate the leg and apply ice for the first 24 hours. Tell him to bear only partial weight — using crutches, a walker, or a cane — for 48 hours.

1. Before colonoscopy, the patient should avoid:
  A. a soap-suds enema.
  B. GoLYTELY.
  C. castor oil.

Answer: A. A soap-suds enema irritates the mucosa and stimulates mucous secretions that may hinder the examination.

2. Your patient is scheduled for an EGD in the morning. When preparing him, you should explain that:
  A. he may have liquids before the procedure.
  B. he must remove his dentures before the procedure.
  C. he may drive home after the procedure.

Answer: B. The endoscope passes through the mouth into the esophagus. Therefore, the patient must remove his dentures before the procedure to prevent airway obstruction.

3. After a bronchoscopy that required a biopsy, you should instruct the patient to:
  A. refrain from clearing his throat.
  B. perform coughing and deep breathing every 4 hours.
  C. resume his diet immediately.

Answer: A. The patient must refrain from clearing his throat and coughing because these actions could dislodge the clot at the biopsy site and cause hemorrhaging.

4. After arthroscopy, you should instruct your patient to:
  A. elevate his leg, apply ice, and bear full weight.
  B. elevate his leg, apply warm soaks, and bear partial weight.
  C. elevate his leg, apply ice, and bear partial weight.

Answer: C. After arthroscopy, the patient should elevate the affected leg and apply ice for 24 hours to reduce swelling. He should bear only partial weight, using crutches, a walker, or a cane, for 48 hours.

5.   Before arthroscopy, you should shave the area:
- A.   2″ (5.1 cm) below the joint.
- B.   3″ (7.6 cm) above the joint.
- C.   5″ (12.7 cm) above and below the joint.

Answer: C. Just before the procedure, shave the area 5″ above and below the joint.

Scoring

☆☆☆   If you answered all five questions correctly, awesome! You're an Expert of Endoscopy!

☆☆   If you answered three or four questions correctly, terrific! The end of endoscopic study is just around the corner!

☆   If you answered fewer than three questions correctly, don't worry! With a little more work, you'll end up acing endoscopy!

10

Ultrasonography

Just the facts

In this chapter, you'll learn:

♦ about ultrasonographic procedures and how they're performed

♦ what patient care is associated with these tests

♦ what factors can interfere with these tests

♦ what ultrasonographic results may indicate.

A look at ultrasonography

Ultrasonography uses high-frequency sound waves to obtain diagnostic information. The sound waves are directed into the targeted tissue and reflect back to a transducer. A computer interprets the waves, some of which appear on a screen for immediate visualization while others are converted to audible sounds. Some waves are recorded for a permanent test record, called a sonogram or echogram.

Before ultrasonography, explain the procedure to the patient in terms he can understand to ease his anxiety.

Cardiovascular system

Echocardiography

Echocardiography examines the size, shape, and motion of cardiac structures using a transducer placed at an acoustic window (an area where bone and lung tissue are absent) on the patient's chest. The transducer directs sound waves toward cardiac structures, which reflect these waves. The transducer picks up the echoes, converts them to electrical impulses, and relays them to an echocardiography machine for display on a screen and for recording on a strip chart or videotape.

On the move with M-mode

The most commonly used echocardiographic techniques are M-mode (motion-mode) and two-dimensional (cross-sectional). In *M-mode echocardiography*, a single, pencil-like ultrasound beam strikes the heart, producing an "ice pick," or vertical, view of cardiac structures; this method is especially useful for precisely recording the motion and dimensions of intra-cardiac structures.

2-D echo

In *two-dimensional echocardiography*, the ultrasound beam rapidly sweeps through an arc, producing a cross-sectional, or fan-shaped, view of cardiac structures; this technique is useful for recording lateral motion and providing the correct spatial relationship between cardiac structures. In many cases, both techniques are performed to complement each other. (See *Comparing two types of echocardiography*.) Recent advances in cardiac stress testing include exercise echocardiography and dobutamine stress echocardiography. (See *Teaching about cardiac stress testing*, page 294.)

What it all means

A normal echocardiogram reveals normal position, size, and movement of the cardiac valves and heart muscle wall and shows normal directional flow of blood within the heart chambers.

Detect heart valve abnormalities

The echocardiogram may detect valvular abnormalities, such as mitral stenosis, mitral valve prolapse, aortic insufficiency, and aortic stenosis. Chamber or valvular abnormalities may indicate a congenital disorder. In coronary artery disease, ischemia or infarction may cause motion abnormalities in the ventricular walls. The echocardiogram is especially sensitive in detecting pericardial effusion. (See *Echocardiography interference*, page 295.)

What needs to be done

• Explain the procedure to the patient.

Echocardiography helps diagnose and evaluate valvular abnormalities and atrial tumors, and it measures the size of the heart's chambers.

If my chambers appear large, I may have cardiomyopathy, valvular disorders, or heart failure. If they appear small, I may have restrictive pericarditis.

Now I get it!

Comparing two types of echocardiography

This illustration shows how M-mode and two-dimensional echocardiography differ. The shaded areas beneath the transducer identify cardiac structures that intercept and reflect the transducer's ultrasonic waves.

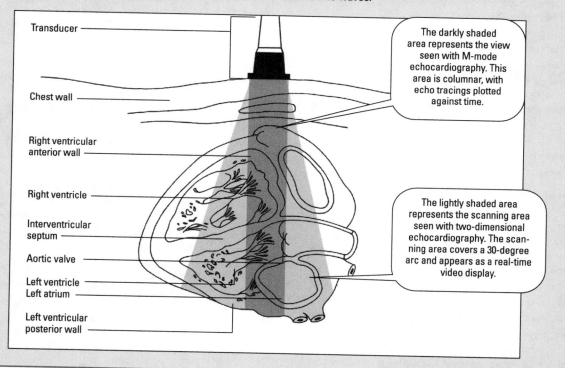

Transducer

Chest wall

Right ventricular anterior wall

Right ventricle

Interventricular septum

Aortic valve

Left ventricle
Left atrium

Left ventricular posterior wall

The darkly shaded area represents the view seen with M-mode echocardiography. This area is columnar, with echo tracings plotted against time.

The lightly shaded area represents the scanning area seen with two-dimensional echocardiography. The scanning area covers a 30-degree arc and appears as a real-time video display.

- Advise the patient to remain still during the test because movement may distort results.

Position is everything

- The patient is placed in the supine position. Conductive gel is applied to the third or fourth intercostal space to the left of the sternum, and the transducer is placed over it. The transducer is systematically angled to direct ultrasonic waves at specific heart regions. During the test, the oscilloscope screen, which displays the returning echoes, is observed; significant findings are recorded on a strip chart recorder (M-mode echocardiography) or videotape recorder (two-dimensional echocardiography).

Teaching about cardiac stress testing

Exercise echocardiography and dobutamine stress echocardiography are types of cardiac stress testing that detect changes in heart wall motion through the use of two-dimensional echocardiography with exercise or a dobutamine infusion. Imaging is done before and after either exercise or dobutamine administration. Usually, these tests are performed to:
• identify the cause of chest pain
• detect heart abnormalities, obstructions, or damage
• determine the heart's functional capacity after myocardial infarction or cardiac surgery
• evaluate myocardial perfusion
• measure the heart chambers
• set limits for an exercise program.

Preparing your patient

When preparing your patient for these tests, cover the following points:
• Explain that this test will evaluate how his heart performs under stress and how specific heart structures work under stress.
• Instruct the patient not to eat, smoke, or drink alcohol or caffeinated beverages for at least 4 hours before the test.
• Advise him to ask his doctor whether he should withhold current medications before the test.
• Tell him to wear a two-piece outfit because he'll be removing all clothing above the waist and will wear a hospital gown.
• Explain that electrodes will be placed on his chest and arms to obtain an initial electrocardiogram (ECG). Mention that the areas where electrodes are placed will be cleaned with alcohol and the skin will be abraded for optimal electrode contact.
• Tell him that an initial echocardiogram will be performed while he's lying down. Conductive gel, which feels warm, will be placed on his chest. Then a special transducer will be placed at various angles on his chest to visualize different parts of his heart. Emphasize that he must remain still to prevent distorting the images.
• Inform the patient that the entire procedure should take 60 to 90 minutes. Explain that the doctor will compare the echocardiograms to diagnose his heart condition.

Explaining exercise echocardiography

If the patient will have an exercise stress test after the initial echocardiogram, cover these teaching points:
• Tell him he'll walk on the treadmill at a prescribed rate for a predetermined time to raise his heart rate. After he reaches the prescribed heart rate, he'll lie down and a second echocardiogram will be done.
• Explain that he may feel tired, sweaty, and slightly short of breath during the test. If his symptoms are severe or chest pain develops, the test will be stopped.
• Reassure him his blood pressure will be monitored during the test. After the test is complete, his ECG and blood pressure will be monitored for 10 minutes.

Describing the dobutamine stress test

If the patient will undergo a dobutamine stress test after the initial echocardiogram, cover these teaching points:
• Explain that an I.V. line will be inserted into his vein for the dobutamine infusion. Tell him this drug will increase his heart rate without exercise. Tell him to expect initial discomfort when the I.V. line is inserted. Mention that during the infusion, he may feel palpitations, shortness of breath, and fatigue.
• Inform the patient that a second echocardiogram will be done during the dobutamine infusion. After the drug is infused and his heart rate reaches the desired level, a third echocardiogram will be obtained.
• Reassure the patient that his blood pressure will be monitored during the test.

A different view

- For a left lateral view of the heart, the patient may be on his left side. To record heart function under various conditions, he is asked to inhale and exhale slowly, hold his breath, or inhale amyl nitrite.
- Doppler echocardiography may also be used in this examination. This technique assesses heart sounds and murmurs as they relate to cardiac hemodynamics.
- After the procedure, remove the conductive gel from the skin.

Warning!

Echocardiography interference

Thickened chest muscles, chronic obstructive pulmonary disease, and chest wall abnormalities may alter test results.

Transesophageal echocardiography

In transesophageal echocardiography, ultrasonography is combined with endoscopy to provide a better view of the heart's structures. A small transducer is attached to the end of a gastroscope and inserted into the esophagus, allowing images to be taken from the posterior aspect of the heart. This causes less tissue penetration and interference from chest wall structures and produces high-quality images of the thoracic aorta (except for the superior ascending aorta, which is shadowed by the trachea).

What it all means

Transesophageal echocardiography can reveal thoracic and aortic disorders, endocarditis, congenital heart disease, intracardiac thrombi, and tumors; it can also evaluate valvular disease or repairs. Findings may include aortic dissection or aneurysm, mitral valve disease, or congenital defects such as patent ductus arteriosus. (See *Transesophageal echocardiography interference*, page 296.)

Is there an echo in here? Transesophageal echocardiography evaluates aortic disorders, valvular heart disease, and problems with prosthetic devices.

What needs to be done

- Explain the procedure to the patient. Tell him he'll need to fast for 6 hours before the test.
- Before the test, have the patient remove dentures or oral prostheses, and note loose teeth. Tell him he'll receive an I.V. sedative before the procedure. Ask the patient about any allergies, and note them on the chart. Make sure the patient or a responsible family member signs a consent form, if required.
- Have resuscitation equipment, including a suction apparatus, readily available.
- Connect the patient to monitors so his blood pressure, heart rate, and pulse oximetry values can be assessed.
- Help the patient lie down on his left side, and administer the ordered sedative. Then the back of his throat is sprayed with a topi-

Warning!

Transesophageal echocardiography interference

• The transthoracic approach prevents unobstructed visualization of the left atrial appendage and the ascending or descending aorta.
• Patients with chronic obstructive pulmonary disease and those on mechanical ventilators aren't good candidates for this test because excessive air in the lungs impedes movement of ultrasound waves.

Transesophageal echocardiography should be avoided in patients with esophageal obstruction or varices, GI bleeding, previous mediastinal radiation therapy, or severe cervical arthritis.

cal anesthetic. A bite block is placed in his mouth, and he's instructed to close his lips around it.
• The doctor introduces the gastroscope and advances it. Ultrasound images are recorded and reviewed after the procedure.
• Monitor the patient's vital signs and oxygenation. Observe the cardiac monitor closely for a vasovagal response, which may occur with gagging.

TEE-time is over

• Keep the patient supine until the sedative wears off.
• Encourage the patient to cough after the procedure, while lying on his side or sitting upright.
• Don't give the patient food or water until his gag reflex returns.
• Advise the outpatient to have someone drive him home.

Doppler ultrasonography

Doppler ultrasonography evaluates blood flow in the major blood vessels of the arms and legs and in the extracranial cerebrovascular system. A handheld transducer directs high-frequency sound waves to the artery or vein being tested. The sound waves strike moving red blood cells and are reflected back to the transducer at frequencies that correspond to bloodflow velocity through the vessel. The transducer then amplifies the sound waves to permit direct listening and graphic recording of blood flow. Measurement of systolic pressure helps detect the presence, location, and extent of peripheral arterial occlusive disease. (See *How the Doppler probe works*.)

Pulse volume recorder testing may be performed along with Doppler ultrasonography to yield a quantitative recording of changes in blood volume or flow in an extremity or organ.

Now I get it!

How the Doppler probe works

The Doppler ultrasonic probe directs high-frequency sound waves through layers of tissue. When these waves strike red blood cells (RBCs) moving through the bloodstream, their frequency changes in proportion to the flow velocity of the RBCs. Recording these waves permits detection of arterial and venous obstruction but not quantitative blood flow measurement.

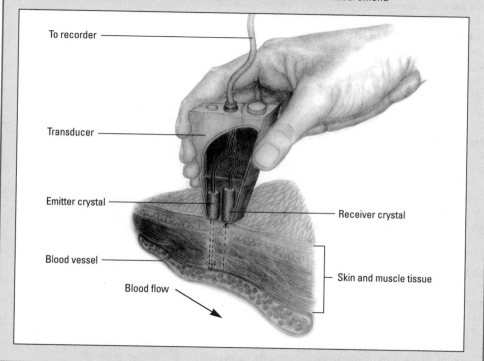

To recorder

Transducer

Emitter crystal

Receiver crystal

Blood vessel

Skin and muscle tissue

Blood flow

Doppler ultrasonography aids diagnosis of peripheral vascular disease and arterial occlusion, detects abnormal carotid blood flow, and monitors patients after arterial reconstruction and bypass grafts.

What it all means

Normally, venous blood flow fluctuates with respiration, so observing changes in sound wave frequency during respiration helps detect venous occlusive disease. Compression maneuvers can also help detect occlusion of the veins as well as occlusion or stenosis of carotid arteries.

Abnormal images and Doppler signals may indicate plaque, stenosis, occlusion, dissection, aneurysm, carotid body tumor, and arteritis.

What needs to be done

• Explain the test to the patient, and tell him that it takes about 20 minutes. Check with the vascular laboratory to determine whether special equipment will be used and whether special instructions are necessary.
• Water-soluble conductive jelly is applied to the tip of the transducer to provide coupling between the skin and the transducer.

Evaluating peripheral arteries

• Peripheral arterial evaluation is always performed bilaterally. The usual test sites in the leg include the common femoral, superficial femoral, popliteal, posterior tibial, and dorsalis pedis arteries; in the arm, the subclavian, brachial, radial, ulnar and, occasionally, palmar arch and digital arteries.
• The patient is instructed to remove all clothing above or below the waist, depending on the test site. After he's placed in the supine position on the examining table or bed, with his arms at his sides, measure his brachial blood pressure and place the transducer at various points along the test arteries. The signals are monitored and the waveforms recorded for later analysis.
• Segmental limb blood pressure is obtained to localize arterial occlusive disease. For lower-extremity tests, a blood pressure cuff is wrapped around the calf, pressure readings are obtained, and waveforms are recorded from the dorsalis pedis and posterior tibial arteries. Then the cuff is wrapped around the thigh, and waveforms are recorded at the popliteal artery. For upper-extremity tests, a blood pressure cuff is wrapped around the forearm, pressure readings are taken, and waveforms are recorded over both the radial and the ulnar arteries. Then the cuff is wrapped around the upper arm, pressure readings are taken, and waveforms are recorded with the transducer over the brachial artery.
• Blood pressure readings and waveform recordings are repeated with the arm in extreme hyperextension and hyperabduction to check for compression factors that may impede arterial blood flow. The upper extremity examination is performed on one arm, with the patient first supine, then sitting. It's repeated on the other arm.

Evaluating peripheral veins

• The usual test sites in the leg are the popliteal, superficial femoral, and common femoral veins and the posterior tibial vein at the ankle; in the arm, the brachial, axillary, subclavian, and jugular veins and, occasionally, the inferior and superior venae cavae.
• Instruct the patient to remove all clothing above or below the waist, depending on the test site. He's placed in the supine posi-

Now I get it!

Detecting thrombi with a Doppler probe

Typically, the Doppler probe is used to detect venous thrombi. Here's how it works.

After the transducer is positioned properly, the blood vessel is occluded by compression, as shown here in a normal leg. Water-soluble conductive jelly is applied to the transducer's tip to provide coupling between the skin and the transducer.

When pressure is released, blood flow resumes. The transducer picks up the sudden augmentation of the flow sound and permits graphic recording of blood blow. If a thrombus is present, compression fails to produce the augmented sound because blood flow, as shown here in the femoral vein, is impaired.

tion and instructed to breathe normally. The transducer is placed over the appropriate vein, waveforms are recorded, and respiratory modulations noted.

• Proximal limb compression maneuvers are performed and augmentation noted after release of compression, to evaluate venous valve competency. Changes in respiration are monitored. For lower-extremity tests, the patient is asked to perform Valsalva's maneuver, and venous blood flow is recorded. The procedure is repeated for the other arm or leg.

Evaluating extracranial cerebrovascular arteries

- The usual test sites include the supraorbital, common carotid, external carotid, internal carotid, and vertebral arteries.
- The patient is placed in the supine position on the examining table or bed, with a pillow beneath his head for support.
- Brachial blood pressure is then recorded, using the Doppler probe. Next, the transducer is positioned over the test artery, and blood flow velocity is monitored and recorded. The influence of compression maneuvers on blood flow velocity is measured, and the procedure is repeated on the opposite side. (See *Detecting thrombi with a Doppler probe*, page 299.)
- After the procedure, remove conductive jelly from the skin.

Miscellaneous tests

Abdominal ultrasonography

During abdominal ultrasonography, the technician guides a transducer over the area of the patient's body being evaluated. The transducer sends sound waves through the targeted tissue. These sound waves travel at various speeds, depending on the density of the tissue they're passing through.

Tissue densities

After passing through the tissue, sound waves reflect back to the transducer, and are converted into electrical impulses. These impulses are amplified and displayed on a screen. Because tissue densities vary, sound waves pass through them at different speeds. Images displayed on the screen reflect these differences. Cross-sectional images show different shades of gray, which depict various tissue densities. Ultrasound can provide images of many abdominal structures, including the gallbladder and biliary system, liver, spleen, and pancreas.

What it all means

A normal abdominal ultrasound shows the normal size, position, and appearance of the liver, gallbladder, bile ducts, pancreas, kidneys, adrenals, and spleen. It also helps visualize the abdominal aorta and inferior vena cava and their major tributaries.

Abdominal ultrasound evaluates organ size and structure, differentiates between cysts and solid tumors, and monitors radiation or chemotherapy effects.

Warning!

Abdominal ultrasonography interference

• Residual contrast media from studies done within the past 24 hours may distort or hinder imaging.
• In a dehydrated patient, body fluid deficiency may prevent ultrasonography from showing the boundaries between organs and tissue structures.
• Obesity interferes with ultrasound transmission, and fatty infiltration of the gland makes distinguishing the pancreas from surrounding tissue difficult.
• Residual barium in the colon or stomach may prevent visualization of the spleen.

Unwelcome guests

Abdominal ultrasound can detect:
• liver abnormalities, such as cysts, abscesses, tumors, and metastases, cirrhosis, and variations in portal venous flow
• gallbladder and bile duct abnormalities, including duct dilation or obstruction, gallstones, cholecystitis, and tumors
• pancreas abnormalities, such as pancreatitis, pseudocyst, and cysts and tumors, including adenocarcinoma
• kidney abnormalities, including hydronephrosis, tumors, cysts, calculi, and abscesses
• adrenal abnormalities, such as pheochromocytoma, adrenal hemorrhage, and metastases
• spleen abnormalities, including splenomegaly, lymph node enlargement, and trauma
• vascular abnormalities, such as abdominal aortic aneurysm, thrombi, and abnormal blood flow patterns
• other abnormalities, including ascites, congenital defects, and hematomas. (See *Abdominal ultrasonography interference*.)

What needs to be done

• Explain the procedure to the patient, and tell him he'll need to put on a hospital gown. Tell him he must remain still during scanning and hold his breath as requested to prevent a distorted image.

If your patient is a smoker, ask him to abstain before the ultrasound. Otherwise, he may swallow air while inhaling, which interferes with test results.

The nose knows

- For a gallbladder and biliary ultrasound, instruct the patient to eat a fat-free meal in the evening and then fast for 8 to 12 hours before the test. This promotes bile accumulation in the gallbladder and enhances ultrasonic visualization. The patient must keep fasting to prevent bile excretion in the gallbladder. Even smelling greasy foods, such as popcorn, can cause the gallbladder to empty.

Fasting before testing

- For ultrasonography of the liver, pancreas, or spleen, the patient must fast for 8 to 12 hours before the test.
- The patient is placed in a supine position.
- The area to be examined is coated with a water-soluble jelly. The transducer then scans the targeted area, projecting the images on the oscilloscope screen. These images are photographed for subsequent examination.
- The patient may be placed in right or left lateral positions for subsequent views and may be repositioned many times to get all necessary scans.
- After the procedure, clean the contact jelly from the skin.
- Tell the patient he may resume his usual diet.

> Transcranial Doppler studies measure blood flow in the brain and detect and monitor cerebral vasospasm progression.

Transcranial Doppler studies

By measuring the velocity of blood flow through cerebral arteries, transcranial Doppler studies provide information about the presence, quality, and changing nature of circulation to an area of the brain. Narrowed blood vessels produce high velocities, indicating possible stenosis or vasospasm. High velocities may also indicate an arteriovenous malformation caused by the accumulated signal from the extra blood flow associated with such lesions.

What it all means

The types of waveforms and velocities obtained indicate whether a pathologic condition exists. Although this test often isn't definitive, it provides diagnostic information noninvasively. Typically, high velocities are abnormal and suggest blood flow is too turbulent or the vessel is too narrow.

What needs to be done

- Explain the purpose of the study to the patient or his family.

Investigating vessels

- Tell the patient the study usually takes less than 1 hour, depending on the number of vessels that will be examined and any interfering factors.
- The patient reclines in a chair or on a stretcher or bed. A small amount of gel is applied to the transcranial "window," an area where bone is thin enough to allow the Doppler signal to enter and be detected. The most common approaches are temporal, transorbital, and through the foramen magnum.
- The technician directs the signal toward the artery being studied and records the velocities detected. A complete study assesses the middle cerebral arteries, anterior cerebral arteries, ophthalmic arteries, carotid siphon, vertebral arteries, and basilar artery.
- The Doppler signal — measured in millimeters — can be transmitted to varying depths. Waveforms may be printed for later analysis. When the study is complete, wipe the gel away.

Quick quiz

1. Which statement about M-mode echocardiography is *true?*
   A. A single ultrasound beam strikes the heart using an "ice pick" view of cardiac structures.
   B. An ultrasound beam sweeps through an arc, producing a fan-shaped view of cardiac structures.
   C. The lateral motion and correct spatial relationships between cardiac structures are recorded.

   Answer: A. In M-mode echocardiography, a single, pencil-like ultrasound beam strikes the heart, producing an "ice pick," or vertical, view of cardiac structures. This method is especially useful for precise recording of the motion and dimensions of intracardiac structures.

2. When used during echocardiography, amyl nitrate:
   A. has no adverse effects.
   B. is administered by inhalation.
   C. is administered I.V.

   Answer: B. A sweet-smelling gas, amyl nitrate is administered by inhalation during echocardiography.

3. When teaching your patient about transesophageal echocardiography, be sure to mention that:
- A.   he doesn't have to restrict his intake before the test.
- B.   he doesn't have to remove his dentures before the test.
- C.   his throat will be sprayed with a topical anesthetic just before the test.

Answer: C. Tell the patient that his throat will be sprayed with a topical anesthetic and that he may gag when the tube is inserted.

4. Which statement about venous thrombosis is *false*?
- A.   It can be detected during Doppler ultrasound.
- B.   It causes no change in venous blood flow velocity in response to Valsalva's maneuver.
- C.   It causes a change in venous blood flow velocity with respirations.

Answer: C. Venous thrombosis is present if venous blood flow velocity is unchanged by respiration, doesn't increase in response to compression or Valsalva's maneuver, or is absent.

5. Before an ultrasound of the gallbladder and biliary system, the patient must:
- A.   fast for 4 to 6 hours.
- B.   eat a high-fat meal.
- C.   avoid greasy food odors.

Answer: C. The odor of greasy foods, such as popcorn, can cause the gallbladder to empty and should be avoided before the test.

Scoring

☆☆☆   If you answered all five items correctly, yahoo! You're an ultrasonic superstar!

☆☆   If you answered three or four items correctly, super! Your comprehension is ultra sound!

☆   If you answered fewer than three correctly, don't dunk your Doppler just yet…you'll get the hang of it before long!

Radiography

Just the facts

In this chapter, you'll learn:

♦ about radiographic procedures and how they're performed

♦ what patient care is associated with these tests

♦ what factors can interfere with these tests

♦ what radiographic results may indicate.

A look at radiography

In radiography, X-ray beams penetrate bone and tissue and react on specially sensitized film. Normal tissue is radiolucent on film, whereas abnormalities appear as densities.

Before radiography, explain the procedure to the patient to ease anxiety. If contrast medium will be used, check the patient's history for hypersensitivity.

Neurologic system

Skull radiography

Skull radiography evaluates the three groups of bones that make up the skull. The bones of the skull form an anatomic structure so complex that several radiologic views of each area are needed for a complete skull examination.

What it all means

A radiologist interprets the radiographs, evaluating the size, shape, thickness, and position of cranial bones as well as the vas-

Skull radiography can detect fractures in patients who have suffered head trauma. It also aids diagnosis of pituitary tumors and detects congenital anomalies.

Positioning the head for skull radiography

The illustrations below show positioning for each view of the skull taken during X-ray.

For the *right lateral* and *left lateral* views, the sagittal plane is parallel to the tabletop and the film. A support, such as a folded towel or the patient's clenched fist, is placed under the chin. (Adequate film shows both halves of the mandible.)

For the *posteroanterior Caldwell's* view, the patient lies in a prone position, his chin supported by a folded towel or his fist. The sagittal plane and canthomeatal line are perpendicular to the tabletop and the film. The X-ray beam is angled 15 degrees toward the feet.

For the *anteroposterior Towne's* view, the patient lies in a supine position, with his chin flexed toward the neck; the canthomeatal line is perpendicular to the tabletop and film. The X-ray beam is angled 30 degrees toward the feet.

For an *axial (base)* view, the patient lies in a prone position, with chin fully extended; his head rests so that the line of the face is perpendicular and the canthomeatal line is parallel to the tabletop and the film.

cular markings, sinuses, and sutures; all should be normal for the patient's age.

Abnormal findings

Skull radiography can confirm fractures, although basilar fractures may not show on the film if the bone is dense. This test may confirm congenital anomalies and may show erosion, enlargement, or decalcification of the sella turcica caused by increased intracranial pressure (ICP).

Skull radiographs may also show abnormal areas of calcification in such conditions as osteomyelitis, with possible calcification of the skull itself, and chronic subdural hematomas. They can detect neoplasms within the brain that contain calcium. Radiography may also detect other changes in bone structure, for example, those associated with such metabolic disorders as acromegaly or Paget's disease.

> Carefully immobilizing the patient's head during skull radiography can increase his comfort while improving results.

What needs to be done

• Explain the procedure to the patient. Inform him that it takes about 15 minutes. Instruct him to remove glasses, dentures, jewelry, and other metal objects in the radiographic field.
• The patient is placed in the supine position on an X-ray table or seated in a chair and is instructed to keep still while radiographs are taken. A head band, foam pads, or sandbags may be used to immobilize his head and increase comfort.
• Routinely, five views are taken: left and right lateral, anteroposterior Towne's, posteroanterior Caldwell's, and axial (or base). Films are developed and checked for quality before the patient leaves the area. (See *Positioning the head for skull radiography*.)

Cerebral angiography

Cerebral angiography allows radiographic examination of the cerebral blood vessels after injection of a contrast medium. Possible injection sites include the femoral, carotid, and brachial arteries. The femoral artery is used most commonly because it allows visualization of four vessels (the carotid and vertebral arteries).

What it all means

Use of contrast medium allows visualization of superficial and deep arteries and arterioles as well as superficial and deep veins. The finding of apparently normal (symmetrical) cerebral blood

Advice from the experts

Comparing cerebral angiograms

The angiograms below show the differences between normal and abnormal cerebral vasculature.

This cerebral angiogram is normal.

This cerebral angiogram shows occluded blood vessels caused by a large arteriovenous malformation.

Cerebral angiography helps detect aneurysms, thrombosis, narrowing, or occlusion. It also helps locate clips applied to blood vessels during surgery and helps evaluate postoperative vessel status.

vessels, however, must be correlated with the patient's history and clinical status. (See *Comparing cerebral angiograms.*)

Suggestive vessels

Changes in the caliber of the vessels lumina suggests vascular disease possibly resulting from spasms, plaques, fistulas, arteriovenous malformation, or arteriosclerosis. Diminished blood flow to vessels may be related to increased ICP.

Vessel displacement may reflect tumor presence and size, areas of edema, or obstruction of the cerebrospinal fluid pathway. Cerebral angiography may also show circulation within a tumor, giving precise information on the tumor's position and nature. Meningeal blood supply originating in the external carotid artery may indicate an extracerebral tumor but usually designates a meningioma. Such a tumor may arise outside the brain substance but still be within the cerebral hemisphere.

What needs to be done

• Explain the procedure to the patient. Tell him it takes 2 to 4 hours, depending on the extent of testing ordered. Instruct him to fast for 8 to 10 hours before the test. If ordered, a sedative and an anticholinergic will be given 30 to 45 minutes before the test. Tell the patient that he'll be asked to wear a hospital gown and to remove jewelry, dentures, hairpins, and other metal objects in the radiographic field.

Historically speaking

• Make sure the patient or responsible family member has signed a consent form if required. Check the patient history for hypersensitivity to iodine, iodine-containing substances (such as shellfish), or other contrast media. Also check for contraindications, such as hepatic, renal, or thyroid disease. Mark hypersensitivities on the patient's chart, and notify the doctor; he may order prophylactic drugs or may cancel the test.

• The patient is placed in the supine position on a radiographic table, and the injection site (femoral, carotid, or brachial artery) is shaved. He's instructed to lie still with his arms at his sides. The skin is cleaned with alcohol and povidone-iodine solution. The local anesthetic is then injected.

• The doctor punctures the artery with the appropriate needle and catheterizes it. If the femoral approach is used, the doctor threads a catheter up the aortic arch. If the carotid artery is used, the patient hyperextends his neck, and a rolled-up towel or a sandbag is placed under his shoulders. His head is then immobilized with a restraint or tape. If the brachial artery (least common) is used, a blood pressure cuff is placed distal to the puncture site and inflated before injection to prevent the contrast medium from flowing into the forearm and hand.

Contrast mediums

• After verifying needle (or catheter) placement, the doctor injects the contrast medium and observes the patient for a reaction, such as urticaria, flushing, and laryngeal stridor. A first series of lateral and anteroposterior radiographs is taken, developed, and reviewed. Depending on results of this series, the doctor may inject more contrast medium and take another series of radiographs. Arterial catheter patency is maintained by continuous or periodic flushing with normal saline solution or

> As in all tests, careful review of the patient history is the key to safe, effective testing. With cerebral angiography, look for iodine hypersensitivity.

heparin solution. Vital and neurologic signs are monitored throughout the test.

• After obtaining an acceptable series of radiographs, the doctor withdraws the needle (or catheter). Firm pressure is applied to the pressure site for 15 minutes.

• The patient is observed for bleeding, distal pulses are checked, and a pressure bandage is applied.

Enforce and observe

• Enforce bed rest for 12 to 24 hours and provide pain medication, as ordered. Monitor vital signs and neurologic status for 24 hours—every hour for the first 4 hours, then every 4 hours.

• Check the puncture site for signs of extravasation, such as redness and swelling. To ease the patient's discomfort and minimize swelling, apply an ice bag to the site. If bleeding occurs, apply firm pressure on the puncture site.

Femoral approach

• If the femoral approach was used, keep the affected leg straight for at least 12 hours, and routinely check pulses distal to the site. Check the temperature, color, and tactile sensations of the affected leg because thrombosis or hematoma can occlude blood flow. Extravasation can also block blood flow by exerting pressure on the artery.

Carotid artery angle

• If a carotid artery was used as the injection site, watch for dysphagia or respiratory distress, which can result from hematoma or extravasation. Also watch for disorientation and weakness or numbness in the extremities (signs of thrombosis or hematoma) and for arterial spasms, which produce symptoms of transient ischemic attacks. Notify the doctor if abnormal signs develop.

Brachial route

• If the brachial approach was used, immobilize the arm for at least 6 hours, and routinely check the radial pulse. Place a sign above the patient's bed warning personnel against taking blood pressure readings from the affected arm. Observe the arm and hand, noting any change in color, temperature, or tactile sensations. If they become pale, cool, or numb, notify the doctor.

• Tell the patient to resume his usual diet.

• For patients who have been receiving aspirin daily, take extra care to compress the puncture site.

Encourage oral fluids after angiography to help the patient flush out the contrast dye.

Myelography

Myelography combines fluoroscopy and radiography to evaluate the spinal subarachnoid space after injection of a contrast medium. Because the contrast medium is heavier than cerebrospinal fluid (CSF), it will flow through the subarachnoid space to the dependent area when the patient, lying prone on a fluoroscopic table, is tilted up or down. The fluoroscope allows visualization of the flow of the contrast medium and the outline of the subarachnoid space. X-rays are taken for a permanent record.

Myelography helps locate a spinal lesion, a ruptured disk, spinal stenosis, or an abscess. It also helps detect arachnoiditis, spinal nerve root injury, and skull tumors.

What it all means

The contrast medium should flow freely through the subarachnoid space, showing no obstruction or structural abnormalities.

Abnormal findings

This test can identify and localize lesions within or surrounding the spinal cord or subarachnoid space. Common extradural lesions include herniated intervertebral disks and metastatic tumors. Common lesions within the subarachnoid space include neurofibromas and meningiomas; within the spinal cord, ependymomas and astrocytomas. This test may also detect syringomyelia, a congenital abnormality marked by fluid-filled cavities in the spinal cord and widening of the cord itself. Myelography may also detect arachnoiditis, spinal nerve root injury, and tumors in the posterior fossa of the skull. Test results must be correlated with the patient's history and clinical status.

What needs to be done

• Explain the procedure to the patient. Instruct him to restrict food and fluids for 8 hours before the test. Tell him the test takes at least 1 hour.

Consenting adults

• Make sure the patient or a responsible family member signs a consent form. Check his history for hypersensitivity to iodine and iodine-containing substances (such as shellfish), contrast media, and drugs associated with the procedure. Also check for such contraindications as increased ICP or an infection at the puncture site. Notify the radiologist of a history of epilepsy or phenothiazine use. If metrizamide is used as the contrast medium, discontinue phenothiazines 48 hours before the test.

Pretest preliminaries

- Before the test, tell the patient that the head of his bed must be elevated for 6 to 8 hours after the test and that he'll remain on bed rest for an additional 6 to 8 hours. If an oil-based contrast agent is used, inform the patient that it will be manually removed after the test and that he'll need to remain flat in bed for 6 to 24 hours.
- Instruct the patient to remove jewelry and metal objects in the X-ray field. Administer pretest medications, and perform pretest procedures, as ordered. If the puncture is to be performed in the lumbar region, an enema may be ordered. A sedative and an anticholinergic, such as atropine sulfate, may be ordered to reduce swallowing during the procedure.

Position and puncture

- The patient is positioned on his side at the edge of the table, with his knees drawn up to his abdomen and his chin on his chest. A lumbar puncture is performed, and the fluoroscope is used to verify proper needle position in the subarachnoid space. Some CSF may be removed for routine laboratory analysis.

Reassure, reposition, and rest

- The patient is then turned to the prone position and is secured with straps across his upper back, under his arms, and across his ankles. His chin is hyperextended to prevent the flow of contrast medium into the cranium; a towel or sponge is placed under his chin for comfort. In this position, the patient may complain of a headache, have trouble swallowing, or feel he isn't inhaling enough oxygen. If so, reassure him that he'll have opportunities during the procedure to rest from this uncomfortable position.
- With the spinal needle in place, the contrast medium is injected and the table tilted so that the contrast flows through the subarachnoid space. The flow of the contrast medium is studied on the fluoroscope, and X-rays are taken.
- When the required X-rays have been obtained, the contrast medium is withdrawn, if necessary, and the needle is removed. The puncture site is cleaned with povidone-iodine solution, and a small adhesive bandage is applied. (See *Removing contrast media after myelography.*)

Special aftercare

- Find out which contrast medium was used for the test, and position the patient accordingly.
- Monitor vital signs and neurologic status at least every 30 minutes for the first 4 hours, then every 4 hours for 24 hours.
- Encourage the patient to drink extra fluids. He should void within 8 hours after returning to his room.

Now I get it!

Removing contrast media after myelography

Some types of contrast media must be removed after myelography, whereas others are left to be absorbed by the body.

When removal is a must

Iophendylate must be removed after the procedure because it isn't water-soluble and won't be excreted. Left in the body, it could cause inflammation or adhesive arachnoiditis.

Two methods may be used to remove iophendylate:

• With the patient in the prone position, the contrast agent pools in the lumbar region and can then be aspirated.

• With the patient on his side (the usual position for lumbar puncture), the dye may be aspirated or allowed to drip from the needle.

Iophendylate removal may cause pain in the buttocks or legs from nerve root irritation. The patient must return to his room on a stretcher and lie flat for 24 hours after myelography.

A more mellow medium

Metrizamide is water-soluble and doesn't have to be removed. After it's absorbed into the bloodstream, the kidneys excrete it. However, the patient must return to his room in a wheelchair or on a stretcher with the head elevated at least 60 degrees. In his room, he must sit in a chair or lie in bed with his head elevated at least 60 degrees. He must not lie flat for at least 8 hours because metrizamide can irritate cervical nerve roots and cranial structures.

• If no complications or adverse reactions occur, the patient may resume his usual diet and activities the day after the test.

• If fever, back pain, or signs of meningeal irritation (headache, irritability, or neck stiffness) develop, keep the room quiet and dark, and provide an analgesic or an antipyretic, as ordered.

Respiratory system

Chest radiography

In chest radiography (commonly known as chest X-ray), X-ray beams penetrate the chest and react on specially sensitized film. Because normal pulmonary tissue is radiolucent, such abnormalities as infiltrates, foreign bodies, fluids, and tumors appear as densities on the film. A chest radiograph is most useful when com-

Advice from the experts

Understanding chest X-ray findings

The table below describes how anatomic structures normally appear on chest X-ray, lists possible abnormalities, and describes the implications of these abnormalities.

Anatomic structure and normal appearance	Abnormality	Implications
Trachea Visible midline in the anterior mediastinal cavity; translucent, tubelike appearance	• Deviation from midline • Narrowing, with hourglass appearance and deviation to one side	• Tension pneumothorax, atelectasis, pleural effusion, consolidation, mediastinal nodes; in children, enlarged thymus • Substernal thyroid • Stenosis secondary to trauma
Heart Visible in the anterior left mediastinal cavity; appears solid because of blood contents; edges may be clear in contrast with surrounding air density of the lung	• Shift • Hypertrophy of right heart • Cardiac borders obscured by stringy densities ("shaggy heart")	• Atelectasis, pneumothorax • Cor pulmonale, heart failure • Cystic fibrosis
Mediastinum (mediastinal shadow) Visible as the space between the lungs; shadowy appearance that widens at the hilum of the lungs	• Deviation to nondiseased side; deviation to diseased side by traction • Gross widening	• Pleural effusion or tumor, fibrosis or collapsed lung • Neoplasms of esophagus, bronchi, lungs, thyroid, thymus, peripheral nerves, lymphoid tissue; aortic aneurysm; mediastinitis; cor pulmonale
Ribs Visible as thoracic cavity encasement	• Break or misalignment • Widening of intercostal spaces	• Fractured sternum or ribs • Emphysema
Mainstem bronchus Visible; part of the hila with translucent, tubelike appearance	• Spherical or oval density	• Bronchogenic cyst
Bronchi Usually not visible	• Visible	• Bronchial pneumonia
Lung fields Usually not visible throughout, except for the blood vessels	• Visible • Irregular, patchy densities	• Atelectasis • Resolving pneumonia, infiltrates, silicosis, fibrosis, metastatic neoplasm

pared with the patient's previous films because it allows the radiologist to detect changes.

What it all means

For normal and abnormal findings, see *Understanding chest X-ray findings*. For accurate diagnosis, radiography findings must be correlated with additional radiologic and pulmonary tests as well as with physical assessment findings. Pulmonary hyperinflation with low diaphragm and generalized increased radiolucency may suggest emphysema but may also appear in a healthy person's radiographs.

What needs to be done

- Describe the procedure to the patient.
- Provide a gown without snaps, and ask the patient to remove all jewelry in the radiographic field. Tell him he'll be asked to take a deep breath and hold it momentarily while the film is being taken, to provide a clear view of pulmonary structures.
- For a stationary radiography machine, the patient stands or sits in front of the machine so that films can be taken of the posteroanterior and left lateral views.
- For a portable radiography machine, used at the patient's bedside, help position the patient. Because an upright chest radiograph is preferable, move the patient to the top of the bed if this position can be tolerated. Elevate the head of the bed for maximum upright positioning. Move cardiac monitoring cables, oxygen tubing, I.V. tubing from subclavian lines, pulmonary artery catheter lines, and safety pins as far out of the radiographic field as possible.
- If the patient is intubated, check that no tubes have been dislodged during positioning.
- To avoid exposure to radiation, leave the room or the immediate area while the films are being taken. If you must stay in the area, wear a lead-lined apron.

Chest X-ray helps detect pneumonia, atelectasis, pneumothorax, pulmonary bullae, and tumors. It also helps assess pulmonary status and determine correct placement of a pulmonary artery catheter, endotracheal tube, or chest tube.

Fluoroscopy

In fluoroscopy, a continuous stream of X-rays passes through the patient, casting shadows of the heart, lungs, and diaphragm on a fluorescent screen. Because fluoroscopy exposes the patient to high levels of radiation and reveals less detail than does standard chest radiography, it's indicated only when diagnosis requires visualization of physiologic or pathologic motion of thoracic contents—for example, to rule out paralysis in patients with diaphragmatic elevation.

What it all means

Normal diaphragmatic movement is synchronous and symmetrical. Normal diaphragmatic excursion ranges from ¾″ to 1⅝″ (2 to 4 cm).

Diminished excursion

Diminished diaphragmatic movement may indicate pulmonary disease. Increased lung translucency (not transparent but permitting light passage) may indicate elasticity loss or bronchiolar obstruction. In elderly people, the lowest part of the trachea may be displaced to the right by an elongated aorta. Diminished or paradoxical diaphragmatic movement may indicate diaphragmatic paralysis, which sometimes occurs after open-heart surgery. However, fluoroscopy may not detect such paralysis if the patient compensates for diminished diaphragm function by forcefully contracting abdominal muscles to aid expiration.

Fluoroscopy can detect bronchiolar obstructions and pulmonary disease. It also aids placement of a tube or catheter such as a pulmonary artery catheter.

What needs to be done

• Describe the procedure to the patient, and explain that this test assesses respiratory structures and their motion. Tell the patient that the test usually takes 5 minutes.
• Instruct the patient to remove all metallic objects, including jewelry, in the X-ray field.
• If necessary, assist with patient positioning. Move cardiac monitoring cables, I.V. tubing from subclavian lines, pulmonary artery catheter lines, and safety pins as far as possible from the X-ray field. During the test, cardiopulmonary motion is observed on a screen.
• If the patient is intubated, check that no tubes have been dislodged during positioning.
• To avoid exposure to radiation, leave the room or the immediate area during the test; if you must stay, wear a lead-lined apron.

Pulmonary angiography

Pulmonary angiography, also known as pulmonary arteriography, is the radiographic examination of the pulmonary circulation after injection of a radiopaque contrast agent into the pulmonary artery or one of its branches. This procedure is usually used to confirm symptomatic pulmonary emboli when scans prove nondiagnostic (especially before anticoagulant therapy) or are contraindicated.

It also provides accurate preoperative evaluation of patients with congenital heart disease.

Complicating factors

Possible complications include arterial occlusion, myocardial perforation or rupture, ventricular arrhythmias from myocardial irritation, and acute renal failure from hypersensitivity to the contrast agent; bleeding, hematoma formation, or infection may occur at the catheter insertion site.

What it all means

The contrast agent should flow symmetrically and without interruption through the pulmonary circulatory system. Interruption of blood flow may result from emboli, vascular filling defects, or stenosis.

What needs to be done

• Explain the procedure to the patient. Instruct him to fast for 8 hours before the test, or as ordered. Tell him the test takes about 90 minutes.

> Pulmonary angiography helps detect pulmonary embolism, locate emboli, and evaluate abnormal pulmonary circulation.

Pretest precautions

• Make sure the patient or a responsible family member has signed the consent form. Check his history for hypersensitivity to anesthetics, iodine, seafood, radiographic contrast agents, or anticoagulants and check for contraindications such as pregnancy. Obtain or check laboratory tests, including prothrombin time, partial thromboplastin time, platelet count, and blood urea nitrogen (BUN) and serum creatinine levels, and notify the radiologist of abnormal results. I.V. hydration may need to be considered, depending on the patient's renal and cardiac status. The radiologist may want to discontinue a heparin infusion 3 to 4 hours before the test.
• Keep emergency equipment available in case of a hypersensitivity reaction to the contrast agent.
• After the patient is placed in a supine position, the local anesthetic is injected and the cardiac monitor is attached to the patient. The doctor makes a puncture at the procedure site and introduces a catheter into the antecubital or femoral vein.

Safe passage

• As the catheter passes through the right atrium, right ventricle, and pulmonary artery, the doctor measures pressures and draws blood samples from various regions of the pulmonary circulation.

- Monitor for ventricular arrhythmias caused by myocardial irritation from passage of the catheter through the heart chambers.
- The doctor injects the contrast agent, which circulates through the pulmonary artery and lung capillaries while X-rays are taken.
- Observe for signs and symptoms of hypersensitivity to the contrast agent, such as dyspnea, nausea, vomiting, sweating, increased heart rate, and numbness of extremities.

When it's over

- Have the patient maintain bed rest for about 6 hours.
- Check blood pressure, pulse rate, and the catheter insertion site every 15 minutes for 1 hour, every hour for 4 hours, and then every 4 hours for 16 hours.

Trouble on the way

- Observe the site for bleeding and swelling. If they occur, maintain pressure at the insertion site for 10 minutes and notify the radiologist.
- Observe for signs of myocardial perforation or rupture by monitoring vital signs as ordered.
- Be alert for signs of acute renal failure, such as sudden onset of oliguria, nausea, and vomiting. Check BUN and serum creatinine levels.
- Report evidence of a delayed hypersensitivity reaction to the contrast agent or local anesthetic — dyspnea, itching, tachycardia, palpitations, hypotension or hypertension, excitation, and euphoria.
- Measure pulmonary artery pressures. Right ventricular end-diastolic pressure is usually less than or equal to 20 mm Hg, and pulmonary artery systolic pressure is usually less than or equal to 70 mm Hg. Pressures greater than this increase the risk of mortality associated with this procedure.

Back to normal

- Advise the patient of any activity restrictions, and tell him he may resume his usual diet.
- Encourage the patient to drink fluids, or give him I.V. fluids to help flush the contrast agent from his body.

Gastrointestinal system

Barium swallow

Barium swallow, also known as esophagography, is the radiographic or fluoroscopic examination of the pharynx and the fluoroscopic examination of the esophagus after ingestion of thick and thin mixtures of barium sulfate. This test, most commonly performed as part of the upper GI series, is indicated for patients with a history of dysphagia and regurgitation. Further testing is usually required for a definitive diagnosis.

Before the barium swallow

However, cholangiography and the barium enema test, if ordered, should precede the barium swallow because ingested barium may obscure anatomic details on the radiographs.

What it all means

After the barium is swallowed, it pours over the base of the tongue into the pharynx. A peristaltic wave propels it through the entire length of the esophagus in about 2 seconds. When the peristaltic wave reaches the base of the esophagus, the cardiac sphincter opens, allowing the barium to enter the stomach. After passage of the barium, the cardiac sphincter closes. Normally, it evenly fills and distends the lumen of the pharynx and esophagus, and the mucosa appears smooth and regular.

Inside view

Barium swallow may reveal hiatal hernia, diverticula, and varices. Although strictures, tumors, polyps, ulcers, and motility disorders, such as pharyngeal muscular disorders, esophageal spasms, and achalasia (cardiospasm), may be detected, a definitive diagnosis commonly requires endoscopic biopsy or, for motility disorders, manometric studies. (See *GI motility study*, page 320.)

What needs to be done

• Explain to the patient that this test evaluates the function of the pharynx and esophagus. Instruct the patient to fast after midnight before the test. If the patient is an infant, delay feeding to ensure complete digestion of barium. Explain that the test takes approximately 30 minutes.

A barium swallow diagnoses hiatal hernia, diverticula, and varices. It also helps detect strictures, ulcers, tumors, polyps, and motility disorders.

Now I get it!

GI motility study

When intestinal disease is strongly suspected, the GI motility study may follow the upper GI and small-bowel series. This study, which evaluates intestinal motility and the integrity of the mucosal lining, records barium passage through the lower digestive tract.

Riding the time line

About 6 hours after barium ingestion, the head of the barium column is usually in the hepatic flexure and the tail is in the terminal ileum. The barium completely opacifies the large intestine by 24 hours after ingestion.

Because the amount of barium passing through the large intestine isn't sufficient to fully extend the lumen, spot films taken 24, 48, or 72 hours after barium ingestion prove inferior to the barium enema. However, when spot films suggest intestinal abnormalities, the barium enema and colonoscopy can provide more specific, confirming diagnostic information.

- Describe the milkshake consistency and chalky taste of the barium preparation the patient will ingest; although it's flavored, it may be unpleasant to swallow.
- Tell him he'll first receive a thick mixture and then a thin one and that he must drink 12 to 14 oz (355 to 414 ml) during the examination. Inform him that he'll be placed in various positions on a tilting radiograph table and that radiographs will be taken.
- If gastric reflux is suspected, withhold antacids, histamine-2 (H_2) blockers, and proton pump inhibitors, as ordered. Just before the procedure, instruct the patient to put on a hospital gown without snap closures and to remove jewelry, dentures, hairpins, and other radiopaque objects from the radiograph field.
- Check the patient history for contraindications to the barium swallow, such as intestinal obstruction and pregnancy. Radiation may have teratogenic effects.
- The patient is placed in an upright position behind the fluoroscopic screen and undergoes examination of his heart, lungs, and abdomen. He's then instructed to take one swallow of the thick barium mixture, after which the pharyngeal action is recorded. The patient is then told to take several swallows of the thin barium mixture. The passage of the barium is examined fluoroscopically, and spot films of the esophageal region are taken.

Location, location, location

- Esophageal strictures and obstruction of the esophageal lumen by the lower esophageal ring are best detected when the patient is upright.
- The patient is then secured to the radiograph table and is rotated to the Trendelenburg position to evaluate esophageal peristalsis or to demonstrate hiatal hernia and gastric reflux. Again, he's instructed to take several swallows of barium while the esophagus is examined fluoroscopically, and spot films of significant findings are taken when indicated.
- After the table is rotated to a horizontal position, the patient is told to take several swallows of barium so that the esophagogastric junction and peristalsis can be evaluated. The passage of barium is then fluoroscopically observed, and spot films of significant findings are taken with the patient in supine and prone positions.
- During fluoroscopic examination of the esophagus, the cardia and fundus of the patient's stomach are also carefully studied because neoplasms in these areas may invade the esophagus and cause obstruction.
- Check that additional spot films and repeat fluoroscopic evaluation haven't been ordered before allowing the patient to resume his usual diet.
- Instruct the patient to drink plenty of fluids, unless contraindicated, and administer a cathartic, if ordered, to help eliminate the barium. (See *After barium swallow.*)
- Check the patient for abdominal distention and absent bowel sounds, which are associated with constipation and may suggest barium impaction.

Upper GI and small-bowel series

The upper GI and small-bowel series test involves the fluoroscopic examination of the esophagus, stomach, and small intestine after the patient ingests barium, a contrast agent. As the barium passes through the digestive tract, fluoroscopy shows peristalsis and the mucosal contours of the respective organs, and spot films record significant findings. This test is indicated for patients who have upper GI symptoms (difficulty swallowing, regurgitation, burning or gnawing epigastric pain), signs of small-bowel disease (diarrhea, weight loss), and signs of GI bleeding (hematemesis, melena).

Before and after

Although this test can detect various mucosal abnormalities, many patients need a biopsy afterward to rule out cancer or to

The upper GI and small-bowel series help detect hiatal hernia, diverticula, varices, and motility disorders. It also aids diagnosis of strictures, ulcers, tumors, and malabsorption syndrome.

distinguish specific inflammatory diseases. Oral cholecystography, barium enema, and routine X-rays should always precede this test because retained barium clouds anatomic detail on X-ray films.

What it all means

After the barium suspension is swallowed, it's propelled by a peristaltic wave through the entire length of the esophagus in about 2 seconds. When the peristaltic wave reaches the base of the esophagus, the cardiac sphincter opens, allowing the barium to enter the stomach. Then the cardiac sphincter closes.

A grand entrance

As barium enters the stomach, it outlines folds called rugae. When the stomach is completely filled with barium, its outline appears smooth and regular without evidence of flattened, rigid areas that suggest lesions.

Looping through the duodenum

After barium enters the stomach, it quickly empties into the duodenal bulb. Although the duodenal bulb mucosa is relatively smooth, circular folds become apparent as barium enters the duodenal loop. These folds deepen and become more numerous in the jejunum. Barium temporarily lodges between these folds, producing a speckled pattern on the X-ray film. As barium enters the ileum, the circular folds become less prominent and, except for their broadness, resemble those in the duodenum. The film also shows that the diameter of the small intestine tapers gradually from the duodenum to the ileum.

Experiencing the esophagus

Radiographic studies of the esophagus may reveal strictures, tumors, hiatal hernia, diverticula, varices, and ulcers (particularly in the distal esophagus). Benign strictures usually dilate the esophagus, whereas malignant ones cause erosive changes in the mucosa. Tumors produce filling defects in the column of barium, but only malignant ones change the mucosal contour. Nevertheless, a biopsy is necessary for a definitive diagnosis of esophageal strictures and tumors.

Erratic behavior

Motility disorders such as esophageal spasm are usually difficult to detect because spasms are erratic and transient. Achalasia is strongly suggested when the distal esophagus appears to narrow. Gastric reflux appears as a backflow of barium from the stomach into the esophagus.

Searching the stomach

Radiographic studies of the stomach may reveal tumors and ulcers. Malignant tumors, usually adenocarcinomas, appear as filling defects and usually disrupt peristalsis. Benign tumors, such as adenomatous polyps and leiomyomas, appear as outpouchings of the gastric mucosa and generally don't affect peristalsis. Ulcers occur most commonly in the stomach and duodenum, particularly in the duodenal bulb. Benign ulcers usually show evidence of partial or complete healing and are characterized by radiating folds extending to the edge of the ulcer crater. Malignant ulcers usually have radiating folds that extend beyond the ulcer crater to the edge of the mass. However, only a biopsy provides a definitive diagnosis of tumors and ulcers.

Radiographic studies of the small intestine may reveal regional enteritis, malabsorption syndrome, and tumors.

What needs to be done

• Explain the procedure to the patient. Instruct him to maintain a low-residue diet for 2 or 3 days before the test and then to fast and avoid smoking after midnight before the test. Because the procedure takes up to 6 hours to complete, encourage him to bring reading material to the radiography department.
• Describe the milkshake consistency and chalky taste of the barium; although it's flavored, he may find its taste unpleasant. Tell him he must drink 16 to 20 oz (473 to 591 ml) for a complete examination.

What to withhold

• As ordered, withhold most oral medications after midnight and anticholinergics and narcotics for 24 hours because these drugs affect small-intestine motility. Antacids, histamine$_2$-receptor antagonists, and proton pump inhibitors are also sometimes withheld for several hours if gastric reflux is suspected.

A lovely gown...but no accessories

• Just before the procedure, instruct the patient to put on a hospital gown without snap closures and to remove jewelry, dentures, hairpins, and other objects that might obscure anatomic detail.
• After the patient is secured in a supine position on the X-ray table, the table is tilted until the patient is erect, and the heart, lungs, and abdomen are examined fluoroscopically.
• Then the patient is instructed to take several swallows of the barium suspension. During fluoroscopic examination, spot films of the esophagus are taken from lateral angles and from right and left posteroanterior angles.

Palpation station

• When barium enters the stomach, the patient's abdomen is palpated or compressed to ensure adequate coating of the gastric mucosa with barium. To perform a double-contrast examination, the patient is instructed to sip the barium through a perforated straw. As he does so, a small amount of air is introduced into the stomach to allow detailed examination of the gastric rugae, and spot films of significant findings are taken. The patient is then instructed to ingest the remaining barium suspension, and filling of the stomach and emptying into the duodenum are observed fluoroscopically. Two series of spot films of the stomach and duodenum are taken, with the patient erect and then supine.

Nearing the end

• Barium passage into the remainder of the small intestine is observed fluoroscopically, and spot films are taken at 30- to 60-minute intervals until the barium reaches the ileocecal valve and the region around it. If small intestine abnormalities are detected, the area is palpated and compressed to help clarify the defect, and a spot film is taken. When the barium enters the cecum, the examination ends.

Finishing up

• Make sure additional X-rays haven't been ordered before allowing the patient food, fluids, and oral medications (if applicable).
• Tell the patient to drink plenty of fluids (unless contraindicated) to help eliminate the barium.
• Administer a cathartic or enema to the patient as ordered. Tell him his stool will be light-colored for 24 to 72 hours. Record and describe any stool that he passes in the hospital. Because barium retention in the intestine may cause obstruction or fecal impaction, notify the doctor if the patient doesn't pass barium within 2 to 3 days.
• Tell the patient to advise the doctor of abdominal fullness or pain or a delay in return to brown stools.

Banish the barium! Have the patient drink fluids galore to flush out the barium.

Barium enema

Barium enema, also known as a lower GI examination, is the radiographic examination of the large intestine after rectal instillation of barium (single-contrast technique) or barium and air (double-contrast technique). This test is indicated for patients with a history of altered bowel habits, lower abdominal pain, or passage of blood, mucus, or pus in the stools. It may also be performed after colostomy or ileostomy; in such patients, barium (or barium and air) is instilled through the stoma.

What to be wary of

Possible complications of barium enema include perforation of the colon, water intoxication, barium granulomas and, in rare cases, intraperitoneal and extraperitoneal extravasation of barium and barium embolism.

What it all means

In a single-contrast test, the intestine is uniformly filled with barium, and colonic haustral markings are clearly apparent. The intestinal walls collapse as the barium is expelled, and the mucosa has a regular, feathery appearance.

In the double-contrast test, the intestine is uniformly distended with air, with a thin layer of barium providing excellent detail of the mucosal pattern. As the patient is assisted to various positions, the barium collects on the dependent walls of the intestine by force of gravity.

Abnormal findings

Barium enema may reveal adenocarcinoma. However, endoscopic biopsy may be necessary to confirm the diagnosis.

Barium enema demonstrates and defines the extent of inflammatory diseases, such as diverticulitis, ulcerative colitis, and granulomatous colitis. This test may also reveal polyps; structural changes in the intestine, such as intussusception, telescoping of the bowel, sigmoid volvulus (360-degree turn or greater), and sigmoid torsion (a turn of up to 180 degrees); gastroenteritis; irritable colon; vascular injury caused by arterial occlusion; and selected cases of acute appendicitis. (See *Barium enema interference*.)

What needs to be done

• Explain the procedure to the patient.

Bowel prep

• Instruct the patient to restrict dairy products and to follow a liquid diet for 24 hours before the test. Tell the patient to drink five 8-oz (237-ml) glasses of water or clear liquids for 12 to 24 hours before the test to ensure adequate hydration. Withhold breakfast before the procedure; if the test is scheduled for late afternoon or is delayed, clear liquids may be allowed. Administer a bowel preparation supplied by the radiography department (A GoLYTE-

> Barium enema aids diagnosis of colorectal cancer and inflammatory disease and detects polyps, diverticula, and structural changes in the large intestine.

Warning!

Barium enema interference

Performing a barium swallow within a few days of a barium enema may impair the quality of radiographic films.

LY preparation isn't recommended because it leaves the bowel too wet and the barium won't coat the walls of the bowel.) An enema or repeat enemas may be ordered until return is clear.

Proceed with caution

Don't give laxatives or enemas to a patient with ulcerative colitis or active GI bleeding.

• Although various diets, laxatives, and enemas may be used, remember that certain conditions, such as ulcerative colitis and active GI bleeding, may prohibit the use of laxatives and enemas, so check the patient history for any of these conditions. Also check for such contraindications as tachycardia, fulminant ulcerative colitis associated with systemic toxicity and megacolon, toxic megacolon, or suspected perforation and pregnancy.

• After the patient is in a supine position on a tilting radiograph table, spot films of the abdomen are taken. The patient is assisted to Sims' position. A well-lubricated rectal tube is inserted through the anus. If the patient can't retain the tube, a rectal tube with a retaining balloon may be inserted. The barium is then administered slowly, and the filling process is monitored fluoroscopically. To aid filling, the table may be tilted or the patient assisted to various positions.

• As the flow of barium is observed, spot films are taken of significant findings. When the intestine is filled with barium, overhead films of the abdomen are taken, and the rectal tube is withdrawn. The patient is escorted to the toilet or given a bedpan and told to expel as much barium as possible. After evacuation, an additional overhead film is taken to record the mucosal pattern of the intestine and evaluate the efficiency of colonic emptying.

Double-contrast time

• A double-contrast barium enema may directly follow this examination or may be performed separately. If it's performed immediately, a thin film of barium remains in the patient's intestine, coating the mucosa, and air is carefully injected to distend the bowel lumen. When the double-contrast technique is performed separately, a colloidal barium suspension is instilled, filling the patient's intestine to either the splenic flexure or the middle of the transverse colon. The suspension is then aspirated, and air is forcefully injected into the intestine.

• The patient is then assisted to erect, prone, supine, and lateral decubitus positions in sequence. Barium filling is monitored fluoroscopically, and spot films are taken of significant findings. After the required films are taken, the patient is escorted to the toilet or provided with a bedpan.

Rest and fluids

- Make sure further studies haven't been ordered before allowing the patient food and fluids. Encourage extra fluid intake as ordered to prevent dehydration and help eliminate the barium.
- Encourage rest because this test and the bowel preparation that precedes it exhaust most patients.
- Because barium retention after this test can cause intestinal obstruction or fecal impaction, administer a mild cathartic or an enema as ordered. Tell the patient his stools will be light-colored for 24 to 72 hours. Record and describe any stools that the patient passes in the hospital.

Endoscopic retrograde cholangiopancreatography

Endoscopic retrograde cholangiopancreatography (ERCP) is the radiographic examination of the pancreatic ducts and hepatobiliary tree after injection of a contrast medium into the duodenal papilla. It's indicated in patients with confirmed or suspected pancreatic disease or with obstructive jaundice of unknown etiology. Complications may include cholangitis and pancreatitis.

What it all means

The duodenal papilla appears as a small, red or sometimes pale erosion extending into the lumen. Its orifice is commonly bordered by a fringe of white mucosa, and a longitudinal fold running perpendicular to the deep circular folds of the duodenum helps mark its location. Although the pancreatic and hepatobiliary ducts usually unite in the ampulla of Vater and empty through the duodenal papilla, separate orifices are sometimes present. The contrast agent uniformly fills the pancreatic duct, the hepatobiliary tree, and the gallbladder.

Abnormal findings

Examination of the hepatobiliary tree may reveal calculi, strictures, or irregular deviations that suggest biliary cirrhosis, primary sclerosing cholangitis, or cancer of the bile ducts. Examination of the pancreatic ducts may show calculi, strictures, and irregular deviations that may indicate pancreatic cysts and pseudocysts, pancreatic tumor, cancer of the head of the pancreas, chronic pancreatitis, pancreatic fibrosis, carcinoma of the duodenal papilla, or papillary stenosis.

ECRP assesses obstructive jaundice; diagnoses cancer of the duodenal papilla, pancreas, and biliary ducts; and locates calculi and stenosis in the hepatobiliary tree and pancreatic ducts.

What needs to be done

- Explain to the patient that this procedure permits examination of the liver, gallbladder, and pancreas through radiographs taken after injection of a contrast medium and that it takes 1 to 2 hours. Instruct him to fast after midnight before the test.
- Just before the test, tell the patient to remove all metal and other radiopaque objects and constricting undergarments and to void to ease the discomfort of urine retention after the test.

Contraindication and consent

- Make sure the patient or responsible family member has signed a consent form. Check the patient history for such contraindications as pregnancy (because of the risk of fetal harm secondary to radiation exposure), infectious disease, pancreatic pseudocysts, stricture or obstruction of the esophagus or duodenum, or acute pancreatitis, cholangitis, or cardiorespiratory disease.
- Obtain baseline vital signs just before the procedure and attach the patient to continuous electrocardiogram monitoring and pulse oximetry.
- An I.V. infusion is started with 150 ml of normal saline solution. First, the local anesthetic is administered as ordered; this usually takes effect in about 10 minutes. If a spray is used, ask the patient to hold his breath while his mouth and throat are sprayed. Then place him in a left lateral position and give him an emesis basin and tissues. Encourage him to let saliva drain from the side of his mouth. Then insert the mouthguard.
- While the patient remains in the left lateral position, diazepam or midazolam is administered I.V. as well as a narcotic analgesic, if needed. When ptosis or dysarthria develops, the patient's head is bent forward, and he's asked to open his mouth. The doctor inserts his left index finger into the patient's mouth and guides the tip of the endoscope. As the endoscope passes through the posterior pharynx, have the patient slowly extend his head to assist the advance of the scope.
- When the scope is advanced well into the esophagus — about 12″ (30.5 cm) — the patient's chin is moved toward the table or a continuous suction catheter is placed in his mouth to allow drainage of saliva. The doctor advances the endoscope through the remainder of the esophagus and into the stomach. When the pylorus is located, the doctor insufflates a small amount of air and angles the tip of the endoscope upward and passes it into the duodenum.

Descending to the duodenum

- After the doctor rotates the endoscope clockwise to enter the descending duodenum, the patient is assisted into the prone position. An anticholinergic or glucagon I.V. is administered. Air is insufflated, and the endoscope is manipulated until the duodenal papilla is located. Then the cannula, filled with contrast medium, is passed through the biopsy channel of the endoscope and into the ampulla of Vater. The pancreas is visualized first.

Getting it on film

• The cannula is repositioned, and the hepatobiliary tree is visualized by injection of 10 to 15 ml of contrast medium. After each injection, rapid-sequence radiographs are taken. Additional films may be taken. When the required films have been obtained, the cannula is removed. Before the endoscope is withdrawn, a tissue specimen may be obtained or fluid aspirated for examination

Postprocedure care

• Observe the patient closely for signs of cholangitis, pancreatitis, and perforation, such as abdominal pain, bleeding, and fever.
• Tell the patient that he may experience a feeling of fullness, some cramping, and passage of flatus several hours after the test.
• Continue to watch for signs of respiratory depression, apnea, hypotension, excessive diaphoresis, bradycardia, and laryngospasm. Be sure to have available emergency resuscitation equipment and a benzodiazepine antagonist such as flumazenil, or a narcotic antagonist such as naloxone.
• Check vital signs every 15 minutes for 4 hours, every hour for 4 hours, then every 4 hours for 48 hours.
• Withhold food and fluids until the gag reflex returns. Test the gag reflex by touching the back of the throat with a tongue blade. When the gag reflex returns, allow fluids and a light meal.
• Discontinue or maintain the I.V. infusion as ordered.
• Check for signs of urine retention. Notify the doctor if the patient hasn't voided within 8 hours.
• If this test is performed on an outpatient basis, make sure that transportation is available. Patients who have undergone anesthesia or sedation shouldn't operate an automobile for at least 12 hours postprocedure. Alcohol should be avoided for 24 hours.

Thumbs down on food and fluids until the patient's gag reflex returns.

Genitourinary and reproductive systems

Kidney-ureter-bladder radiography

Usually the first step in diagnostic testing of the urinary system, kidney-ureter-bladder (KUB) radiography surveys the abdomen to determine the position of the kidneys, ureters, and bladder and to detect gross abnormalities. This test, also known as a scout film or flat plate of the abdomen, doesn't require intact renal function and may aid differential diagnosis of urologic and GI diseases, which commonly produce similar signs and symptoms. However, KUB radiography has many limitations and nearly always must be followed by more elaborate tests, such as excretory urography or renal computed tomography. KUB radiography shouldn't follow recent instillation of barium, which obscures the urinary system.

What it all means

The shadows of the kidneys appear bilaterally, the right slightly lower than the left. Both kidneys should be approximately the same size. The ureters are only visible when an abnormality such as calcification is present. Visualization of the bladder depends on the density of its muscular wall and on the amount of urine in it. Generally, the bladder's shadow can be seen but not as clearly as the kidneys' shadows.

KUB abnormality

Bilateral renal enlargement may result from polycystic kidney disease, multiple myeloma, lymphoma, amyloidosis, hydronephrosis, or compensatory renal hypertrophy. A tumor, a cyst, or hydronephrosis may cause unilateral enlargement. Abnormally small kidneys may suggest end-stage glomerulonephritis or bilateral atrophic pyelonephritis. An apparent decrease in the size of one kidney suggests possible congenital hypoplasia, atrophic pyelonephritis, or ischemia. Renal displacement may be caused by a retroperitoneal tumor such as an adrenal tumor.

Congenital anomalies

Congenital anomalies, such as abnormal location or absence of a kidney, may be suggested by renal axes that parallel the vertebral column, especially if the inferior poles of the kidneys can't be clearly distinguished. A lobulated edge or border may indicate polycystic kidney disease or patchy atrophic pyelonephritis.

Opaque bodies may reflect calculi or vascular calcification caused by aneurysm or atheroma; they may also suggest cystic tumors, fecaliths, foreign bodies, or abnormal fluid collection. (See *KUB interference*.)

What needs to be done

• Explain to the patient that the test shows the position of the urinary system organs and helps detect abnormalities in them. Explain that the test takes only a few minutes.

Check me out! KUB helps evaluate my size, structure, and position. It's used to screen for abnormalities, such as calcifications, soft-tissue masses, and malformations.

Warning!

KUB interference

The following factors may prevent clear visualization of the urinary system:

• gas, feces, contrast medium, or foreign bodies in the intestine

• calcified uterine fibromas or ovarian lesions

• obesity or ascites.

• Place the patient on an adjustable X-ray table in the supine position and in correct body alignment. Tell him to extend his arms overhead, and then check for symmetrical positioning of the iliac crests. If the patient can't extend his arms or stand, he may lie on his left side with his right arm up. A single radiograph is taken.
• The male patient should have gonadal shielding to prevent irradiation of the testes. The female patient's ovaries can't be shielded because they're too close to the kidneys, ureters, and bladder.

Excretory urography

The cornerstone of a urologic workup, excretory urography allows visualization of the renal parenchyma, calyces, and pelvis as well as the ureters, bladder and, in some cases, the urethra after I.V. administration of a contrast medium.

What it all means

The kidneys, ureters, and bladder show no gross evidence of soft- or hard-tissue lesions. Prompt visualization of the contrast medium in the kidneys demonstrates bilateral renal parenchyma and pelvicaliceal systems of normal conformity. The ureters and bladder should be outlined, and the postvoiding should show no mucosal abnormalities and little residual urine.

System abnormalities

Excretory urography can demonstrate many urinary system abnormalities, including renal and ureteral calculi; abnormal size, shape, or structure of the kidneys, ureters, or bladder; supernumerary or absent kidney; polycystic kidney disease associated with renal hypertrophy; redundant pelvis or ureter; space-occupying lesions; pyelonephritis; renal tuberculosis; hydronephrosis; and renovascular hypertension. (See *Abnormal excretory urogram*, page 332, and *Excretory urography interference*, page 332.)

What needs to be done

• Explain the procedure to the patient. After ensuring he's well hydrated, instruct him to fast for 8 hours before the test.
• Make sure the patient or responsible family member has signed a consent form. Check the patient history for hypersensitivity to iodine, iodine-containing foods, or contrast media containing iodine. Mark any sensitivities on the chart, and notify the doctor. Premedication with corticosteroids may be indicated for patients with severe asthma or a history of sensitivity to the contrast medium.

Excretory urography evaluates the structure and excretory function of the kidneys, ureters, and bladder.

Advice from the experts

Abnormal excretory urogram

In a patient with suspected renal hypertension, an excretory urogram taken 8 minutes after injection of a contrast medium shows normal filling of the right kidney but delayed filling of the left kidney and ureter (see below).

This impaired excretion of the contrast material commonly results from narrowing of the renal artery feeding the subject kidney. Constriction hinders blood flow to the glomerulus and leads to increased renal absorption of water and decreased urine output. Demonstration of delayed filling can distinguish unilateral renal hypertension from essential hypertension.

• The patient is placed in the supine position on the table. A KUB radiograph is performed to detect gross abnormalities of the urinary system. If no such abnormalities are found, the contrast medium is injected, and the patient is observed for signs and symptoms of hypersensitivity. The first radiograph, visualizing the renal parenchyma, is obtained about 1 minute after the injection. (This may be supplemented by tomography if small, space-occupying masses — such as cysts or tumors — are suspected.) Films are then exposed at regular intervals — usually 5, 10, and 15 or 20 minutes after the injection.

On to the inflated bladders

- Ureteral compression is performed after the 5-minute film is exposed. This is accomplished through inflation of two small rubber bladders placed on the abdomen on both sides of the midline, secured by a fastener wrapped around the patient's torso. The inflated bladders occlude the ureters without causing discomfort, and promote retention of the contrast medium by the upper urinary tract. (Ureteral compression is contraindicated in ureteral calculi, aortic aneurysm, pregnancy, or recent abdominal trauma or surgical procedure.) After the 10-minute film is exposed, ureteral compression is released. As the contrast flows into the lower urinary tract, another film is taken of the lower halves of both ureters an followed by a film of the bladder.
- At the end of the procedure, the patient voids, and another film is taken immediately to visualize residual bladder contents or mucosal abnormalities of the bladder or urethra.

Aftercare

- After the procedure, monitor vital signs and observe for delayed reactions to the contrast medium.
- Continue I.V. fluids or provide oral fluids to increase hydration.

Renal angiography

Renal angiography permits radiographic examination of the renal blood vessels and parenchyma after arterial injection of a contrast medium. As the contrast agent goes through the renal blood vessels, rapid-sequence radiographs show the vessels during three phases of filling: arterial, nephrographic, and venous.

What it all means

Renal arteriographs show normal formation of the vascular tree and renal parenchyma.

Abnormal findings

Renal tumors usually show hypervascularity; renal cysts typically appear as clearly delineated masses. Renal artery stenosis caused by arteriosclerosis produces a noticeable constriction in the blood vessel; this is a crucial finding in confirming renal hypertension.

In renal infarction, blood vessels may appear to be absent or cut off and the normal tissue replaced by scar tissue. Another typical finding is the appearance of triangular areas of infarcted tissue near the periphery of the affected kidney. The kidney itself may appear shrunken because of tissue scarring.

Renal angiography assesses renal vessels before surgery and helps determine the cause of renal hypertension. It's also used to evaluate chronic renal disease, assess renal masses and trauma, and detect complications after a kidney transplant.

Renal angiography

Renal angiography may also detect renal artery aneurysms (saccular or fusiform), severe or chronic pyelonephritis, renal abscesses or inflammatory masses. When angiography is used to evaluate renal trauma, it may detect intrarenal hematoma, parenchymal laceration, shattered kidney, and areas of infarction; it may also be useful in evaluating donors and recipients before and after kidney transplantation. (See *Renal angiography interference.*)

What needs to be done

- Explain the procedure to the patient. Instruct him to fast for 8 hours before the test and to drink extra fluids the day before the test and after the test to maintain adequate hydration (or he may have an I.V. line started, if needed). Tell him the test takes about 1 hour and that he may receive a laxative or an enema the evening before the test.
- Before the test, instruct the patient to put on a hospital gown and to remove all metallic objects that may interfere with test results.
- Check the patient's history for hypersensitivity to iodine-based contrast media or iodine-containing foods such as shellfish.
- Make sure the patient or a responsible family member has signed a consent form. Administer medication, if ordered (usually a narcotic analgesic and a sedative, such as midazolam or diazepam). Record baseline vital signs. Ensure that recent laboratory test results (BUN, serum creatinine, bleeding studies) are documented on the patient's chart. Verify adequate renal functioning and adequate clotting ability. Evaluate peripheral pulse sites, and mark them for easy access in postprocedure assessment.
- The patient is placed in the supine position, and a peripheral I.V. infusion is started. The skin over the arterial puncture site is cleaned with antiseptic solution, and a local anesthetic is injected.
- Using the Seldinger technique, the femoral artery is punctured and, with the aid of fluoroscopy, cannulated. (If a femoral pulse is absent or the artery is otherwise inaccessible, another approach may be used.) After passing the flexible guide wire through the artery, the cannula is withdrawn, leaving several inches of wire in the lumen.

Here comes the catheter

- Next, a catheter is passed over the wire and advanced up the femoroiliac vessels to the aorta. The guide wire is removed, and the catheter is flushed with heparin flush solution to prevent clotting in the catheter tip. At this juncture, the contrast medium is injected and screening aortograms are taken before proceeding. On

Warning!

Renal angiography interference

The following factors may interfere with the quality of radiographs and their interpretation:
- patient movement during the test
- recent contrast studies such as a barium enema
- presence of feces or gas in the GI tract.

completion of the aortographic study, a renal catheter is exchanged for the former one.
• To determine the position of the renal arteries and to ensure that the tip of the catheter is in the lumen, a test bolus (3 to 5 ml) of contrast dye is injected immediately. This prevents subintimal injection or arterial spasm that may mimic a renal artery lesion. If the patient has no adverse reaction, 20 to 25 ml of contrast dye is injected just below the origin of the renal arteries so that it doesn't reach the mesenteric vessels first, obscuring the renal arteries. After this injection, a series of rapid-sequence films of the filling of the renal vascular tree is exposed.
• If further selective studies are needed, the catheter remains in place while the films are examined. If the films are satisfactory, the catheter is removed and a sterile dressing is firmly applied to the puncture site for 15 minutes. Before the patient returns to his room, the puncture site is observed for hematoma.

Wait and watch

• Keep the patient flat in bed; keep the leg on the affected side straight for at least 6 hours or as ordered.
• Check vital signs every 15 minutes for 1 hour, every 30 minutes for 2 hours, and then every hour until they stabilize. Monitor popliteal and dorsalis pedis pulses for adequate perfusion at least every hour for 4 hours. Note the color and temperature of the involved extremity, and compare them with those of the uninvolved extremity. Watch for pain or paresthesia in the involved limb.
• Watch for bleeding or hematomas at the injection site. Keep the pressure dressing in place, and check for bleeding when you check all vital signs. If bleeding occurs, notify the doctor promptly and apply direct pressure or a weighted sandbag to the site.
• Apply cold compresses to the puncture site to lessen edema and pain.
• Provide extra fluids (2,000 to 3,000 ml in the 24-hour period after the test) to prevent nephrotoxicity from the contrast medium.

Mammography is used for breast cancer screening and to monitor breast cancer patients who have been treated with breast-conserving surgery and radiation.

Mammography

Mammography is a radiographic technique used to detect breast cysts or tumors, especially those not palpable on physical examination. In xeromammography, a specially charged plate records the radiographic images and transfers them to a special paper. Biopsy of suspicious areas may be required to confirm malignancy. Although 90% to 95% of malignant breast tumors can be detected by mammography, this test produces many false-positive results. Mammography may follow such screening procedures as ultrasonography or thermography. (See *Using ultrasound to detect breast cancer*, page 336, and *Understanding ductal lavage*, page 337.)

Now I get it!

Using ultrasound to detect breast cancer

Ultrasonography — especially useful for diagnosing tumors less than ¼" (0.6 cm) in diameter — also helps distinguish cysts from solid tumors in dense breast tissue. As in other ultrasound techniques, a transducer is used to focus a beam of high-frequency sound waves through the patient's skin and into the breast. The sound waves bounce back to the transducer as an echo that varies in strength with density of the underlying tissues. A computer processes these echoes and displays the resulting image on a screen for interpretation.

Ultrasound can show all breast areas, including the difficult area close to the chest wall, which is hard to study with X-rays. When used as an adjunct to mammography, ultrasound increases diagnostic accuracy. When used alone, it's more accurate than mammography in examining the denser breast tissue of young patients.

Listen up!

Mammography screening advice

Tell your patient that the American Cancer Society (ACS) recommends that all women have a screening mammogram between ages 35 and 39 as well as a clinical physical breast examination every 3 years from ages 20 to 39. For women age 40 and older, the ACS recommends a yearly mammogram and a yearly physical breast examination.

The American College of Radiologists and the American Cancer Society have established separate guidelines for the use and potential risks of mammography. (See *Mammography screening advice.*) Both groups agree that despite low radiation levels (0.1 to 0.3 rad), the test is contraindicated during pregnancy.

Magnetic resonance imaging is becoming a more popular method of breast imaging; it tends to be highly sensitive but not very specific, leading to biopsies of many benign lesions.

What it all means

A normal mammogram reveals normal ducts, glandular tissue, and fat architecture. No abnormal masses or calcifications should appear.

Benign or malignant?

Well-outlined, regular, and clear spots suggest benign cysts; irregular, poorly outlined, and opaque areas suggest a malignant tumor. Malignant tumors are generally solitary and unilateral, whereas benign cysts tend to occur bilaterally. Findings that suggest cancer require further tests, such as biopsy, for confirmation. (See *Mammography follow-up probe* and *Mammography interference.*)

What needs to be done

• Assess the patient's understanding of the test, answer her questions, and correct any misconceptions. Assure her that the test is usually painless. Tell the patient not to use underarm deodorant or powder the day of her examination to avoid having confusing

Now I get it!

Understanding ductal lavage

Ductal lavage is a new procedure that can identify cancerous and precancerous cells in the milk ducts of the breast. The technique uses a nonsurgical approach to identify abnormal cells — possibly before they become cancerous.

In step one of this two-step procedure, a breast pump applies gentle suction to the patient's nipple. This may cause a drop of fluid to appear at the duct opening. Fluid is more likely to appear at the opening of a duct with abnormal cells than a duct with normal cells.

Under pressure

If ductal fluid is present, ductal lavage progresses to step two. After an anesthetic is applied to the nipple, a flexible catheter is inserted about ½" into the nipple's duct opening. Then saline solution is infused through the catheter into the duct and aspirated back out. Cells collected in the aspirated fluid are analyzed.

Warning!

Mammography interference

• Highly glandular breasts (common under age 30), previous breast surgery, and active lactation can impair readability of films.
• Breast implants may prevent detection of masses.

shadows on the film. If she has breast implants, tell her to inform the staff when she schedules the mammogram so that a technologist familiar with imaging breast implants is on duty.
• Inform her that although the test takes only about 15 minutes, she may be asked to wait while the films are checked to make sure they're readable. Advise her that the test has a high rate of false-positive results. Give her a gown that opens in the front and ask her to remove all jewelry and clothing above the waist.
• The patient is asked to rest one of her breasts on a table above a radiograph cassette. The technician places the compressor on the breast and tells the patient to hold her breath.
• A radiograph is taken of the craniocaudal view. The machine is rotated, the breast is compressed again, and a radiograph of the lateral view is taken. The procedure is repeated on the other breast. After the films are developed, they're checked to make sure they're readable.

Mammography follow-up probe

TransScan Medical's T-Scan 2000 probe can be used as follow-up examination for women with ambiguous mammograms. Suspicious areas are evaluated with a handheld probe that displays the image on a computer screen. Possible cancers are identified as bright spots with electrical impedance values that differ from those of normal tissue. These impedance values are consistent with those of malignant tissue.

Quick quiz

1. During skull radiography, all of the following are monitored *except:*
   A.   vital signs.
   B.   neurologic status.
   C.   ECG.

Answer: C. Vital signs and neurologic status are monitored throughout the test.

2. Perforation is a complication associated with ERCP. Signs and symptoms suggesting that perforation has occurred include:
   A.   shortness of breath, abdominal pain, and fever.
   B.   abdominal pain, bleeding, and fever.
   C.   cramping, hypertension, and fever.

Answer: B. Signs and symptoms of perforation include abdominal pain, bleeding, and fever.

3. When the contrast medium is injected during excretory urography, the patient may experience all of the following *except:*
   A.   transient burning sensation.
   B.   metallic taste.
   C.   headache.

Answer: C. When the contrast medium is injected, the patient may experience a transient burning sensation and a metallic taste.

4. After renal angiography, nursing responsibilities include:
   A.   keeping your patient flat in bed, with the affected side straight for at least 6 hours.
   B.   comparing the color and temperature of the involved and uninvolved extremities.
   C.   applying warm compresses to the puncture site to lessen edema and pain.

Answer: C. After renal angiography, you should apply cold compresses to the puncture site to lessen edema and pain.

Scoring

☆☆☆   If you answered all four items correctly, you nailed it! X-ray marks the spot!

  ☆☆   If you answered two or three items correctly, stellar! Your knowledge of radiography rules!

   ☆   If you answered fewer than two correctly, hang tight! You're bound to catch the radiography ride next time it comes around!

Computed tomography and magnetic resonance imaging

Just the facts

In this chapter, you'll learn:

♦ about computed tomography and magnetic resonance imaging

♦ what patient care is associated with each procedure

♦ what factors can interfere with test results

♦ what test results may indicate.

A look at CT and MRI

Computed tomography (CT) records detailed internal images of a predetermined plane of body tissue to produce thin, cross-sectional images. Multiple X-rays pass through this body area and are measured, while detectors measure differences in tissue densities. A computer processes and reconstructs this data as a two-dimensional image on a video monitor. Because CT images avoid superimposition of structures, this technique permits doctors to make fine distinctions among various tissues and organs.

Before the procedure, explain the test to the patient to ease his anxiety. Make sure the patient or a responsible family member has signed a consent form, if required. If the patient is restless or apprehensive, notify the doctor, who may order a sedative. Tell the patient he'll need to remove all metal objects and jewelry before the test.

After a procedure involving contrast medium, observe the patient for evidence of an allergic reaction (itching, increased or decreased blood pressure, diaphoresis, tachycardia, and urticaria).

A message about a medium

If the patient will receive a contrast medium (which accentuates tissue density differences), check his chart for hypersensitivity to shellfish, iodine, or radiographic contrast agents. Then start an I.V. saline lock. Tell him he may experience, warmth, facial flushing, and a salty taste when the contrast medium is injected.

Of magnets and spinning atoms

Magnetic resonance imaging (MRI) relies on the atom's magnetic properties. The MRI scanner uses a powerful magnetic field and radiofrequency (RF) energy to produce images based on hydrogen content of body tissues. Exposed to an external magnetic field, positively charged electrons align uniformly. RF energy directed at the atoms knocks them out of magnetic alignment and causes them to precess, or spin. When the RF pulse stops, the atoms re-align themselves with the magnetic field, emitting RF energy as a tissue-specific signal based on the relative density of nuclei and the realignment time. A computer processes these signals and displays information as a high-resolution video image.

Before MRI, explain the procedure to the patient to ease his anxiety. Tell him that although MRI is painless, he may feel uncomfortable while remaining still inside a small space. Tell him he'll be positioned on a narrow bed, which slides into a large cylinder housing MRI magnets. Mention that the scanner will make clicking, whirring, and thumping noises as it moves inside its housing to obtain different images; note that he may receive earplugs.

Ask if claustrophobia might be an issue; if so, the patient may not be able to tolerate the procedure or might need sedation. Although open scanners have been developed for patients with ex-

Memory jogger

The simple pneumonic SIC will help you remember what allergies to ask the patient about before a CT scan or MRI that requires contrast medium.

Shellfish

Iodine

Contrast media (prior sensitive reaction)

Now I get it!

Open MRI: A better choice for claustrophobes

With an open magnetic resonance imaging (MRI) unit, the patient isn't completely enclosed in a tunnel. This is ideal for patients with claustrophobia. Open MRI units are low-field units (0.2 to 0.5 Tesla), whereas closed MRI units are typically high-field units (1.0 to 1.5 or greater Tesla).

But not ideal

Image quality is almost always better in a high-field unit because of field strength, gradient speed and strength, surface coils, and software. Also, accurate diagnosis may be difficult unless the interpreting radiologist has experience reading low-field units.

MRI and metals don't mix

Before your patient undergoes magnetic resonance imaging (MRI), make sure he doesn't have a pacemaker or a surgically implanted joint, pin, clip, valve, or pump containing metal. Such objects could be attracted to the strong MRI magnet. Also ask whether he has ever worked with metals or has metal in his eyes. (Some facilities may have a checklist that covers all pertinent questions regarding metals, clips, pins, pacemakers, and other devices.) If he does have such a device, he won't be able to undergo the test.

treme claustrophobia or morbid obesity, tests using such machines take longer. (See *Open MRI: A better choice for claustrophobes.*) Reassure the patient that he'll be able to communicate with the technician at all times and that the procedure will be stopped if he feels claustrophobic.

Check your metal at the door

Immediately before the test, instruct the patient to remove all metal objects. (See *MRI and metals don't mix.*)

At the scanner room door, the patient is checked one last time for metal objects. Discontinue I.V. infusion pumps, feeding tubes with metal tips, pulmonary artery catheters, and similar devices before the test.

Computed tomography

CT of the intracranium

CT of the intracranium provides a series of images that represent cross-sectional images of various brain layers. This technique can reconstruct cross-sectional, horizontal, sagittal, and coronal plane images. (See *Intracranial computed tomography*, pages 348 and 349.)

What it all means

The density of tissue determines the amount of radiation that passes through it. Tissue densities appear as black, white, or shades of gray on the CT image.

Check me out! A CT scan of the intracranium helps diagnose lesions and abnormalities and helps monitor the effects of cancer treatment.

White, gray, or black

Bone, the densest tissue, appears white; brain matter appears in shades of gray; ventricular and subarachnoid cerebrospinal fluid (CSF)—the least dense—appears black. Structures are evaluated according to their density, size, shape, and position.

CT scans may indicate intracranial tumor, hematoma, cerebral atrophy, infarction, edema, or congenital anomalies such as hydrocephalus.

What needs to be done

• Explain the procedure to the patient. If no contrast enhancement is scheduled, tell him he need not restrict food or fluids. If contrast enhancement is scheduled, instruct him to fast for 4 hours before the test. Inform him that the test takes 15 to 30 minutes. (See *Teaching about CT scans.*)
• The patient is placed in a supine position on an X-ray table, with his head immobilized by straps. The head of the table is moved into the scanner, which rotates around the patient's head, taking radiographs at 1-degree intervals in a 180-degree arc.
• When this series of radiographs is complete, contrast medium is administered, if ordered. Usually, 50 to 100 ml of contrast medium are injected by I.V. infusion or by I.V. drip over 1 to 2 minutes.
• After injection of the contrast medium, another series of scans is taken.
• No specific posttest care is necessary if the test was performed without contrast enhancement. If a contrast agent was used, watch for residual adverse reactions after the test.

> **Memory jogger**
>
> To remember the signs and symptoms of a hypersensitivity reaction to contrast media, think of the mnemonic PURR.
>
> Pruritus
>
> Urticaria
>
> Rash
>
> Respiratory distress

Listen up!

Teaching about CT scans

Cover the following points if your patient will undergo a computerized tomography (CT) scan:
• Tell the patient he'll have to lie still during the procedure.
• Inform him that he'll be placed supine on an X-ray table and that the table will be advanced into the opening of the scanner.
• Explain that the scanner will revolve around him and make clicking noises as it takes the films.
• Tell him that after the first film series, he'll receive an I.V. injection, if a contrast medium is necessary.
• Warn him that he may experience a feeling of warmth during the injection and experience a salty, metallic taste in his mouth, which will last about 2 minutes.
• Instruct him to notify you immediately if he experiences nausea, vomiting, dizziness, headache, hives, or itching.

CT of the biliary tract and liver

In CT of the biliary tract and liver, multiple X-rays pass through the upper abdomen and are measured while detectors record differences in tissue attenuation. A computer reconstructs this data as a two-dimensional image on a monitor. CT scanning distinguishes the biliary tract and the liver if the ducts are large. Use of an I.V. contrast medium can further emphasize differences in tissue density.

What it all means

Normally, the liver has a uniform density that's slightly greater than that of the pancreas, kidneys, and spleen. Areas of slightly lower density, representing hepatic vessels, may interrupt this uniform appearance. The portal vein is usually visible; the hepatic artery usually isn't. I.V. contrast medium enhances both vessels and the main portion of the liver, and they become dense.

Obstruction detective

CT scan of the biliary tract and liver can detect small lesions, hepatic abscesses and cysts, and hepatic hematoma. Dilation of the biliary ducts indicates obstructive jaundice. If the biliary ducts aren't dilated, then nonobstructive jaundice is present. Use of an I.V. contrast medium helps detect biliary dilation, especially when the ducts are only slightly dilated. CT scans can usually identify the cause of obstruction, such as calculi or pancreatic carcinoma.

What needs to be done

• Explain the procedure to the patient. Tell him he'll be given a contrast medium to drink and should fast until after the examination. If contrast won't be used, fasting isn't necessary. Tell him the test takes about 1 hour.
• Give the patient the oral contrast agent supplied by the radiology department.

Photo op

• The patient is placed in the supine position on an X-ray table and then positioned in the opening of the scanner. A series of radiographs is taken and recorded on magnetic tape.
• When the first series of films is completed, I.V. contrast enhancement may be ordered. After the contrast medium is injected, a second series of films is taken.
• Observe for a delayed allergic reaction to the contrast dye. (See *Biliary tract and liver CT scan interference.*)

> It says here that a CT of the biliary tract and liver can be used to detect abscesses, cysts, and hematomas and that it also helps distinguish between obstructive and nonobstructive jaundice.

Warning!

Biliary tract and liver CT scan interference

• An oral or I.V. contrast medium excreted in the bile in previous diagnostic studies can interfere with detection of biliary dilation.
• Barium studies performed within 4 days before a computed tomography (CT) scan may obscure the image.

CT of the pancreas

In CT of the pancreas, multiple X-rays penetrate the upper abdomen while a detector records differences in tissue density, which are then displayed as an image on a monitor. A series of cross-sectional views can provide a detailed look at the pancreas. CT scanning accurately distinguishes the pancreas and surrounding organs and vessels if enough fat is present between the structures. Use of an I.V. or oral contrast medium can further accentuate differences in tissue density.

CT of the pancreas is used to detect pancreatic cancer, pseudocysts, and pancreatitis.

What it all means

The pancreas generally lies obliquely across the upper abdomen, and its parenchyma shows a uniform density (particularly if an I.V. contrast medium is used). The gland normally thickens from tail to head and generally has a smooth surface. An oral contrast medium opacifies the adjacent stomach and duodenum and helps outline the pancreas, particularly in persons with little peripancreatic fat, such as children and very thin adults. (See *Normal CT scan of the pancreas.*)

Because the tissue density of pancreatic cancer resembles that of the normal pancreatic tissue, changes in pancreas size and shape help demonstrate carcinoma and pseudocysts. Use of an I.V. contrast medium helps detect metastases by highlighting the pancreatic and hepatic tissues.

What needs to be done

• Explain the procedure to the patient. Instruct him to fast after administration of the oral contrast medium. Tell him the test takes about 1½ hours. Inform him that he may be given a contrast medium I.V. or orally to aid pancreas visualization. Describe possible adverse effects of the contrast agent, and tell him to report these.
• Check the patient history for recent barium studies. Give him the oral contrast agent as ordered.
• The patient is placed in the supine position on an X-ray table, and the table is positioned in the opening of the scanner.
• A series of transverse radiographs is taken and recorded on magnetic tape. After the first series of films is completed, I.V. contrast enhancement may be ordered.
• After the I.V. contrast medium is administered, another series of films is taken. (See *Pancreatic CT scan interference.*)

Advice from the experts

Normal CT scan of the pancreas

This normal computed tomography (CT) scan shows the pancreas highlighted by contrast medium.

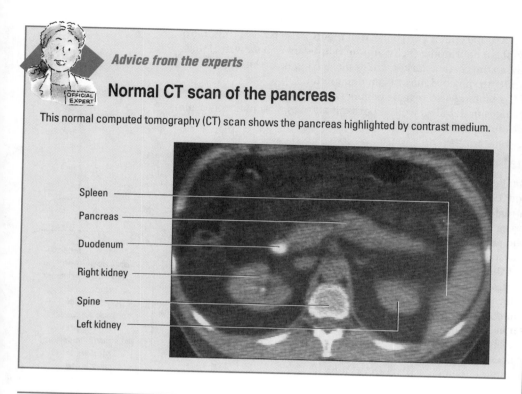

Spleen

Pancreas

Duodenum

Right kidney

Spine

Left kidney

Warning!

Pancreatic CT scan interference

Barium retained in the GI tract from an earlier test may obscure visualization.

CT of the spine

CT scans of the spine provide detailed images in the cross-sectional, longitudinal, sagittal, and lateral planes. Multiple X-ray beams from a computerized body scanner are directed at the spine from different angles; they pass through the body and strike radiation detectors, producing electrical impulses. A computer converts these impulses into digital information, which appears as a three-dimensional image on a monitor.

What it all means

In the CT image, spinal tissue appears black, white, or gray, depending on its density. Vertebrae, the densest tissues, are white; soft tissues appear in shades of gray; CSF is black.

A dense crowd

By highlighting areas of altered density and depicting structural malformation, CT scanning can reveal spinal lesions and abnormalities. It's particularly useful in detecting and localizing tumors, which appear as masses of varying density. Measuring this density and noting the configuration and location

You learn something new every day! It says here that CT of the spine helps diagnose spinal lesions and abnormalities and helps monitor the effects of surgery and treatment.

relative to the spinal cord can often identify the type of tumor. For example, a neurinoma (schwannoma) appears as a spherical mass dorsal to the cord; a darker, wider mass lying more laterally or ventrally to the cord may be a meningioma.

CT scanning also reveals degenerative processes and structural changes in detail as well as paraspinal cysts, vascular malformations, and congenital spinal malformations.

What needs to be done

• Explain the procedure to the patient. Unless contrast dye is ordered, tell the patient that he need not restrict food or fluids. If a contrast dye will be used, instruct him to fast for 4 hours before the test. Tell the patient the test takes 30 to 60 minutes.
• The patient is placed in the supine position on an X-ray table and is told to lie still. The table is then slid into the circular opening of the body CT scanner. The scanner revolves around the patient, taking radiographs at preselected intervals.
• After the first set of scans, the patient is removed from the scanner and a contrast medium (usually, 50 to 100 ml) is administered. Then he's moved back into the scanner, and another series of scans is taken.
• If necessary, administer analgesics before the scan, if ordered, so the patient can lie still comfortably.

> Bone CT detects and assesses the extent of primary bone tumors, skeletal metastases, soft-tissue tumors, ligament or tendon injuries, and fractures.

CT of bone

CT scanning of bone provides a series of tomograms, translated by a computer and displayed on a monitor, that represent cross-sectional images of various bone layers. This technique can reconstruct cross-sectional, horizontal, sagittal, and coronal plane images.

What it all means

The scan should reveal no pathology in the bones or joints.

Because of its ability to display cross-sectional anatomy, CT scanning can obtain images of the shoulder, spine, hip, and pelvis. It can reveal primary bone and soft-tissue tumors as well as skeletal metastases. It can also reveal joint abnormalities that other methods can't detect.

(Text continues on page 351.)

Incredibly Easy miniguide: Echocardiography

An echocardiograph uses ultrahigh-frequency waves to help examine the size, shape, and motion of the heart's structures. Here's how it works.

Electrocardiograph screen

A special transducer is placed over an area on the chest where bone and lung tissues are absent. It directs sound waves to the heart structures and converts them to electrical impulses.

These electrical impulses are sent to the echocardiograph and displayed on a screen. The image is then recorded on a strip chart or videotaped.

Incredibly Easy miniguide: Intracranial computed tomography

Intracranial computed tomography provides a series of tomograms, or radiographs, of a selected layer of the body (in this case, the brain). These tomograms, which are translated by a computer and displayed on a screen, represent cross-sectional images of various layers (or slices) of the brain. Intracranial tumors and other brain lesions may be identified.

The patient is placed in a supine position on an X-ray table with her head immobilized. The head of the table moves into the scanner, which rotates around the patient's head, taking radiographs at 1-degree intervals in a 180-degree arc.

This image shows a normal brain. Whew!

Incredibly Easy miniguide: Intracranial computed tomography

The density of tissue determines the amount of radiation that passes through it. Areas of altered density or displaced vasculature or other structures may indicate a tumor, an infarction, or a hematoma. Let's take a look at a few abnormal intracranial computed tomography scans.

Incredibly Easy miniguide: Endoscopic ultrasound

Endoscopic ultrasound combines ultrasonography with endoscopy to visualize the GI tract. An ultrasound probe, incorporated at the end of an endoscope, allows ultrasonic imaging in addition to typical endoscopy.

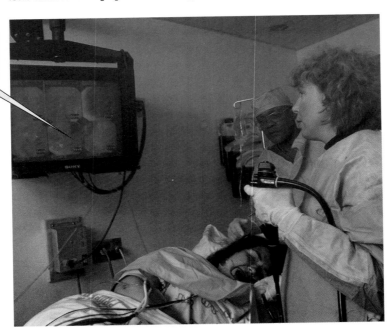

Images can be transmitted onto a screen for better visualization.

The doctor passes the endoscope through the esophagus. When examination of the esophagus and the cardiac sphincter is complete, she advances it into the stomach...

...After examining the stomach lining, the doctor advances the endoscope into the duodenum. She examines the duodenum and then slowly withdraws the endoscope.

What needs to be done

• Explain the procedure to the patient. Tell him he need not restrict food or fluids unless contrast medium is ordered, in which case he must fast for 4 hours before the test. Explain that the procedure takes 30 to 60 minutes.
• The patient is placed in a supine position on a radiograph table and told to lie as still as possible. The table is then moved into the circular opening of the CT scanner. The scanner revolves around the patient, taking scans at preselected intervals.
• After the first set of scans is taken, the patient is removed from the scanner and a contrast medium is administered, if ordered.

Pete and repeat

• After the injection, the patient is moved back into the scanner and another series of scans is taken.
• Urge the patient to drink lots of fluids to help eliminate the contrast agent.
• Tell the patient that he may resume his usual activities and diet.
• If necessary, give analgesics, as ordered, so the patient can lie still comfortably during the scan.

CT of the thorax

Thoracic CT scanning provides cross-sectional views of the chest by passing an X-ray beam from a computerized scanner through the body at different levels. CT scanning may be done with or without an injected contrast agent, which is used primarily to highlight blood vessels and to allow greater visualization.

What it all means

Black and white areas on a thoracic CT scan refer, respectively, to air and bone densities. Shades of gray correspond to fluid, fat, and soft-tissue densities.

Abnormal thoracic CT scan findings include tumors, nodules, cysts, aortic aneurysms, enlarged lymph nodes, pleural effusions, and accumulations of blood, fluid, or fat.

What needs to be done

• Explain the procedure to the patient. If contrast enhancement will be used, instruct him to fast for 4 hours before the test. Tell him the procedure usually takes 1 hour.
• After the patient is placed in a supine position on the X-ray table and while the contrast agent is being injected, the machine scans the patient at different levels.

CT of the thorax helps locate tumors, plan radiation treatment, and evaluate lymph nodes, aortic aneurysms, and lung disease severity.

• Encourage fluid intake if a contrast agent was used.

CT of the kidney

Renal CT scanning provides an image of the kidneys from a series of tomograms, which are translated by a computer and displayed on a special screen. The image reflects the amount of radiation absorbed by renal tissue and permits identification of masses and other lesions. An I.V. contrast medium may be injected to highlight tissue density and help differentiate renal masses.

What it all means

Normal renal tissue is slightly more dense than the liver but less dense than bone, which appears white on a CT scan. The collecting system usually exhibits low (black) density, unless contrast medium is used to enhance it to a higher (whiter) density. Kidney position is evaluated according to the surrounding structures; kidney size and shape are determined by counting cuts between the superior and inferior poles and following the kidney's contour.

Demonstrating densities

Renal masses appear as areas of different density than normal tissue, possibly altering the kidneys' shape or projecting beyond their margins. Renal cysts, for example, appear as smooth, sharply defined masses, with thin walls and a lower density than normal tissue. Such tumors as renal cell carcinoma usually have thick walls and nonuniform density. (See *Abnormal renal CT scan.*)

When contrast medium is used, solid tumors show a higher density than renal cysts but a lower density than normal tissue. Tumors with hemorrhage, calcification, or necrosis show higher densities. Vascular tumors are more clearly defined with contrast enhancement. Adrenal tumors are confined masses that are usually detached from the kidneys and other retroperitoneal organs.

Renal CT scans may also identify obstructions, calculi, polycystic kidney disease, congenital anomalies, and abnormal fluid accumulation around the kidneys, such as from hematomas, lymphoceles, and abscesses.

What needs to be done

• Explain the procedure to the patient. If contrast medium will be used, tell him he must fast for 4 hours before the test. Mention that the test takes about an hour.
• The patient is placed in the supine position on the scanning table and is secured with straps. The table is moved into the scan-

How revealing! A renal CT scan can show all my secrets: renal tumor, obstruction, calculi, polycystic kidney disease, congenital anomalies, and abnormal fluid accumulation.

Advice from the experts

Abnormal renal CT scan

This photograph of a renal computed tomography (CT) scan reveals a renal adenocarcinoma that has displaced and distorted the right kidney and that now exceeds the kidney in size. The left kidney appears normal, the spine is sharp and white in the center of the photograph, and the stomach is equally clear at the top.

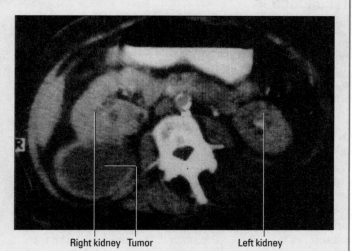

Right kidney Tumor   Left kidney

Warning!

Kidney CT scan interference

Artifacts may result from many factors, such as recent contrast studies, foreign bodies, catheters, and surgical clips.

ner, and the patient is instructed to lie still. The scanner rotates around the patient, taking multiple images at different angles.
• When one series of tomograms is complete, an I.V. contrast medium may be administered. Another series of tomograms is then taken. (See *Kidney CT scan interference*.)

Magnetic resonance imaging

MRI of bone and soft tissue

A noninvasive technique, MRI produces clear, sensitive tomographic images of bone and soft tissue. It provides superior contrast of body tissues and allows imaging of multiple planes in regions that can't be easily visualized with X-rays or CT scans.

Magnetic resonance images are easily generated from the proton of the hydrogen atom. Each water molecule has two hydrogen atoms, but the distribution of water molecules varies with the specific body tissue. For example, bone is considered

MRI of bone and soft tissue helps evaluate tumors and identify changes in the bone marrow cavity. It also helps identify spinal disorders.

"dry" because it contains little hydrogen. Consequently, bone produces a weak signal and can't be visualized. Normal bone marrow has the brightest signal and can be seen well.

What it all means

MRI should reveal no pathology in bone, muscles, and joints.

MRI is an excellent method for visualizing disease of the spinal canal and cord and for identifying primary and metastatic bone tumors. It's useful in providing anatomic delineation of muscles, ligaments, and bones. The images show superior contrast of body tissues and sharply define healthy, benign, and malignant tissues.

What needs to be done

• First, make sure the scanner can accommodate the patient's weight and abdominal girth. Explain to the patient that this test assesses bone and soft tissue. Tell him that the test takes 30 to 90 minutes. Explain that a contrast medium may be used.
• The patient is placed on a narrow, padded table that moves into the scanner tunnel. Fans continuously circulate air in the tunnel, and an intercom is used to maintain verbal contact with the technician. The patient must remain still.
• While the patient lies within the strong magnetic field, the area to be studied is stimulated with RF waves. The MRI computer measures resulting energy changes at these body sections and uses them to generate images. The images resemble two-dimensional slices through the tissues, bone, or organs.
• Provide comfort measures and pain medication, as needed, because of prolonged positioning in the scanner.
• If the patient is unstable, make sure all equipment is compatible with MRI imaging. If necessary, monitor his oxygen saturation, cardiac rhythm, and respiratory status during the test.

Cardiac MRI helps detect congenital heart disease, valvular heart disease, and vascular disease such as thoracic aneurysm. It also helps detect cardiac tumors and structural anomalies.

MRI of the cardiovascular system

A great asset in diagnosing cardiac disorders, MRI can see through bone and delineate fluid-filled soft tissue in great detail as well as produce images of organs and vessels in motion. For this noninvasive procedure, the patient is placed in a magnetic field and cross-sectional images of the anatomy are viewed in multiple planes and recorded for a permanent record.

What it all means

MRI should reveal no anatomic or structural dysfunctions in cardiovascular tissue.

MRI can detect cardiomyopathy and pericardial disease as well as atrial or ventricular septal defects and other congenital defects. The test also can be used to identify paracardiac or intracardiac masses and evaluate the extent of pericardial or vascular disease.

What needs to be done

• Explain the procedure to the patient. Tell him the test takes up to 90 minutes.
• The patient is placed supine on a padded, nonmetallic bed, which slides to the desired position inside the scanner. RF energy is directed at the patient's chest. The resulting images appear on a monitor and are recorded on film or magnetic tape. During the procedure, the patient must remain still.
• Monitor the sedated patient's hemodynamic, cardiac, respiratory, and mental status until the sedative effects have worn off.
• If the patient is unstable, make sure that all equipment is compatible with MRI imaging. If necessary, monitor the patient's oxygen saturation, cardiac rhythm, and respiratory status during the test.

MRI of the neurologic system

Like CT, MRI produces cross-sectional images of the brain and spine in multiple planes. The greatest advantage of an MRI is its ability to "see through" bone and to delineate fluid-filled soft tissue. The magnetic fields and RF energy used for MRI are imperceptible to the patient; no harmful effects have been documented.

What it all means

MRI can show details of the normal central nervous system anatomy in any plane, without interference from bone. Brain and spinal cord structures should appear distinct and sharply defined.

Represents dense tissues

Because the MRI signal represents the proton density (water content) of tissue, MRI shows structural changes resulting from disorders that increase tissue water content, such as cerebral edema, demyelinating disease, and pontine and cerebellar tumors.

What needs to be done

• Explain the procedure to the patient. Tell him it takes up to 90 minutes and that a radioactive contrast dye may be used.

MRI of the neurologic system helps identify intracranial lesions and diagnose spinal lesions and soft-tissue abnormalities.

• The patient is placed in the supine position on a narrow bed, which moves to the desired position inside the scanner. RF energy is directed at his head or spine; the resulting images are displayed on a monitor and recorded on film or magnetic tape. The patient must remain still during the procedure.

Quick quiz

1. Before CT involving a contrast medium, you should ask the patient whether he's allergic to:
    A.   shellfish.
    B.   nuts.
    C.   penicillin.

Answer: A. Before CT, you should question the patient about allergies to shellfish, iodine, and contrast media.

2. Hypersensitivity reactions to I.V. contrast medium, such as respiratory distress, urticaria, and rash, usually develop within:
    A.   10 minutes.
    B.   30 minutes.
    C.   60 minutes.

Answer: B. Hypersensitivity reactions usually develop within 30 minutes of contrast medium injection.

3. You're caring for a comatose, head-injured patient who requires mechanical ventilation. Which test is most appropriate for evaluating this patient's brain tissues?
    A.   Skull X-rays
    B.   MRI of the neurologic system
    C.   CT of the intracranium

Answer: C. Although MRI has surpassed CT scanning in diagnosing neurologic disorders, CT can be performed when the patient is on a ventilator, whereas MRI can't.

Scoring

☆☆☆   If you answered all three questions correctly, congratulations on a magnetic and resounding success!

☆☆   If you answered two questions correctly, super! You've done a good job of computing tomographies!

☆   If you answered just one question correctly, don't let it affect your self-image! You'll get the hang of it in no time!

(13)

Nuclear medicine scans

Just the facts

In this chapter, you'll learn:

♦ about nuclear medicine scans

♦ what patient care is associated with each procedure

♦ what factors can interfere with test results

♦ what test results may indicate.

A look at nuclear medicine scans

In nuclear medicine scans, a radiopharmaceutical agent is inhaled or injected. A specialized camera detects the amount and changing distribution of the agent in the area or organ, and feeds the information into a computer. The computer then processes the data and produces two-dimensional images for immediate visualization, which are analyzed to diagnose certain conditions.

Explain the procedure to the patient in easily understood terms. Make sure he or a responsible family member has signed a consent form, if necessary.

Lung perfusion scan

A lung perfusion scan produces a visual image of pulmonary blood flow after I.V. injection of a macroaggregated albumin bonded to technetium. This test is useful for confirming pulmonary vascular obstruction such as pulmonary or septic emboli. When performed in addition to a lung ventilation scan, this scan assesses ventilation-perfusion ratios.

A lung perfusion scan helps assess arterial perfusion. It's also useful for detecting pulmonary emboli and evaluating lung function before resection.

Warning!

Lung perfusion scan interference

• Scheduling the patient for more than one radionuclide test per day (especially if different trace substances are used) can inhibit diffusion of the radioactive substance in the second test.
• I.V. injection of the radiopharmaceutical while the patient is sitting can produce abnormal images because many particles settle to the lung bases.
• Such conditions as chronic obstructive pulmonary disease, vasculitis, pulmonary edema, tumor, sickle cell disease, and parasitic disease may cause abnormal perfusion, affecting the accuracy of test results.

Memory jogger

How can you remember the difference between hot spots and cold spots? Simple: Think about the weather. When it's **hot** outside, the temperature is **high**. So, **hot spots** have a **high** uptake of radioactive substance. Similarly, when it's **cold** outside, the temperature is **low**. So **cold spots** have **low** radioactive substance uptake.

What it all means

Hot spots (areas of high radioactive substance uptake) indicate normal blood perfusion. A normal lung shows a uniform uptake pattern. Cold spots (areas of low radioactive substance uptake) indicate poor perfusion, suggesting an embolism; however, a ventilation scan is necessary to confirm the diagnosis. Decreased regional blood flow that occurs without vessel obstruction may indicate pneumonitis.

What needs to be done

• Explain the procedure to the patient. Tell him it takes about 30 minutes.

Smile...you're on candid camera!

• Inform the patient that a radiopharmaceutical will be injected into a vein in his arm.
• With the patient supine and taking moderately deep breaths, the radiopharmaceutical is injected slowly over 5 to 10 seconds.
• After uptake of the radiopharmaceutical, the camera takes a series of single stationary images of the various views of the chest. Images projected on a special screen show the distribution of radioactive particles.
• If a hematoma develops at the injection site, apply warm soaks. (See *Lung perfusion scan interference*.)

Lung ventilation scan

A lung ventilation scan—a nuclear scan performed after inhalation of air mixed with radioactive gas—delineates areas of the lung ventilated during respiration. During the scan, the distribu-

Advice from the experts

Comparing normal and abnormal ventilation scans

The normal ventilation scan on the left, taken 30 minutes to 1 hour after the wash-out phase, shows equal gas distribution. The abnormal scan on the right, taken 1½ to 2 hours after the start of the wash-out phase, shows unequal gas distribution, represented by the area of poor wash-out on both the left and right sides.

Normal scan

Abnormal scan

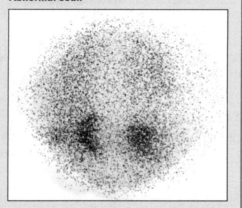

tion of the gas is recorded in three phases: during the buildup of radioactive gas (wash-in phase), after the patient rebreathes from a bag and the radioactivity reaches a steady level (equilibrium phase), and after removal of the radioactive gas from the lungs (wash-out phase). (See *Comparing normal and abnormal ventilation scans.*) In a patient on mechanical ventilation, krypton gas must be substituted for xenon gas, which is usually used during the test. This test is performed in combination with a lung perfusion scan.

What it all means

Gas should be equally distributed in both lungs, and wash-in and wash-out phases should be normal.

It's a gas, gas, gas

Unequal gas distribution in both lungs indicates poor ventilation or airway obstruction in areas with low radioactivity. When compared with a lung perfusion scan, in vascular obstructions such as

Hmmmm…it says here that a lung ventilation scan can help diagnose pulmonary emboli, atelectasis, obstructing tumors, and chronic obstructive pulmonary disease.

pulmonary embolism, perfusion to the embolized area is decreased, but ventilation to this area is maintained; in parenchymal diseases such as pneumonia, both ventilation and perfusion are abnormal within the areas of consolidation.

What needs to be done

• Explain the procedure to patient. Tell him it takes 15 to 30 minutes.
• Instruct the patient to remove all metal objects in the scanning field. Tell him that he'll be asked to hold his breath for a short time after inhaling gas and to remain still while a machine scans his chest.
• After the patient inhales air mixed with a small amount of radioactive gas through a mask, its distribution in the lungs is monitored on a nuclear scanner. The patient's chest is scanned as the gas is exhaled.

Radioactive iodine uptake test

The radioactive iodine uptake (RAIU) test evaluates thyroid function by measuring the amount of orally ingested radioactive isotopes of iodine, ^{123}I or ^{131}I, that accumulate in the thyroid gland after 2, 6, and 24 hours. An external single-counting probe measures the radioactivity in the thyroid as a percentage of the original dose, thus indicating the ability of the gland to trap and retain iodine.

What it all means

After 2 hours, 4% to 12% of the radioactive iodine should have accumulated in the thyroid; after 6 hours, 5% to 20%; after 24 hours, 8% to 29%. The remaining radioactive iodine is excreted in the urine.

Comprehending percentages

Local variations in the normal range of iodine uptake may stem from regional differences in dietary iodine intake or procedural differences among individual laboratories.

Below-normal percentages of iodine uptake may indicate hypothyroidism, subacute thyroiditis, or iodine overload. Above-normal percentages may indicate hyperthyroidism, early Hashimoto's disease, hypoalbuminemia, ingestion of lithium, or iodine-deficient goiter.

However, in hyperthyroidism, the rate of turnover may be so rapid that the 24-hour measurement appears falsely normal.

RAIU testing evaluates thyroid function and, when used with other tests, helps distinguish between primary and secondary thyroid disorders.

Warning!

RAIU test interference

- Renal failure, diuresis, severe diarrhea, radiographic contrast media studies, ingestion of iodine preparations (including iodized salt, cough syrups, and some multivitamins), and other drugs (thyroid hormones, thyroid hormone antagonists, salicylates, penicillins, antihistamines, anticoagulants, corticosteroids, and phenylbutazone) decrease iodine uptake.
- An iodine-deficient diet or phenothiazine use increase iodine uptake.

What needs to be done

- Explain the procedure to the patient. Instruct him to fast from midnight before the test.
- Check the patient history for past or present iodine exposure, which may interfere with test results. If the patient previously had radiologic tests using contrast media or nuclear medicine procedures or if he's currently receiving iodine preparations or thyroid medications, note this on the request.
- At 2, 6, and 24 hours after an oral dose of radioactive iodine is administered, the patient's thyroid is scanned by placing the anterior portion of the patient's neck in front of an external single counting probe. The amount of radioactivity that the probe detects is compared to the amount in the original dose to determine the percentage of radioactive iodine retained by the thyroid.
- As ordered, instruct the patient to resume a light diet 2 hours after taking the oral dose of ^{123}I or ^{131}I. (See *RAIU test interference*.)

Radionuclide thyroid imaging assesses thyroid size, structure, and position and helps evaluate thyroid function.

Radionuclide thyroid imaging

Radionuclide thyroid imaging allows visualization of the thyroid gland by a gamma camera after administration of a radioisotope—usually ^{123}I, ^{131}I, or technetium-99m (^{99m}Tc) pertechnetate. The first two radioisotopes are used most often because of their short half-lives (which limit exposure to radiation) and because of their ability to measure thyroid function.

This test is usually performed concurrently with measurement of serum triiodothyronine (T_3) and serum thyroxine levels and thyroid uptake tests.

Listen up!

Getting ready for radionuclide thyroid imaging

If your patient will undergo radionuclide thyroid imaging, cover the following points to help prepare him for the test.
• Instruct him to stop taking thyroid hormones, thyroid hormone antagonists, iodine preparations (Lugol's solution, some multivitamins, and cough syrups), phenothiazines, and corticosteroids at least 2 to 3 weeks before the test as ordered.
• Tell him to avoid iodized salt, iodinated salt substitutes, and seafood for 14 to 21 days.
• Instruct him to discontinue liothyronine, propylthiouracil, and methimazole 3 days before the test and to discontinue thyroxine 10 days before the test.

What it all means

Radionuclide thyroid imaging should reveal a thyroid gland that's about 2″ (5 cm) long and 1″ (2.5 cm) wide, with a uniform uptake of the radioisotope and without tumors. The gland should be butterfly-shaped, with the isthmus located at the midline. Occasionally, a third lobe called the pyramidal lobe may be present; this is a normal variant.

Where's the hot spot?

During radionuclide thyroid imaging, hyperfunctioning nodules (areas of excessive iodine uptake) appear as black regions called hot spots. The presence of hot spots requires a follow-up T_3 (Cytomel) thyroid suppression test to determine whether the hyperfunctioning areas are autonomous.

Hey, cool!

Hypofunctioning nodules (areas of little or no iodine uptake) appear as white or light gray regions called cold spots. If a cold spot appears, thyroid ultrasonography may be performed later to rule out cysts; in addition, fine-needle aspiration and biopsy of such nodules may be performed to rule out a malignant tumor.

What needs to be done

• Explain the procedure to the patient. If he's scheduled to receive an oral dose of ^{123}I or ^{131}I, instruct him to fast after midnight the night before the test. Tell him the actual imaging takes only 30 minutes.

Warning!

Thyroid imaging interference

• An iodine-deficient diet and phenothiazine use increase radioactive iodine uptake.
• Renal disease, iodized salt, iodinated salt substitutes, cough syrups containing inorganic iodides, multivitamins, seafood, and use of thyroid hormones, thyroid hormone antagonists, and corticosteroids decrease radioactive iodine uptake.
• Severe diarrhea and vomiting also can decrease uptake (by impairing GI absorption of radioiodine).

• Check the patient history for tests within the past 60 days that used radiographic contrast media. Note such tests or the use of drugs that may interfere with iodine uptake on the radiograph request. (See *Getting ready for radionuclide thyroid imaging*.)
• The test is performed 24 hours after oral administration of ^{123}I or ^{131}I or 20 to 30 minutes after I.V. injection of ^{99m}Tc pertechnetate. Just before the test, tell the patient to remove his dentures and any jewelry that could interfere with visualization of the thyroid.
• The patient's thyroid gland is palpated. Then, with the patient in a supine position and his neck extended, the gamma camera is placed over the anterior portion of his neck. The radioactive substance within the thyroid gland projects an image of the gland on a display screen and X-ray film. Three views of the thyroid are obtained: one straight-on anterior view and two bilateral oblique views. (See *Thyroid imaging interference*.)

Technetium-99m pyrophosphate scanning

Technetium-99m (99mTc) pyrophosphate scanning (also known as hot spot myocardial imaging and infarct avid imaging) is used to detect recent myocardial infarction (MI) and to determine its extent. In this test, an I.V. tracer isotope (99mTc pyrophosphate) is injected into a vein. The isotope accumulates in damaged myocardial tissue (possibly by combining with calcium in the damaged myocardial cells), where it forms a hot spot on a scan.

What it all means

A normal technetium scan shows no isotope in the myocardium. The isotope is taken up by the sternum and ribs, and activity there is compared with the heart's; 2+, 3+, and 4+ activity (equal to or greater than bone) indicates a positive myocardial scan. The technetium scan can reveal areas of isotope accumulation (hot spots) in damaged myocardium, particularly 48 to 72 hours after onset of acute MI; however, hot spots are apparent as early as 12 hours after acute MI. In most MI patients, hot spots disappear after 1 week; in some, they persist for several months if necrosis continues in the infarction area.

What needs to be done

• Explain the procedure to the patient. Tell him who will perform the 30- to 60-minute test.
• Usually, 20 mCi of ^{99m}Tc pyrophosphate is injected into the antecubital vein. After 2 to 3 hours, the patient is placed in the supine position, and electrocardiogram (ECG) electrodes are attached for

Deductive reasoning is powerful, but sometimes you need a technetium scan! This test confirms and defines the size and location of a recent MI.

continuous monitoring during the test. Scans are usually taken with the patient in several positions, including anterior, left anterior oblique, right anterior oblique, and left lateral. Each scan takes 10 minutes. (See *99mTc pyrophosphate scan interference*.)

Thallium imaging

Thallium imaging (also called cardiac nuclear imaging, cold spot myocardial imaging, or myocardial perfusion scan) evaluates blood flow after I.V. injection of the radioisotope thallium-201 or Cardiolyte. Areas with poor blood flow and ischemic cells fail to take up the isotope and thus appear as cold spots on a scan.

What it all means

Thallium imaging should show normal distribution of the isotope throughout the left ventricle and no defects (cold spots). The results may be normal if the patient has narrowed coronary arteries but adequate collateral circulation.

Persistent defects indicate MI; transient defects (those that disappear after a 3- to 6-hour rest) indicate ischemia caused by coronary artery disease. After coronary artery bypass surgery, improved regional perfusion suggests patency of the graft. Increased perfusion after ingestion of antianginal drugs can show that the drugs relieve ischemia. Improved perfusion after balloon angioplasty suggests increased coronary flow.

What needs to be done

- The procedure varies with the type of imaging.
- Explain to the patient that this test helps determine whether any areas of the heart muscle aren't receiving an adequate supply of blood. (See *Teaching about thallium imaging*.)

Thallium imaging assesses the location and extent of an MI. It also evaluates graft patency and the effectiveness of antianginal therapy or balloon angioplasty.

Stressin' out

- For stress imaging, instruct the patient to restrict alcohol, tobacco, and nonprescription medications for 24 hours and to have nothing by mouth after midnight the night before the test. Tell him that initial testing takes 45 to 90 minutes and that additional scans may be required.
- Tell the patient he'll receive a radioactive tracer I.V. and that multiple images of his heart will be scanned.
- For stress imaging, instruct the patient to wear walking shoes during the treadmill exercise and to report fatigue, pain, or shortness of breath immediately.

Stress imaging

- The patient, wired with electrodes, walks on a treadmill at a regulated pace that's gradually increased while his ECG, blood pressure, and heart rate are monitored. When the patient reaches peak stress, the examiner injects thallium into the antecubital vein, then flushes it with normal saline solution or an infusion of Cardiolyte. The patient exercises an additional 45 to 60 seconds to permit circulation and uptake of the isotope and then lies on his back under the camera. If the patient is asymptomatic, the precordial leads are removed. Scanning begins after 10 minutes, with the patient in anterior, left anterior oblique, and left lateral positions. Additional scans may be taken after the patient rests and occasionally after 24 hours. Taking a scan after the patient rests is helpful in differentiating between an ischemic area and an infarcted or scarred area of the myocardium.

> Thallium imaging is contraindicated in pregnancy, impaired neuromuscular function, acute MI or myocarditis, aortic stenosis, acute infection, unstable metabolic conditions, digoxin toxicity, and recent pulmonary infarction.

Listen up!

Teaching about thallium imaging

Explain to the patient that the thallium imaging test can be performed either in a resting state or after stress.

   Resting imaging can detect acute myocardial infarction (MI) within the first few hours of symptoms but doesn't distinguish an old from a new infarct. *Stress imaging* is performed after the patient exercises on a treadmill to the point of angina or rate-limiting fatigue. It can assess known or suspected coronary artery disease and evaluate the effectiveness of antianginal therapy or balloon angioplasty. It's also used to determine graft patency after coronary artery bypass surgery. Complications of stress testing include arrhythmias, angina pectoris, and MI.

Warning!

Thallium scan interference

- Cold spots may result from sarcoidosis, myocardial fibrosis, cardiac contusion, attenuation caused by soft tissue and artifacts (for example, diaphragm, implants, breast, electrodes), apical cleft, or coronary spasm.
- Absence of cold spots in a patient with coronary artery disease may result from an insignificant obstruction, inadequate stress, delayed imaging, single-vessel disease (particularly the right or left circumflex coronary arteries), or collateral circulation.

Resting imaging

- Within the first few hours of MI symptoms, the patient receives an injection of thallium I.V. or Cardiolyte. Scanning begins after 10 minutes, with the patient positioned as described previously.
- If further scanning is required, have the patient rest and restrict foods and beverages other than water. (See *Thallium scan interference.*)

Bone scan

A bone scan permits imaging of the skeleton by a scanning camera after I.V. injection of a radioactive tracer compound. The tracer of choice, ^{99m}Tc diphosphonate, collects in bone tissue in increased concentrations at sites of abnormal metabolism. When scanned, these sites appear as hot spots that are often detectable months before radiography can reveal a lesion.

What it all means

The tracer concentrates on bone tissue at sites of new bone formation or increased metabolism. The epiphyses of growing bone are normal sites of high concentration. (See *Comparing normal and abnormal bone scans.*)

Although a bone scan demonstrates hot spots that identify sites of bone formation, it doesn't distinguish between normal and abnormal bone formation. However, scan results can identify all types of bone cancer, infection, fracture, and other disor-

> A bone scan can detect bone cancer, bone trauma associated with pathologic fractures, and infection. It also helps stage cancer and monitor degenerative bone disorders.

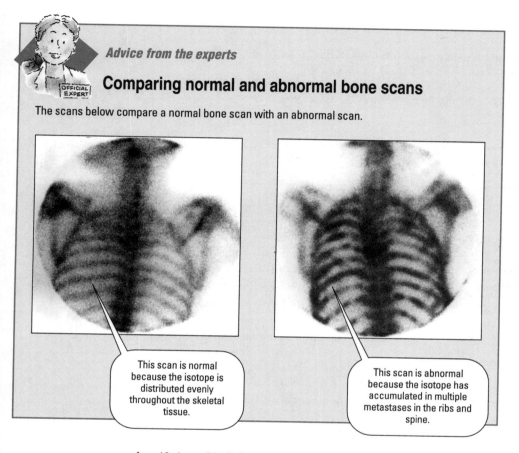

Advice from the experts

Comparing normal and abnormal bone scans

The scans below compare a normal bone scan with an abnormal scan.

> This scan is normal because the isotope is distributed evenly throughout the skeletal tissue.

> This scan is abnormal because the isotope has accumulated in multiple metastases in the ribs and spine.

ders if viewed in light of the patient's medical and surgical history, radiographic findings, and laboratory test results.

What needs to be done

• Explain the procedure to the patient. In the interval between tracer injection and actual scanning (about 1 to 3 hours), advise him to drink lots of fluids.

• Position the patient on the scanner table.

• As the scanner head moves over the patient's body, it detects low-level radiation emitted by the skeleton and translates this into a film or paper chart, or both, to produce two-dimensional pictures of the area scanned. The patient may have to be repositioned several times during the test to obtain adequate views.

• Check the injection site for redness and swelling.

• Don't schedule other radionuclide tests for this patient for the next 24 to 48 hours.

Hydration station

• Instruct the patient to drink lots of fluids and to empty his bladder frequently for the next 24 to 48 hours.
• Provide analgesics, as needed, for pain resulting from positioning on the scanning table. (See *Bone scan interference*.)

Warning!

Bone scan interference

• Antihypertensives may affect test results.
• A distended bladder may obscure pelvic detail.

Quick quiz

1. A lung perfusion scan is useful for detecting:
  A. obstructing tumors.
  B. chronic obstructive pulmonary disease.
  C. pulmonary emboli.

Answer: C. A lung perfusion scan helps assess arterial perfusion of the lungs. Therefore, it's useful for detecting pulmonary emboli.

2. What dietary instructions should you give the patient who will be undergoing RAIU testing?
  A. Resume a light diet 2 hours after taking the oral dose of ^{123}I or ^{131}I.
  B. Fast after midnight before the test.
  C. No dietary restrictions are necessary before the test.

Answer: A. As ordered, instruct the patient to resume a light diet 2 hours after taking the oral dose of ^{123}I or ^{131}I. After the complete study, he can resume his normal diet.

3. In most patients who have had an MI, hot spots on a technetium scan disappear after:
  A. 12 hours.
  B. 72 hours.
  C. 1 week.

Answer: C. Typically, hot spots disappear 1 week after MI. In some patients, they persist for several months if necrosis continues in the infarction area.

Scoring

☆☆☆ If you answered all three questions correctly, outstanding! You're a nuclear power plant!
☆☆ If you answered two questions correctly, not bad! You know how to tell fact from fission!
☆ If you answered only one question correctly, don't worry! You just need to build on the nucleus of knowledge you already have!

Monitoring, catheterization, and miscellaneous tests

Just the facts

In this chapter, you'll learn:

♦ about monitoring, catheterization, and miscellaneous tests

♦ what patient care is associated with each procedure

♦ what factors can interfere with test results

♦ what test results may indicate.

A look at monitoring, catheterization, and miscellaneous tests

Monitoring, catheterization, and miscellaneous tests help diagnose various disorders, evaluate the effectiveness of treatment, and identify complications. Before the patient undergoes testing, explain the procedure in terms he can easily understand. Make sure an informed consent form has been signed, if necessary. These tests may cause anxiety, so be sure to provide emotional support.

Monitoring tests

External fetal monitoring

In external fetal monitoring, a noninvasive test, an electronic transducer and a cardiotachymeter amplify and record the fetal heart rate (FHR) while a pressure-sensitive transducer—the toko-dynamometer—simultaneously records uterine contractions. This procedure records the baseline FHR (average FHR over two contraction cycles or 10 minutes), periodic fluctuations in the baseline FHR, and beat-to-beat heart rate variability.

What it all means

Normally, FHR baseline ranges from 120 to 160 beats/minute, with 5 to 25 beats/minute variability.

Low fetal heart rate

Bradycardia—an FHR of less than 120 beats/minute—may indicate fetal heart block, malposition, or hypoxia. Fetal bradycardia may also be drug-induced.

Rapid fetal heart rate

Tachycardia—an FHR of more than 160 beats/minute—may result from vagolytic drugs; maternal fever, tachycardia, or hyperthyroidism; early fetal hypoxia; or fetal infection or arrhythmia.

External fetal monitoring helps measure FHR and the frequency of uterine contractions. It also evaluates fetal health during stressful and nonstressful situations.

Less fluctuation

Decreased variability—FHR fluctuation of less than 5 beats/minute—may stem from fetal cardiac arrhythmia or heart block, vagolytic drugs, fetal hypoxia, central nervous system (CNS) malformation, or infection. FHR accelerations may result from early hypoxia. They may precede or follow variable decelerations and may indicate a breech position.

Nonstressful situation

During an antepartum nonstress test, the fetus is considered healthy and should remain so for another week if two fetal movements associated with FHR acceleration of more than 15 beats/minute from baseline occur within 20 minutes. Nonstress testing is also done for postdate fetal well-being. A normal healthy fetus usually has three FHR rises in 10 to 15 minutes, but a fetus may sleep up to 45 minutes at a time. A positive nonstress test result (fewer than two FHR accelerations of more than 15 seconds each, with a heart rate acceleration over 15 beats/minute) indicates an exaggerated risk of perinatal morbidity and mortality and usually necessitates a contraction stress test (CST). However, the CST produces a high rate of false-positive results.

What needs to be done

• Explain the procedure to the patient. If monitoring will be performed antepartum, instruct her to eat a meal just before the test to increase fetal activity, which decreases the test time. If the patient is still smoking, advise her to abstain for 2 hours before testing because smoking decreases fetal activity.

- Place the patient in the semi-Fowler or left lateral position with her abdomen exposed. Cover the ultrasonic transducer with ultrasound transmission gel. After palpating the abdomen to identify the fetal chest area, locate the most distinct fetal heart sounds and secure the ultrasound transducer over this area with the elastic band, stockinette, or abdominal strap. Check the recordings to ensure an adequate printout, and verify the fetal monitor's alarm boundaries.

Chasin' the baseline

- If the patient is undergoing antepartum monitoring with a nonstress test, tell her to hold the pressure transducer in her hand and push it each time she feels the fetus move. Within a 20-minute period, monitor the baseline FHR until you record two fetal movements of more than 15 seconds each and cause heart rate accelerations of more than 15 beats/minute from the baseline. If you can't obtain two FHR accelerations, wait 30 minutes, shake the patient's abdomen to stimulate the fetus, and repeat the test.

Contraction action

- If the patient is undergoing intrapartum monitoring, secure the pressure transducer with an elastic band, stockinette, or abdominal strap over the area of greatest uterine electrical activity during contractions (usually the fundus). Adjust the machine to record 0 to 10 mm Hg pressure between palpable contractions. Review the tracing frequently. Record maternal movement, drug administration, and procedures performed directly on the tracing so tracing changes can be evaluated in view of these activities. Report abnormalities immediately. (See *External fetal monitoring interference*.)
- As labor progresses, reposition the pressure transducer as needed so it remains on the fundal portion of the uterus. You may also need to reposition the ultrasonic transducer as fetal position changes.

Warning!

External fetal monitoring interference

- Maternal obesity or excessive maternal or fetal activity may inhibit recording of uterine contractions or fetal heart rate (FHR).
- Drugs that affect the sympathetic and parasympathetic nervous systems may depress FHR.

Internal fetal monitoring

For internal fetal monitoring, an invasive procedure, an electrode attached directly to the fetal scalp measures the FHR—especially its beat-to-beat variability—and a fluid-filled catheter placed in the uterine cavity measures the frequency and pressure of uterine contractions. This procedure is performed exclusively during labor, after the membranes have ruptured and the cervix has dilated 1¼″ (3.2 cm), with the fetal head lower than the –2 station.

Maternal risks (perforated uterus or intrauterine infection) and fetal risk (scalp abscess or hematoma) are minimal.

What it all means

Normally, FHR ranges from 120 to 160 beats/minute, with a variability of 5 to 25 beats/minute from FHR baseline. (See *Normal intrauterine pressure readings during labor.*)

Slowin' down

Bradycardia—an FHR below 120 beats/minute—may indicate fetal heart block, malposition, hypoxia, or maternal ingestion of certain drugs, such as propranolol or narcotic analgesics.

Speedin' up

Tachycardia—an FHR above 160 beats/minute—may result from maternal use of vagolytic drugs, early fetal hypoxia, fetal infection or arrhythmia, prematurity, or maternal fever, tachycardia, or hyperthyroidism.

Even-keeled

Decreased variability—fluctuation of fewer than 5 beats/minute from FHR baseline—may result from maternal use of vagolytic drugs, fetal cardiac arrhythmia or heart block, or fetal hypoxia, CNS malformation, or infection.

Slowin' down early

Early decelerations (FHR slowing at contraction onset, with recovery to baseline not greater than 15 seconds after completion of

A valuable tool for evaluating intrapartal fetal health, internal fetal monitoring helps assess FHR and the frequency and pressure of uterine contractions.

Advice from the experts

Normal intrauterine pressure readings during labor

Stage of labor	Contractions per 10 minutes	Baseline pressure	Pressure during contraction
Prelabor	1 to 2	None	25 to 40 mm Hg
First stage	3 to 5	8 to 12 mm Hg	30 to 40 mm Hg (or higher)
Second stage	5	10 to 20 mm Hg	50 to 80 mm Hg

the uterine contraction) are related to fetal head compression and usually mean the fetus is healthy.

Slowin' down late

Late decelerations (FHR slowing, with onset after the contraction starts, a lag time greater than 20 seconds, and a recovery time greater than 15 seconds) may indicate uteroplacental insufficiency, fetal hypoxia, or acidosis.

What needs to be done

- Prepare for two separate procedures: electrode insertion for fetal heart rate monitoring and probe insertion for monitoring contractions.
- Explain the procedure to the patient.

Picking up the FHR

- Place the patient in the dorsal lithotomy position, and prepare her perineal area for a vaginal examination. After the vaginal examination, the fetal scalp is palpated and an area not over a fontanel is identified. Then the plastic guide tube surrounding the small corkscrew-type electrode is introduced into the cervix, pressed firmly against the fetal scalp, and rotated 180 degrees clockwise to insert the electrode into the scalp. After the electrode wire is tugged slightly to make sure it's attached properly, the tube is withdrawn, leaving the electrode in place.
- Next, a leg plate with a conduction medium is strapped to the mother's thigh. Electrode wires are attached to the leg plate, and a cable from the leg plate is plugged into the fetal monitor. To check proper placement of the scalp electrode, the monitor is turned on and the electrocardiogram (ECG) button is pressed; an FHR signal indicates proper electrode attachment. (See *Understanding internal fetal monitoring,* page 374.)

Converting contractions

- *To measure uterine contractions:* Before inserting the uterine catheter, fill it with sterile normal saline solution to prevent air emboli. Ask the patient to breathe deeply through her mouth and relax her abdominal muscles. After the vagina has been examined and the fetal presenting part has been palpated, the fluid-filled catheter and catheter guide are inserted ⅜" to ¾" (1 to 2 cm) into the cervix, usually between the fetal head and the posterior cervix. The catheter is then gently inserted into the uterus until the black mark on the catheter is flush with the vulva. (The catheter guide should *never* be passed deeply into the uterus.) Next, the guide is removed and the catheter is connected to a transducer that converts the intrauterine pressure, as measured

374

Now I get it!

Understanding internal fetal monitoring

In internal fetal monitoring, an electrode is attached to the fetal scalp. The resultant fetal electrocardiograms (FECGs) are transmitted to an amplifier. A cardiotachometer then measures the interval between FECGs and plots a continuous fetal heart rate (FHR) graph, which is displayed on a two-channel oscilloscope screen. Intrauterine catheters attached to a transducer in the leg plate measure the frequency and pressure of uterine contractions, which are plotted below the FHR graph.

Warning!

Internal fetal monitoring interference

Drugs that affect the parasympathetic and sympathetic nervous systems may influence fetal heart rate.

by fluid in the catheter, to an electrical signal. To standardize pressure readings, the transducer is exposed to air (it should measure zero pressure). The system is then closed to the air, and intrauterine pressure readings are checked.

• After removal of the fetal scalp electrode, apply antiseptic or antibiotic solution to the attachment site and watch for signs of fetal scalp abscess or maternal intrauterine infection. (See *Internal fetal monitoring interference.*)

Contraction stress test

The contraction stress test (CST), also known as the oxytocin challenge test, measures the fetus's ability to withstand decreased oxygen supply and the stress of contractions induced before actual labor begins. Oxytocin is infused to stimulate uterine contractions while the FHR is assessed to evaluate the placenta's ability to provide sufficient oxygen to the fetus.

What it all means

A negative result occurs when FHR is within normal range (120 to 160 beats/minute), indicating that the fetus can tolerate the stress of labor.

Asphyxia indicator

Late FHR decelerations during two or more contractions or late decelerations that are inconsistent indicate risk of fetal asphyxia.

What needs to be done

• Explain the procedure to the patient. Inform her that food and fluid will be restricted for 4 to 8 hours before the test.
• Have the patient empty her bladder.
• Assist the patient into a semi-Fowler, side-lying position, and drape her for privacy.
• Monitor the patient's blood pressure before and every 10 minutes during the procedure.
• Place the fetal monitor on her abdomen to monitor FHR and the tokodynamometer on the lower abdomen to monitor contractions. A baseline recording is made, and then the FHR is monitored and recorded continuously for 20 minutes.
• An I.V. line is inserted, and I.V. oxytocin (Pitocin) is administered via I.V. pump as ordered. The FHR and contractions are monitored and recorded, and the infusion is discontinued to determine the FHR response to the contractions.
• Encourage the patient to use deep-breathing and relaxation skills while the oxytocin is administered and she feels the contractions.
• Continue to monitor FHR for 30 minutes as uterine movements return to normal.
• If premature labor begins, note the frequency, strength, and length of contractions and prepare for labor or cesarean delivery. (See *CST interference*.)

The CST helps evaluate the fetus's hypoxia risk and ability to withstand uterine contractions. It also helps assess whether the placenta can supply sufficient oxygen to the fetus.

Warning!

CST interference

• Maternal hypotension can produce false-positive results.
• A full bladder can displace the uterus, interfering with monitoring.

Electroencephalography

In EEG, electrodes attached to standard areas of the patient's scalp record a portion of the brain's electrical activity. These electrical impulses are transmitted to an electroencephalograph, which magnifies them 1 million times and records them as brain waves on moving strips of paper.

EEG diagnoses epilepsy and intracranial lesions and confirms brain death.

What it all means

EEG records a portion of the brain's electrical activity as waves; some are irregular, whereas others demonstrate common patterns. Among the basic waveforms are the alpha, beta, theta, and delta rhythms. (See *Comparing EEG tracings.*) Usually, a 100′ to 200′ (30.5- to 61-m) strip of the recording is evaluated, with special focus on basic waveforms, symmetry of cerebral activity, transient discharges, and response to stimulation. A specific diagnosis depends on the patient's clinical status.

Losing consciousness

EEG may reveal epilepsy, absence seizures, generalized tonic-clonic seizures, temporal lobe epilepsy, focal seizures, intracranial lesions (such as tumors or abscesses), or vascular lesions (such as cerebral infarcts and intracranial hemorrhages). Generally, any condition that causes a diminishing level of consciousness alters the EEG pattern in proportion to the degree of consciousness lost.

What needs to be done

• Explain the procedure to the patient. Tell him to restrict caffeine intake before the test.
• Thoroughly wash and dry the patient's hair to remove hair sprays, creams, or oils. Check his medication history for drugs that may interfere with test results.
• If a sleep EEG is ordered, keep the patient awake the night before the test and, as ordered for some patients, administer a sedative (such as chloral hydrate) to help him sleep during the test.
• The patient is positioned comfortably, and electrodes are attached to his scalp. Before the recording procedure begins, the patient is instructed to close his eyes, relax, and remain still. During the recording, the patient is carefully observed through a window in an adjoining room. Blinking, swallowing, talking, or other movements that may cause artifacts are noted. The recording may be stopped periodically to let the patient reposition himself and get comfortable. (See *Wrap your brain around EEG techniques*, page 378.)

Advice from the experts

Comparing EEG tracings

The EEG tracings below compare a normal tracing with tracings associated with various seizure types.

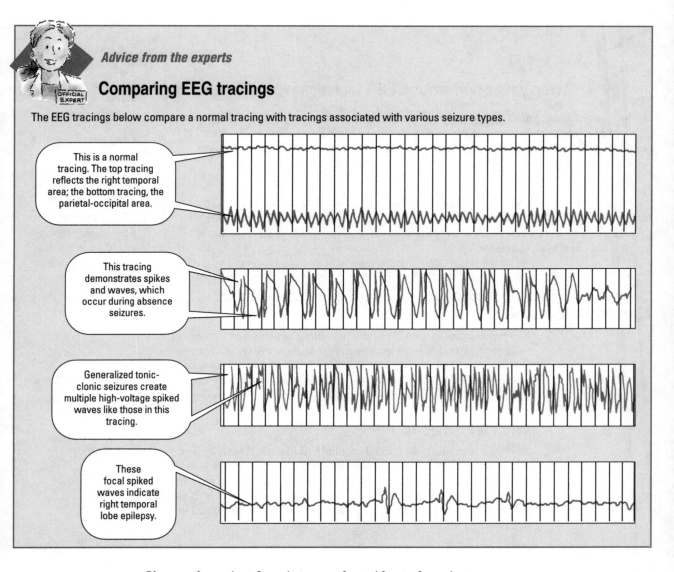

This is a normal tracing. The top tracing reflects the right temporal area; the bottom tracing, the parietal-occipital area.

This tracing demonstrates spikes and waves, which occur during absence seizures.

Generalized tonic-clonic seizures create multiple high-voltage spiked waves like those in this tracing.

These focal spiked waves indicate right temporal lobe epilepsy.

• Observe the patient for seizures, and provide a safe environment.
• If the test is done to confirm brain death in a comatose patient, provide emotional support for the family. (See *EEG interference,* page 378.)

Now I get it!

Wrap your brain around EEG techniques

During an EEG, your patient may be asked to perform certain stress-producing activities so brain wave patterns can be documented. For example, he may be asked to hyperventilate (breathe deeply and rapidly for 3 minutes) to produce brain wave patterns typical of seizure disorders or other abnormalities. This technique is commonly used to detect absence seizures.

Light the way
Photic stimulation, another EEG technique, tests central cerebral activity in response to bright light, accentuating abnormal activity in the absence of myoclonic seizures. In this procedure, a strobe light in front of the patient flashes 1 to 20 times per second. Recordings are made with the patient's eyes opened and closed.

Warning!

EEG interference

• Anticonvulsants, tranquilizers, barbiturates, and other sedatives may cause inaccurate test results.
• Acute drug intoxication or severe hypothermia resulting in loss of consciousness causes a flat EEG.

Electromyography

Electromyography (EMG) is the recording of electrical activity of selected skeletal muscle groups at rest and during voluntary contraction. In this test, a needle electrode is inserted percutaneously into a muscle. The muscle's electrical discharge (or motor unit potential) is then measured and displayed on an oscilloscope screen.

What it all means

At rest, a normal muscle exhibits minimal electrical activity. During voluntary contraction, however, electrical activity increases markedly. A sustained contraction or one of increasing strength produces a rapid "train" of motor unit potentials that can be heard as a crescendo of sounds, similar to the sound of an outboard motor, over the audio amplifier.

Catching a wave

Closely spaced waveforms indicate a high frequency; widely spaced waveforms signify a low frequency. In primary muscle disease, such as muscular dystrophies, motor unit potentials are short (low amplitude), with frequent, irregular discharges. In such disorders as amyotrophic lateral sclerosis and peripheral nerve disorders, motor unit potentials are isolated and irregular but show increased amplitude and duration. In myasthenia gravis, motor unit potentials may be normal initially but diminish in amplitude progressively with continuing contractions. The interpreter

EMG is used to diagnose neuromuscular disorders and spinal nerve disorders.

distinguishes waveforms that indicate a muscle disorder from those indicating denervation.

What needs to be done

• Explain the procedure to the patient. The doctor may forbid cigarettes, coffee, tea, and cola for 2 to 3 hours before the test.
• Tell the patient the test takes at least 1 hour.
• Check his history for medications that may interfere with test results.

That's some signal!

• The patient lies on a stretcher or bed or sits on a chair, depending on the muscles to be tested. The arm or leg is positioned so the muscle to be tested is at rest. The skin is cleaned with alcohol, the needle electrodes are quickly inserted into the selected muscle, and a metal plate is placed under the patient to serve as a reference electrode. The muscle's resulting electrical signal (motor unit potential), recorded during rest and contraction, is amplified 1 million times and displayed on an oscilloscope screen or computer screen. Recorder leadwires are usually attached to an audio-amplifier so voltage fluctuations within the muscle can be heard.
• If the patient experiences residual pain, apply warm compresses and administer analgesics, as ordered. (See *EMG interference*.)

Warning!

EMG interference

Drugs that affect myoneural junctions, such as cholinergics, anticholinergics, and skeletal muscle relaxants, interfere with electromyography (EMG) results.

Electrocardiography

ECG, the most commonly used test for evaluating cardiac status, graphically records the electrical current (electrical potential) generated by the heart. This current radiates from the heart in all directions and, on reaching the skin, is measured by electrodes connected to an amplifier and strip chart recorder. The standard resting ECG uses five electrodes to measure the electrical potential from 12 different leads: the standard limb leads (I, II, III), the augmented limb leads (aV_F, aV_L, and aV_R), and the precordial, or chest, leads (V_1 through V_6).

ECG tracings normally consist of three identifiable waveforms: the P wave, the QRS complex, and the T wave. The P wave depicts atrial depolarization; the QRS complex, ventricular depolarization; and the T wave, ventricular repolarization.

Computerized ECG machines use small electrode tabs that peel off a sheet and adhere to the patient's skin. The entire ECG tracing is displayed on a screen so ab-

ECG helps identify primary conduction abnormalities, cardiac arrhythmias, cardiac hypertrophy, pericarditis, electrolyte imbalance, myocardial ischemia, and myocardial infarction site and extent. It also helps evaluate the effectiveness of cardiac drugs.

Advice from the experts

Normal ECG waveforms

Because each electrocardiogram (ECG) lead takes a different view of heart activity, it generates its own characteristic tracing. The traces shown here represent each of the 12 leads. Leads aV_R, V_1, V_2, and V_3 normally show strong negative deflections below the baseline. Negative deflections indicate that the electrical current flows away from the positive electrode; positive deflections, that the current flows toward the positive electrode.

normalities can be corrected before printing; then it's printed on one sheet of paper. Electrode tabs can remain on the patient's chest, arms, and legs to provide continuous lead placement for serial ECG studies.

What it all means

The lead II waveform, known as the rhythm strip, depicts the heart's rhythm more clearly than any other waveform. (See *Normal ECG waveforms*.)

In lead II, the normal P wave doesn't exceed 2.5 mm (0.25 mV) in height or last longer than 0.11 second. The PR interval, which includes the P wave and PR segment, persists for 0.12 to 0.2 second for cardiac rates over 60 beats/minute. The QT interval varies with the cardiac rate and lasts 0.4 to 0.52 second for rates above 60; R wave voltage in the V_1 through V_6 leads doesn't exceed 27 mm. The total QRS interval lasts 0.06 to 0.1 second.

The lowdown on levels

An abnormal ECG may show myocardial infarction, right or left ventricular hypertrophy, arrhythmias, right or left bundle-branch block, ischemia, conduction defects or pericarditis, electrolyte abnormalities such as hypokalemia, or the effects of cardioactive drugs. Sometimes, an ECG reveals abnormal waveforms only during episodes of angina or during exercise.

What needs to be done

- Explain the procedure to the patient.
- Place the patient in the supine or semi-Fowler position. Expose his chest, both ankles, and both wrists for electrode placement. Drape the female patient's chest until chest leads are applied.
- Place electrodes on the inner aspect of the wrists, the medial aspect of the lower legs, and on the chest. (For the proper chest positions, see *Standard 12-lead ECG*, page 382.) Then connect the leadwires after all electrodes are in place.
- Press the START button and input any required information. The machine will produce a printout showing all 12 leads simultaneously.
- If the wave peaks beyond the top edge of the recording grid, adjust the machine to bring the wave inside the boundaries

Setting the pace

- If the patient has a pacemaker, the ECG may be performed with or without a magnet. Indicate on the request and the patient's record that a pacemaker is present and whether a magnet is used. Many pacemakers function only when the heart rate falls below a

Standard 12-lead ECG

In a standard 12-lead electrocardiogram (ECG), 10 electrodes (4 limb, 6 chest) record the heart's electrical potential from 12 different views, or leads. Lead I connects the left and right arms. Lead II connects the left leg and right arm. Lead III connects the left leg and left arm.

Mind your limbs and Vs

Unipolar augmented limb leads (aV_F, aV_L, and aV_R), which use the same electrode placement as standard limb leads, measure electrical potential between one augmented limb lead and the electrical midpoint of the remaining two leads (determined electronically by the ECG machine). Both standard and augmented leads measure electrical potential while viewing the heart from the front, in a vertical plane.

All walled off

The six unipolar chest leads (V_1 through V_6) shown at right depict the electrical potential from a horizontal plane that helps locate disorders in the heart's lateral, anterior, and posterior walls. The ECG machine averages the electrical potentials of all three limb lead electrodes. Recordings made with the V connection show electrical potential variations that occur under the chest electrode as its position changes.

preset level; a magnet makes the pacemaker fire regularly, which permits evaluation of pacemaker performance.

Exercise electrocardiography

Exercise ECG, commonly known as a stress test, evaluates heart action during physical stress—when oxygen demand increases—and thus provides important diagnostic information that can't be obtained from a resting ECG alone.

In this test, ECG and blood pressure readings are taken while the patient walks on a treadmill or pedals a stationary bicycle and his response to a constant or an increasing workload is observed. Unless complications develop, the test continues until the patient reaches the target heart rate, determined by an established protocol (usually 85% of maximum predicted heart rate for the patient's age and gender) or experiences chest pain or fatigue.

What it all means

In a normal exercise ECG, the P, QRS, and T waves and the ST segment change slightly; a slight ST-segment depression occurs in some patients, especially women. The heart rate rises in direct proportion to the workload and metabolic oxygen demand; systolic blood pressure also rises as workload increases. The normal patient attains endurance levels appropriate for his age and the exercise protocol.

Hypotension resulting from exercise, ST-segment depression of 3 mm or more, downsloping ST segments, and ischemic ST segments appearing within the first 3 minutes of exercise and lasting 8 minutes into the posttest recovery period may indicate multivessel or left coronary artery disease (CAD). ST-segment elevation may indicate dyskinetic left ventricular wall motion or severe transmural ischemia. This test's value in predicting CAD varies with the patient's history and gender.

What needs to be done

- Explain the procedure to the patient. Tell him not to eat, smoke, or drink alcoholic or caffeine-containing beverages for 3 hours before the test. Instruct him to continue his drug regimen unless the doctor directs otherwise.
- Tell the patient to wear comfortable clothing for the procedure.
- The electrode sites are thoroughly cleaned and prepared.
- Electrodes are placed for 12-lead ECG monitoring. The leadwire cable is placed over the patient's shoulder, and the leadwire box is placed on his chest. The cable is secured and the leadwires are connected to the chest electrodes.
- The monitor is started, and a stable baseline tracing is obtained. A blood pressure reading is taken, and the patient is auscultated for S_3 or S_4 gallops and crackles.

Exercise ECG helps screen for asymptomatic CAD, set limitations for an exercise program, and evaluate myocardial perfusion.

Steppin' up

- For the treadmill test, the treadmill is turned on to a slow speed, and the patient is shown how to step onto it and use the support railings to maintain balance but not to support weight. He's instructed to step onto the treadmill, and is kept on a slow speed until he gets used to walking on it. Exercise intensity is increased every 3 minutes by slightly increasing the treadmill speed while raising the incline 3%.

Biking to nowhere

- For the bicycle test, the patient is instructed to sit on the bicycle, not to grip the handlebars tightly, and to pedal until he reaches the desired speed, as shown on the speedometer.

Peak technique

When to stop an exercise ECG

You should stop an exercise electrocardiogram (ECG) test immediately if:
• the ECG shows three consecutive premature ventricular contractions (PVCs) or a significant increase in ectopy
• the patient's systolic blood pressure falls below the resting level
• the patient's heart rate falls 10 beats/minute or more below the resting level
• the patient becomes exhausted.

Other dicey situations
Depending on the patient's condition, the test may be stopped in the following situations:
• the ECG shows bundle-branch block ST-segment depression exceeding 1.5 mm, or frequent or complicated PVCs
• blood pressure fails to rise above resting level
• systolic pressure exceeds 220 mm Hg
• the patient experiences angina.
    Also, the test will be halted if the examiner suspects persistent ST-segment elevation may indicate transmural myocardial ischemia.

Combo-test

• In both tests, a monitor is observed continuously for changes in the heart's electrical activity. The rhythm strip is checked at preset intervals for arrhythmias, premature ventricular contractions (PVCs), ST-segment changes, and T-wave changes. The test level and the amount of time it toook to reach that level are marked on each strip. Blood pressure is monitored, and systolic changes are noted. Common responses to maximal exercise are dizziness, light-headedness, leg fatigue, dyspnea, diaphoresis, and a slightly ataxic gait.
• If symptoms become severe, the test is stopped. Usually, testing stops when the patient reaches the target heart rate. As the treadmill speed slows, he may be instructed to keep walking for several minutes to prevent nausea or dizziness. (See *When to stop an exercise ECG*.)
• Assist the patient to a chair, and continue monitoring heart rate and blood pressure for 10 to 15 minutes or until the ECG returns to baseline.
• Auscultate for S_3 or S_4 gallops. In many patients, an S_4 gallop develops after exercise from increased blood flow volume and turbulence. However, an S_3 gallop, indicating transient left ventricular dysfunction, is more significant than an S_4 gallop.
• Remove the electrodes, and clean the electrode sites. (See *Exercise ECG interference*.)

Warning!

Exercise ECG interference

• Use of beta-adrenergic blockers may make test results hard to interpret.
• Wolff-Parkinson-White syndrome, electrolyte imbalance, or use of digoxin may cause false-positive results.
• Conditions that cause left ventricular hypertrophy may interfere with ischemia testing.

Holter monitoring

Holter monitoring, also called ambulatory ECG or dynamic monitoring, is the continuous recording of heart activity as the patient follows his normal routine, usually for 24 hours, or about 100,000 cardiac cycles. The patient wears a small cassette tape recorder connected to chest electrodes and keeps a diary of activities and associated symptoms. At the end of the recording period, the tape is analyzed and a report is printed, permitting correlation of cardiac irregularities, such as arrhythmias and ST-segment changes, with the patient's activities.

It's versatile! Holter monitoring can help detect cardiac arrhythmias, evaluate chest pain, and monitor the effectiveness of therapy.

What it all means

When evaluated along with the patient's diary, a normal ECG pattern shows no significant arrhythmias or ST-segment changes. Heart rate changes normally occur during various activities.

Abnormalities

Cardiac abnormalities detected by Holter monitoring include PVCs, conduction defects, tachyarrhythmias, bradyarrhythmias, and bradycardia-tachycardia syndrome.

What needs to be done

• Explain the procedure to the patient.
• Show him how to position the recorder when he lies down. Tell him to continue his routine activities during the monitoring period. Instruct him to keep a log of these activities as well as emotional upsets, physical symptoms, and drug use; show the patient a sample diary. Demonstrate how to mark the tape at the symptom onset, if applicable. (If a patient-activated monitor is being used, show him how to press the EVENT button to activate the monitor when he experiences unusual sensations.)

Magnetic attraction

• Instruct the patient to wear loose-fitting clothing with front-buttoning tops during monitoring and not to tamper with the monitor. Provide bathing instructions. Instruct him to avoid magnets, metal detectors, high-voltage areas, and electric blankets. Show him how to check the recorder to make sure it's working properly. Tell him to notify you if an electrode comes off.
• Clean the electrode sites with an alcohol pad and gently abrade them until they redden. Apply the electrodes to the correct sites, and press the sides and bottom of each electrode firmly. Then press the center of the electrode lightly to promote good contact between the jelly and the patient's skin. Attach the electrode cable

Warning!

Holter monitoring interference

Physiologic variation in arrhythmia frequency and severity may cause an arrhythmia to be missed during 24-hour Holter monitoring.

securely to the monitor, and position the monitor (and case) as the patient will wear it; then attach the leadwires to the electrodes.
• Install a new or fully charged battery in the recorder, insert the tape, and turn on the recorder. Test the electrode attachment circuit by connecting the recorder to a standard ECG machine. (See *Holter monitoring interference*, page 385.)

Catheterization tests

Cardiac catheterization

Simply stated, cardiac catheterization is the passing of a catheter into the right or left side or both sides of the heart. This procedure can determine blood pressure and blood flow in the chambers of the heart, permit blood sample collection, and record films of the ventricles (contrast ventriculography) and arteries (coronary arteriography or angiography).

What it all means

Cardiac catheterization should reveal no abnormalities of heart chamber size or configuration, wall motion or thickness, or direction of blood flow or valve motion. Coronary arteries should have a smooth and regular outline. (For more information on normal findings, see *Maximum normal cardiac pressures*.)

Common abnormalities and defects that can be confirmed by cardiac catheterization include CAD, myocardial incompetence, valvular heart disease, and septal defects.

What needs to be done

• Explain the procedure to the patient. Tell him to restrict food and fluids for at least 6 hours before the test. Inform him that the test takes 1 to 2 hours. Tell him that he may receive a mild sedative but will remain conscious during the procedure.
• Have the patient void just before the procedure.
• Check the patient history for hypersensitivity to shellfish, iodine, or contrast media used in other diagnostic tests. Discontinue any anticoagulant therapy as ordered.

> Cardiac catheterization evaluates valvular insufficiency or stenosis, septal defects, congenital anomalies, myocardial function and blood supply, and cardiac wall motion.

Advice from the experts

Maximum normal cardiac pressures

This chart shows the upper limits of normal pressure in the cardiac chambers and great vessels of recumbent (lying down) adults.

Chamber or vessel	Pressure
Right atrium	6 mm Hg (mean)
Right ventricle	30/6 mm Hg*
Pulmonary artery	30/12 mm Hg* (mean, 18)
Left atrium	12 mm Hg (mean)
Left ventricle	140/12 mm Hg*
Ascending aorta	140/90 mm Hg* (mean, 105)
Pulmonary artery wedge	Almost identical to left atrial mean pressure (±1 to 2 mm Hg)

Peak systolic and end-diastolic

Supine is fine

• The patient is placed in the supine position. ECG leads are applied, and an I.V. line is started. After the local anesthetic is injected at the catheterization site, a small incision or percutaneous puncture is made into the artery or vein, depending on where studies will be performed, and the catheter is passed through the sheath into the vessel. The catheter is guided to the cardiac chambers or coronary arteries using fluoroscopy. When the catheter is in place, the contrast medium is injected through it to visualize the cardiac vessels and structures. Vital signs are monitored frequently.

• After the procedure, the catheter is removed and direct pressure is applied to the incision site for 30 minutes; a dressing is applied when hemostasis occurs.

• Monitor vital signs every 15 minutes for 2 hours, every 30 minutes for the next 2 hours, and then every hour for 2 hours. If no hematoma or other problems arise, check every 4 hours. If signs are unstable, check every 5 minutes and notify the doctor.

• Observe the insertion site for a hematoma or blood loss, and reinforce the pressure dressing, as needed.
• Check the patient's color, skin temperature, and peripheral pulse below the puncture site. The brachial approach carries a higher incidence of vasospasm (characterized by cool fingers and hand and weak pulses on the affected side); this usually resolves within 24 hours.
• Enforce bed rest for 8 hours. If the femoral route was used for catheter insertion, keep the patient's leg extended for 6 to 8 hours; if the antecubital fossa route was used, keep the arm extended for at least 3 hours.
• Resume medications withheld before the test as ordered. Administer analgesics as ordered.
• Obtain a posttest ECG to check for possible myocardial damage. (See *Cardiac catheterization interference.*)

Warning!

Cardiac catheterization interference

Patient anxiety increases the heart rate and cardiac chamber pressures.

Pulmonary artery catheterization

Pulmonary artery (PA) catheterization (also known as Swan-Ganz catheterization) uses a balloon-tipped, flow-directed catheter to provide intermittent occlusion of the pulmonary artery. (See *A primer on PA catheters.*)

When the catheter is in place, this procedure permits measurement of both pulmonary artery pressure (PAP) and pulmonary artery wedge pressure (PAWP).

The PAWP reading accurately reflects left atrial pressure and left ventricular end-diastolic pressure, although the catheter itself never enters the left side of the heart.

What it all means

Normal pressures are as follows:
• *right atrial pressure:* 1 to 6 mm Hg
• *systolic right ventricular pressure:* 20 to 30 mm Hg
• *end-diastolic right ventricular pressure:* < 5 mm Hg
• *systolic PAP:* 20 to 30 mm Hg
• *diastolic PAP:* 10 to 15 mm Hg
• *mean PAP:* < 20 mm Hg
• *PAWP:* 6 to 12 mm Hg
• *left atrial pressure:* about 10 mm Hg.

High, low, and in between

An abnormally high right atrial pressure can indicate pulmonary disease, right-sided heart failure, fluid overload, cardiac tamponade, tricuspid stenosis and insufficiency, or pulmonary hypertension.

> PA catheterization helps assess right- and left-sided heart failure. It also helps monitor fluid status in patients who have suffered serious burns or who have renal disease, noncardiogenic pulmonary edema, or adult respiratory distress syndrome.

Now I get it!

A primer on PA catheters

The flexible pulmonary artery (PA) catheter used in PA catheterization comes in two-lumen, three-lumen, and four-lumen (thermodilution) models and in various lengths.

Can you make do with two?

In the two-lumen catheter, one lumen contains the balloon, 1 mm behind the catheter tip. The other lumen, which opens at the tip, measures pressure in front of the balloon. The two-lumen catheter measures pulmonary artery pressure and pulmonary artery wedge pressure and can be used to sample mixed venous blood and to infuse I.V. solutions.

Three gives you CVP

The three-lumen catheter has an additional proximal lumen that opens 12″ (30.5 cm) behind the tip. When the tip is in the main pulmonary artery, the proximal lumen lies in the right atrium, permitting fluid administration or monitoring of right atrial pressure (central venous pressure [CVP]).

Four means a thermistor

The four-lumen type includes a transistorized thermistor for monitoring blood temperature and allows cardiac output measurement. A four-lumen catheter with thermodilution and pacer port mode is used to allow pacing, if necessary. The introducer part of the system may also be used to infuse large amounts of fluids.

Elevated right ventricular pressure can result from pulmonary hypertension, pulmonary valvular stenosis, right-sided heart failure, pericardial effusion, constrictive pericarditis, chronic heart failure, or ventricular septal defects.

An abnormally high PAP is characteristic of increased pulmonary blood flow, as in a left-to-right shunt secondary to atrial or ventricular septal defect; increased pulmonary arteriolar resistance, as in pulmonary hypertension or mitral stenosis; chronic obstructive pulmonary disease; pulmonary edema or embolus; and left-sided heart failure from any cause.

PA systolic pressure is the same as right ventricular systolic pressure. PA diastolic pressure is the same as left atrial pressure, except in patients with severe pulmonary disease causing pulmonary hypertension; in such patients, catheterization is still important diagnostically.

Elevated PAWP can result from left-sided heart failure, mitral stenosis and insufficiency, cardiac tamponade, or cardiac insufficiency; depressed PAWP, from hypovolemia.

What needs to be done

• Explain the procedure to the patient.
• Set up the equipment according to the manufacturer's directions and the facility's procedure. Place the patient in the supine posi-

Now I get it!

PA catheter insertion sites and waveforms

As the pulmonary artery (PA) catheter advances through the chambers on the right side of the heart to its wedge position, it produces distinctive waveforms that reflect the catheter's position in the heart.

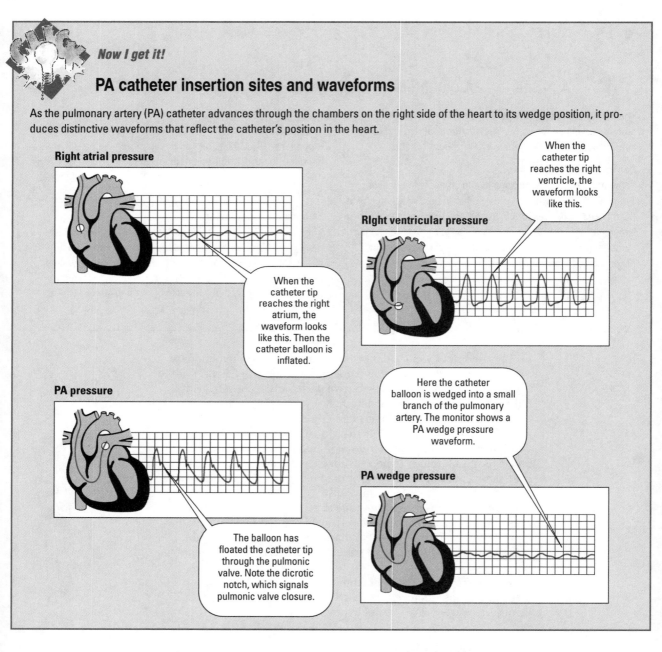

Right atrial pressure

When the catheter tip reaches the right atrium, the waveform looks like this. Then the catheter balloon is inflated.

When the catheter tip reaches the right ventricle, the waveform looks like this.

Right ventricular pressure

PA pressure

The balloon has floated the catheter tip through the pulmonic valve. Note the dicrotic notch, which signals pulmonic valve closure.

Here the catheter balloon is wedged into a small branch of the pulmonary artery. The monitor shows a PA wedge pressure waveform.

PA wedge pressure

tion, and position head, arms and shoulders according to catheter insertion site. If the patient can't tolerate the supine position, assist him to semi-Fowler's position. During the test, all pressures are monitored with the patient in the same position.

- The catheter balloon is checked for defects using sterile technique, and all ports are flushed to ensure patency.
- The catheter is introduced into the vein percutaneously and directed to the right atrium. The catheter balloon is inflated so that venous flow carries the catheter tip through the right atrium and tricuspid valve into the right ventricle and into the pulmonary artery. While the catheter is being directed, the monitor screen is observed for characteristic waveform changes and the location of the catheter tip is found. (See *PA catheter insertion sites and waveforms.*)
- Observe the monitor for any arrhthymias caused by catheter irritation. If this occurs, the catheter may be partially withdrawn or medication administered.
- To record PAWP, the catheter balloon is inflated with the specified amount of air (no more than 1.5 cc); the catheter tip should float into the wedge position, as indicated by an altered waveform on the monitor screen; then the pressure is recorded. If a PAWP waveform occurs with less than the recommended inflation volume, the balloon shouldn't be inflated further. Then the air from the balloon is allowed to return to the syringe, which is then deflated, allowing the catheter to float back into the pulmonary artery. The monitor screen is observed for a PA waveform. Then the system is flushed and recalibrated.

No overinflation

- The balloon catheter shouldn't be overinflated. Overinflation could distend the pulmonary artery, causing vessel rupture.
- When the catheter's correct positioning and function have been established, the catheter is sutured to the skin and antimicrobial ointment and an airtight dressing are applied to the insertion site according to facility policy.
- Obtain a chest X-ray to confirm catheter placement. (See *PA catheterization interference.*)

Warning!

PA catheterization interference

Mechanical ventilators with positive pressure cause increased intrathoracic pressure, raising catheter pressure.

Miscellaneous tests

Electrophysiology studies

Electrophysiology (EPS) studies permit measurement of discrete conduction intervals by recording electrical conduction during slow withdrawal of a bipolar or tripolar electrode catheter from the right ventricle through the His bundle to the sinoatrial node. The catheter is introduced into the femoral vein, passing through the right atrium and across the septal leaflet of the tricuspid valve.

Possible complications of these studies include arrhythmias, phlebitis, pulmonary emboli, thromboemboli, and catheter-site hemorrhage.

What it all means

Normal conduction intervals in adults are as follows: HV interval, 35 to 55 msec; AH interval, 45 to 150 msec; and PA interval, 20 to 40 msec.

His or hers?

A prolonged HV interval (the conduction time from the His bundle to the Purkinje fibers) can result from acute or chronic disease. Atrioventricular nodal (AH interval) delays can stem from atrial pacing, chronic conduction system disease, carotid sinus pressure, recent myocardial infarction, and use of certain drugs. Intra-atrial (PA interval) delays can result from acquired, surgically induced, or congenital atrial disease and atrial pacing.

What needs to be done

• Explain to the patient that EPS studies evaluate the heart's conduction system. Instruct him to restrict food and fluids for at least 6 hours before the test. Inform him that the studies take 1 to 3 hours.

A close shave

• Tell the patient that after the groin area is shaved, a catheter will be inserted into the femoral vein and an I.V. line may be started.
• Have him void before the test.
• The patient is placed in the supine position. Limb electrodes and precordial leads are applied for ECG recording, and the insertion site is shaved, scrubbed, and sterilized. The local anesthetic is injected, and a J-tip electrode is introduced I.V. into the femoral vein (occasionally, into a vein in the antecubital fossa). Guided by fluoroscopy, the catheter is advanced until it crosses the tricuspid valve and enters the right ventricle. Then the catheter is slowly withdrawn from the tricuspid area, and recordings of conduction intervals are made from each pole of the catheter, either simultaneously or sequentially. After recordings and measurements are completed, the catheter is removed and a pressure dressing is applied to the site.
• Monitor the patient's vital signs as ordered. If they're unstable, check every 15 minutes and alert the doctor. Observe for shortness of breath, chest pain, pallor, or changes in pulse rate or blood pressure. Enforce bed rest for 4 to 6 hours.

EPS studies help diagnose arrhythmias and conduction defects and determine the need for an implanted pacemaker, an internal cardioverter-defibrillator, and cardioactive drugs. Also, they evaluate the effects of these treatments.

- Check the catheter insertion site for bleeding as ordered; apply a pressure bandage until the bleeding stops.
- Advise the patient that he may resume his usual diet.
- Make sure a 12-lead resting ECG is scheduled to assess for changes.

Pulse oximetry

Pulse oximetry is a continuous noninvasive study of arterial blood oxygen saturation (SaO_2) using a clip or probe attached to a sensor site (usually an earlobe or a fingertip). The percentage expressed is the ratio of oxygen to hemoglobin (Hb).

What it all means

SaO_2 levels are normally greater than 95%. Hypoxemia with levels less than 95% indicates impaired cardiopulmonary function or abnormal gas exchange.

What needs to be done

- Explain to the patient that this test assesses oxygen content in the Hb.
- Make sure the patient has no false fingernails or nail polish.
- Place the probe or clip over the finger or other intended sensor site so that the light beams and sensors are opposite each other.
- Turn on the monitor and ensure that it accurately detects the patient's pulse and reads the percentage of oxygen.
- If the monitor is to remain on continuously, ensure that the skin remains intact under the probe or clip and that the circulation is adequate.
- After the test is performed, remove the probe and clean it with alcohol. (See *Pulse oximetry interference.*)

> Pulse oximetry monitors oxygenation perioperatively, during an acute illness, and during testing for sleep apnea. It also helps determine bronchodilator effectiveness.

Pulmonary function tests

Pulmonary function tests (PFTs)—including volume, capacity, and flow rate tests—are a series of measurements that evaluate ventilatory function through spirometric measurements; they're performed on patients with suspected pulmonary dysfunction. Of the seven tests that are performed to determine volume, tidal volume (V_T) and expiratory reserve volume (ERV) are direct spirographic measurements; minute volume, carbon dioxide response, inspiratory reserve volume, and residual volume are calculated from the results of other PFTs; and thoracic gas volume (TGV) is calculated from body plethysmography.

Warning!

Pulse oximetry interference

Anemic conditions, vasoconstriction, certain drugs (such as vasopressors), hypotension, vessel obstruction, nail polish or false nails, and lipid emulsions may interfere with test results.

Of the pulmonary capacity tests, vital capacity (VC), inspiratory capacity (IC), functional residual capacity (FRC), total lung capacity, and forced expiratory flow (FEF) may be measured directly or calculated from the results of other tests. Forced vital capacity, flow-volume curve, forced expiratory volume (FEV), peak expiratory flow rate, and maximal voluntary ventilation are direct spirographic measurements. The diffusing capacity for carbon monoxide is calculated from the amount of carbon monoxide exhaled.

PFTs determine the cause of dyspnea, assess treatment effectiveness, and allow preoperative evaluation.

What it all means

Normal values are predicted for each patient based on age, height, weight, and sex and are expressed as a percentage:
- V_T: 5 to 7 mg/kg of body weight
- *ERV:* 25% of VC
- *IC:* 75% of VC
- FEV_1: 83% of VC (after 1 second)
- FEV_2: 94% of VC (after 2 seconds)
- FEV_3: 97% of VC (after 3 seconds).

Reading results

Values such as these can be calculated at bedside with a portable spirometer. Results are usually considered abnormal if they're less than 80% of these values. (See *Interpreting pulmonary function tests.*)

What needs to be done

- Pulmonary function testing requires several areas of testing. Each requires its own procedure.
- Explain the procedure to the patient. Tell him not to eat a heavy meal before the test and not to smoke for 12 hours beforehand.
- Teach the patient how to operate the spirometer, and inform him that the accuracy of the tests depends on his cooperation. Just before the test, tell him to void and to loosen tight clothing.
- Inform the laboratory if the patient is taking an analgesic that depresses respiration. As ordered, withhold bronchodilators for 8 hours.

Tidal volume

- The patient is told to breathe normally into the mouthpiece 10 times.

Expiratory reserve volume

- The patient is told to breathe normally for several breaths and then to exhale as completely as possible.

Advice from the experts

Interpreting pulmonary function tests

Test	Implications
Tidal volume (VT): amount of air inhaled or exhaled during normal breathing	Decreased V_T may indicate restrictive disease.
Minute volume (MV): total amount of air expired per minute	Normal MV can occur in emphysema; decreased MV may indicate other diseases such as pulmonary edema. Increased MV can occur with acidosis, increased carbon dioxide (CO_2), decreased partial pressure of oxygen (Pao_2), exercise, and low compliance states.
CO_2 response: increase or decrease in MV after breathing various CO_2 concentrations	Reduced CO_2 response may occur in emphysema, myxedema, obesity, hypoventilation syndrome, and sleep apnea.
Inspiratory reserve volume (IRV): amount of air inspired after normal inspiration	IRV decreases during normal exercise.
Expiratory reserve volume (ERV): amount of air exhaled after normal expiration	ERV decreases in obese people.
Residual volume (RV): amount of air remaining in the lungs after forced expiration	RV greater than 35% of total lung capacity (TLC) after maximal expiratory effort may indicate obstructive disease.
Vital capacity (VC): total volume of air that can be exhaled after maximum inspiration	Normal or increased VC with decreased flow rates may indicate any condition that reduces functional pulmonary tissue, such as pulmonary edema. Decreased VC with normal or increased flow rates may indicate decreased respiratory effort resulting from neuromuscular disease, drug overdose, or head injury; decreased thoracic expansion; or limited movement of diaphragm.
Inspiratory capacity (IC): amount of air that can be inhaled after normal expiration	Decreased IC indicates restrictive disease.
Thoracic gas volume (TGV): total volume of gas in lungs from both ventilated and nonventilated airways	Increased TGV indicates air trapping.
Functional residual capacity (FRC): amount of air remaining in lungs after normal expiration	Increased FRC indicates lung overdistention.
TLC: total volume of lungs when maximally inflated	Low TLC indicates restrictive disease; high TLC indicates lung overdistention.

(continued)

Interpreting pulmonary function tests *(continued)*

Test	Implications
Forced vital capacity (FVC): measurement of the amount of air exhaled forcefully and quickly after maximum inspiration	Decreased FVC indicates flow resistance in respiratory system from obstructive or restrictive disease.
Flow-volume curve (also called flow-volume loop): greatest rate of flow (Vmax) during FVC maneuvers versus lung volume change	Decreased flow rates at all volumes during expiration indicate obstructive disease. A plateau of expiratory flow near TLC, a plateau of inspiratory flow at mid-VC, and a square wave pattern through most of VC indicate obstructive disease. Normal or increased peak expiratory flow, decreased flow with decreasing lung volumes, and markedly decreased VC indicate restrictive disease.
Forced expiratory volume (FEV): volume of air expired in the 1st, 2nd, and 3rd second of FVC maneuver	Decreased FEV_1 and increased FEV_2 and FEV_3 may indicate obstructive disease; decreased or normal FEV_1 may indicate restrictive disease.
Forced expiratory flow (FEF): average rate of flow during middle half of FVC	Low FEF (25% to 75%) indicates obstructive disease.
Peak expiratory flow rate (PEFR): Vmax during forced expiration	Decreased PEFR may indicate a mechanical problem. PEFR is usually normal in restrictive disease but decreases in severe cases. Because PEFR is effort-dependent, it's also low in a person who has poor expiratory effort or who doesn't understand the procedure.
Maximal voluntary ventilation (MVV) (also called maximum breathing capacity, or MBC): greatest volume of air breathed per unit of time	Decreased MVV may indicate obstructive disease; normal or decreased MVV may indicate restrictive disease.
Diffusing capacity for carbon monoxide (DLco): milliliters of carbon monoxide diffused per minute across the alveolocapillary membrane	Decreased DLco occurs in interstitial pulmonary diseases and emphysema.

Vital capacity

- The patient is told to inhale as deeply as possible and to exhale into the mouthpiece as completely as possible. This procedure is repeated three times, and the test result showing the largest volume is used.

Inspiratory capacity

- The patient is instructed to breathe normally for several breaths and then to inhale as deeply as possible.

Functional residual capacity

• The patient is told to breathe normally into a spirometer that contains a known concentration of an insoluble gas (usually helium or nitrogen) in a known volume of air. After a few breaths, the concentrations of gas in the spirometer and the lungs reach equilibrium. The FRC is calculated by subtracting the spirometer volume from the original volume.

Thoracic gas volume

• The patient is put in an airtight box or body plethysmograph and told to breathe through a tube connected to a transducer. At end-expiration, the tube is occluded, the patient is told to pant, and changes in intrathoracic and plethysmographic pressure are measured. The results are used to calculate total TGV and FRC.

Forced vital capacity and forced expiratory volume

• The patient is instructed to inhale as slowly and deeply as possible and then is asked to exhale into the mouthpiece as quickly and completely as possible. This procedure is repeated three times, and the largest volume is recorded. The volume of air expired at 1 second (FEV_1), at 2 seconds (FEV_2), and at 3 seconds (FEV_3) during all three repetitions is also recorded.

Maximal voluntary ventilation

• The patient is instructed to breathe into the mouthpiece as quickly and deeply as possible for 15 seconds.

Diffusing capacity for carbon monoxide

• The patient is told to inhale a gas mixture with a low concentration of carbon monoxide and then to hold his breath for 10 to 15 seconds before exhaling. (See *Pulmonary function test interference*.)

Warning!

Pulmonary function test interference

• A narcotic analgesic or sedative can decrease inspiratory and expiratory forces.
• Bronchodilators may temporarily improve pulmonary function.
• Lack of patient cooperation, hypoxia, and metabolic disturbances can make testing difficult or impossible.
• Pregnancy or gastric distention may displace lung volume.

Quick quiz

1. A patient is undergoing external fetal monitoring. Which heart rate indicates fetal tachycardia?
   A. 140 beats/minute
   B. 165 beats/minute
   C. 115 beats/minute

398

MONITORING, CATHETERIZATION, AND MISCELLANEOUS TESTS ....

Answer: B. Normal fetal heart rate is 120 to 160 beats/minute. Fetal heart rate less than 120 beats/minute indicates bradycardia; fetal heart rate above 160 beats/minute indicates tachycardia.

2. Which instruction should you give the patient before exercise ECG?

    A.   Avoid caffeinated beverages for 3 hours before the test.

    B.   Avoid smoking for 24 hours before the test.

    C.   Avoid alcoholic beverages for 12 hours before the test.

Answer: A. Instruct the patient not to eat, smoke, or drink alcoholic or caffeinated beverages for 3 hours before exercise ECG.

3. After cardiac catheterization, how long should the patient remain on bed rest?

    A.   12 hours

    B.   8 hours

    C.   24 hours

Answer: B. Bed rest should be enforced for 8 hours after cardiac catheterization.

4. Elevated right atrial pressure may indicate:

    A.   pulmonary hypertension.

    B.   constrictive pericarditis.

    C.   ventricular septal defect.

Answer: A. Abnormally high right atrial pressure may indicate pulmonary disease, right-sided heart failure, fluid overload, cardiac tamponade, tricuspid stenosis and insufficiency, or pulmonary hypertension.

5. A PA catheter balloon should be inflated with no more than:

    A.   1 cc of air.

    B.   2 cc of air.

    C.   1.5 cc of air.

Answer: C. A PA catheter balloon should be inflated with no more than 1.5 cc of air.

Scoring

☆☆☆ If you answered all five questions correctly, outstanding! You're a testing titan!

☆☆ If you answered three or four questions correctly, not bad! You've passed the test!

☆ If you answered fewer than three questions correctly, don't get testy! Just keep at it!

Appendices and index

○ **Appendix A: Normal laboratory test values**   **400**

○ **Appendix B: Guide to uncommon diagnostic tests** **401**

○ **Index**   **406**

Appendix A

Normal laboratory test values

Hematology

Erythrocyte sedimentation rate
Males: 0 to 15 mm/hour (SI, 0 to 15 mm/hour)
Females: 0 to 20 mm/hour (SI, 0 to 20 mm/hour)

Fibrin split products
Screening assay: < 10 μg/ml (SI, < 10 mg/L)
Quantitative assay: < 3 μg/ml (SI, < 3 mg/L)

Fibrinogen, plasma
200 to 400 mg/dl (SI, 2 to 4 g/L)

Hematocrit
Males: 42% to 52% (SI, 0.42 to 0.52)
Females: 36% to 48% (SI, 0.36 to 0.48)

Hemoglobin (Hb), total
Males: 14 to 17.4 g/dl (SI, 140 to 174 g/L)
Females: 12 to 16 g/dl (SI, 120 to 160 g/L)

Partial thromboplastin time
21 to 35 seconds (SI, 21 to 35 s)

Platelet count
140,000 to 400,000/μl (SI, 140 to 400 10^9/L)

Prothrombin time
11 to 13 seconds (SI, 11 to 13 s); international normalized ratio for patients on warfarin therapy, 2 to 2.5 (those with prosthetic heart valve, 3 to 4.5)

Red blood cell (RBC) count
Males: 4.5 to 5.5 million/μl venous blood (SI, 4.5 to 5.5 10^{12}/L)
Females: 4 to 5 million/μl venous blood (SI, 4 to 5 10^{12}/L)

Thrombin time, plasma
7 to 12 seconds (SI, 7 to 12 s)

White blood cell (WBC) count
4,000 to 10,000 μl (SI, 4 to 10 x 10^9/L)

WBC differential, blood
Neutrophils: 47.6% to 76.8% (SI, 0.476 to 0.768)
Lymphocytes: 16.2% to 43% (SI, 0.162 to 0.43)
Monocytes: 0.6% to 9.6% (SI, 0.006 to 0.096)
Eosinophils: 0.3% to 7% (SI, 0.003 to 0.07)
Basophils: 0 to 1% (SI, 0 to 0.01)

Blood chemistry

Amylase, serum
> age 18: 25 to 85 U/L (SI, 0.39 to 1.45 μkat/L)

Arterial blood gases
pH: 7.35 to 7.45 (SI, 7.35 to 7.45)
$Paco_2$: 35 to 45 mm Hg (SI, 4.7 to 5.3 k Pa)
Pao_2: 80 to 100 mm Hg (SI, 10.6 to 13.3 k Pa)
HCO_3^-: 22 to 26 mEq/L (SI, 22 to 26 mmol/L)
Sao_2: 94% to 100% (SI, 0.94 to 1)

Bilirubin, serum
Adults, total: 0.3 to 1.2 mg/dl (SI, 5 to 20 mmol/L)
Neonates, total: 2 to 6 mg/dl (SI, 34 to 102 mmol/L)

Blood urea nitrogen
8 to 20 mg/dl (SI, 2.9 to 7.5 mmol/L)

Calcium, serum
8.2 to 10.2 mg/dl (SI, 2.05 to 2.54 mmol/L)

Carbon dioxide, total, blood
22 to 26 mEq/L (SI, 22 to 26 mmol/L)

Chloride, serum
100 to 108 mEq/L (SI, 100 to 108 mmol/L)

Cholesterol, total, serum
Adults: < 205 mg/dl (SI, < 5.30 mmol/L)

Creatinine, serum
Males: 0.8 to 1.2 mg/dl (SI, 62 to 115 mmol/L)
Females: 0.6 to 0.9 mg/dl (SI, 53 to 97 mmol/L)

Glucose, plasma, fasting
70 to 110 mg/dl (SI, 3.9 to 6.1 mmol/L)

Glucose, plasma, 2-hour postprandial
< 145 mg/dl (SI, < 8 mmol/L)

Lactate dehydrogenase
Total: 71 to 207 U/L (SI, 1.2 to 3.52 μkat/L)

Lipase
< 160 U/L (SI, < 2.72 μkat/L)

Magnesium, serum
1.3 to 2.1 mEq/L (SI, 0.65 to 1.05 mmol/L)
Atomic absorption: 1.7 to 2.1 mg/dl

Phosphates, serum
1.8 to 2.6 mEq/L
Atomic absorption: 2.7 to 4.5 mg/dl (SI, 1.45 to 1.78 mmol/L)

Potassium, serum
3.5 to 5 mEq/L (SI, 3.5 to 5 mmol/L)

Protein, total, serum
6.4 to 8.3 g/dl (SI, 64 to 83 g/L)

Sodium, serum
135 to 145 mEq/L (SI, 135 to 145 mmol/L)

Triglycerides, serum
Males > 20 years: 40 to 180 mg/dl (SI, 0.11 to 2.01 mmol/L)

Females > 20 years: 10 to 190 mg/dl (SI, 0.11 to 2.21 mmol/L)

Troponin I
< 0.35 μg/L (SI, < 0.35 μg/L)

Troponin T
< 0.1 μg/L (SI, < 0.1 μg/L)

Uric acid, serum
Males: 3.4 to 7 mg/dl (SI, 202 to 416 μmol/L)
Females: 2.3 to 6 mg/dl (SI, 143 to 357 μmol/L)

Urine chemistry

Amylase, urine
10 to 80 U/hour (SI, 265 to 680 u/d)

Chloride, urine
140 to 250 mEq/L (SI, 140 to 250 mmol/d)

Sodium, urine
40 to 220 mEq/L/24 hours (SI, 40 to 220 mmol/d)

Urinalysis, routine
Color: straw
Appearance: clear
Specific gravity: 1.005 to 1.035
pH: 4.5 to 8
Epithelial cells: few
Casts: occasional hyaline casts
Crystals: present

Urine osmolality
24-hour urine: 300 to 900 mOsm/kg (SI, 300 to 900 mmol/kg)
Random urine: 50 to 1,400 mOsm/kg (SI, 50 to 1,400 mmol/kg)

WBC count, urine
0 to 4 per high-power field

Appendix B

Guide to uncommon diagnostic tests

Test and purpose	Description	Finding
Dexamethasone suppression test • Screens for Cushing's syndrome • Helps diagnose major depression and monitors its treatment	The patient receives an oral dexamethasone dose. Normally, dexamethasone suppresses blood levels of adrenal steroid hormones. In patients with Cushing's syndrome and some forms of depression, the drug fails to suppress these levels.	**Normal findings** Serum cortisol value normally is below 5 g/dl (SI, 140 nmol/L), indicating dexamethasone suppression. (However, a normal test result doesn't rule out major depression.) **Abnormal findings** Values above 5 g/dl indicate suppression failure, as in Cushing's syndrome, severe stress, and clinical depression.
Folic acid • Helps diagnose megaloblastic anemia • Helps assess folate stores in pregnant women	The patient's blood is tested for folic acid level after an overnight fast. A water-soluble vitamin, folic acid influences red blood cell formation, deoxyribonucleic acid synthesis, and overall body growth. This test is commonly performed with serum vitamin B_{12} testing.	**Normal findings** Normal serum folic acid values range from 1.8 to 9 ng/ml (SI, 4 to 20 nmol/L). **Abnormal findings** Values below 1.8 ng/ml indicate hematologic abnormalities, such as anemia (especially megaloblastic anemia), leukopenia, or thrombocytopenia; hypermetabolic states such as hyperthyroidism; inadequate dietary intake; chronic alcoholism; small-bowel malabsorption syndrome; or pregnancy. Values above 20 ng/ml (SI, above 42 nmol/L) indicate excessive dietary intake of folic acid or folic acid supplements.
Gallium scanning • Detects primary or metastatic neoplasms and inflammatory lesions • Evaluates malignant lymphoma and identifies recurrent tumors after chemotherapy or radiation therapy	The patient undergoes a total body scan 24 to 48 hours after I.V. injection of radioactive gallium Ga 67 citrate. Certain neoplasms and inflammatory lesions attract gallium; however, exact diagnosis requires additional tests.	**Normal findings** Normally, gallium activity appears in the liver, spleen, bones, and large bowel. Bowel activity results from mucosal uptake and fecal excretion of gallium. **Abnormal findings** Gallium scanning may reveal inflammatory lesions, discrete abscesses, or diffuse infiltration.

(continued)

Guide to uncommon diagnostic tests *(continued)*

Test and purpose	Description	Findings
Gastric culture • Aids diagnosis of mycobacterial infections • Identifies the infecting bacteria in neonatal septicemia	Gastric contents are aspirated and cultivated for microbes. This test is performed in conjunction with a chest X-ray and a purified protein derivative skin test. It's especially useful when a sputum sample can't be obtained by expectoration or nebulization.	***Normal findings*** The culture specimen normally is free from pathogenic mycobacteria. ***Abnormal findings*** Identification of *Mycobacterium tuberculosis* indicates active tuberculosis. Testing also may identify other *Mycobacterium* species, such as *M. bovis, M. kansasii,* and *M. avium-intracellulare* complex as well as pathogenic bacteria that cause neonatal septicemia.
Liver-spleen scanning • Screens for hepatic metastasis and hepatocellular disease, such as cirrhosis and hepatitis • Detects focal disease in the liver and spleen, such as tumors, cysts, and abscesses • Demonstrates hepatomegaly, splenomegaly, and splenic infarcts • Assesses liver and spleen condition after abdominal trauma	A gamma camera records radioactivity distribution in the liver and spleen after I.V. injection of a radioactive colloid, most commonly technetium 99m. This substance concentrates in reticuloendothelial cells through phagocytosis. About 80% to 90% is taken up by Kupffer's cells in the liver, 5% to 10% by the spleen, and 3% to 5% by bone marrow. Without moving, the gamma camera images the liver or spleen instantaneously.	***Normal findings*** Because the liver and spleen contain equal numbers of reticuloendothelial cells, they normally appear equally bright on the image. However, radioactive colloid generally has a more uniform distribution in the liver than the spleen. Although liver-spleen scanning may not detect early liver disease, it shows characteristic, distinct patterns as the disease progresses. ***Abnormal findings*** Metastasis to the liver or spleen may appear as a focal defect; confirmation requires biopsy. Because cysts, abscesses, and tumors fail to take up the radioactive colloid, they appear as solitary or multiple focal defects. Ultrasonography can confirm hepatic or splenic cysts. All abscesses require a computed tomography (CT) scan to confirm the diagnosis. Liver-spleen scanning can verify palpable abdominal masses and distinguish splenomegaly from hepatomegaly. Scanning can assess hepatic or splenic injury after abdominal trauma.
Percutaneous liver biopsy • Diagnoses hepatic parenchymal disease, malignant tumors, and granulomatous infections	Under local or general anesthesia using a Menghini needle, a core of liver tissue is aspirated for histologic analysis. Such analysis can identify hepatic disorders after ultrasonography, CT scans, and radionuclide studies have failed to detect them.	***Normal findings*** Normally, the liver consists of sheets of hepatocytes supported by a framework. ***Abnormal findings*** Tissue examination may reveal diffuse hepatic disease, such as cirrhosis or hepatitis, or infections such as tuberculosis. Primary malignant tumors may be present but hepatic metastasis are more common. Nonmalignant findings with a known focal lesion require further studies, such as laparotomy or laparoscopy with biopsy.

Guide to uncommon diagnostic tests (continued)

Test and purpose	Description	Findings
Serum antidiuretic hormone (ADH) • Aids differential diagnosis of central diabetes insipidus, nephrogenic diabetes insipidus (congenital or familial), and syndrome of inappropriate ADH (SIADH)	A fasting blood sample is withdrawn and measured for ADH levels. The patient should limit physical activity for 10 to 12 hours before the test, and should be relaxed and recumbent for 30 minutes before the test. This test may be ordered as part of dehydration or hypertonic saline infusion testing, which determines the body's response to hyperosmolality states.	***Normal findings*** ADH values range from 1 to 5 pg/ml (SI, 1 to 5 ng/L). ADH may be evaluated along with serum osmolality; if serum osmolality is less than 285 mOsm/kg (SI, 285 mmol/kg), ADH normally is less than 2 pg/ml (SI, 2 ng/L). If serum osmolality exceeds 290 mOsm/kg (SI, 290 mmol/kg), ADH may range from 2 to 12 pg/ml (SI, 2 to 12 ng/L). ***Abnormal findings*** Absent or below-normal ADH levels indicate central diabetes insipidus caused by a neurohypophysial or hypothalamic tumor, viral infection, metastatic disease, sarcoidosis, tuberculosis, Hand-Schüller-Christian disease, syphilis, neurosurgical procedures, or head trauma. 　　Normal ADH levels in a patient with signs of diabetes insipidus, such as polydipsia, polyuria, and hypotonic urine, may indicate the nephrogenic form of the disease (marked by renal tubular resistance to ADH); however, levels may rise if the pituitary gland tries to compensate. 　　Elevated ADH levels also may indicate SIADH, possibly resulting from bronchogenic carcinoma, acute porphyria, hypothyroidism, Addison's disease, cirrhosis of the liver, infectious hepatitis, severe hemorrhage, or circulatory shock.
Serum prolactin • Aids diagnosis of pituitary dysfunction that may result from pituitary adenoma • Aids diagnosis of hypothalamic dysfunction regardless of cause • Evaluates secondary amenorrhea and galactorrhea	A blood sample is withdrawn and measured for serum prolactin level. The patient should restrict foods and fluids and limit physical activity for 12 hours before the test. He should be in a relaxed state during blood withdrawal.	***Normal findings*** Normal values range from undetectable to 23 ng/ml (SI, 23 µg/L) in nonlactating females. Serum prolactin levels normally rise tenfold to twentyfold during pregnancy and correspond to rises in human placental lactogen levels. After delivery, prolactin secretion falls to basal levels in mothers who don't breast-feed. However, prolactin secretion increases during breast-feeding. ***Abnormal findings*** Abnormally high prolactin levels, 100 to 300 ng/ml (SI, 100 to 300 IU/L), suggest autonomous prolactin production by a pituitary adenoma (Forbes-Albright syndrome). Rarely, hyperprolactinemia may result from severe endocrine disorders such as hypothyroidism. Idiopathic hyperprolactinemia may be associated with infertility. 　　Decreased prolactin levels in a lactating mother cause lactation failure and may be linked to postpartum pituitary infarction (Sheehan's syndrome).

(continued)

Guide to uncommon diagnostic tests *(continued)*

Test and purpose	Description	Findings
Serum vitamin B_{12} • Helps diagnose megaloblastic anemia • Helps identify central nervous system (CNS) disorders affecting peripheral and spinal myelinated nerves	A fasting blood sample is withdrawn and measured for serum vitamin B_{12} level. This test usually is performed with serum folic acid testing because deficiencies of vitamin B_{12} and folic acid are the two most common causes of megaloblastic anemia.	*Normal findings* Serum vitamin B_{12} values ranges from 200 to 900 pg/ml (SI, 148 to 664 pmol/L). *Abnormal findings* Decreased values indicate inadequate dietary vitamin B_{12} intake, with malabsorption syndrome; hypermetabolic states such as hyperthyroidism; pregnancy; and CNS damage, such as posterolateral sclerosis or funicular degeneration. Elevated values may result from excessive dietary intake, hepatic disease, and myeloproliferative disorders such as myelocytic leukemia.
Serum vitamin D_3 • Aids diagnosis of skeletal diseases, such as rickets and osteomalacia • Helps identify hypercalcemia and vitamin D toxicity	A fasting blood sample is tested for serum 25-hydroxycholecalciferol level after this substance is separated from other vitamin D metabolites and contaminants. This test commonly is combined with serum calcium and alkaline phosphatase tests.	*Normal findings* Normally, serum vitamin D_3 values range from 10 to 60 ng/ml (SI, 25 to 150 nmol/L) *Abnormal findings* A low or undetectable level may reflect vitamin D deficiency, which can cause rickets or osteomalacia (as from poor diet, decreased sun exposure, or impaired vitamin D absorption secondary to hepatobiliary disease, pancreatitis, celiac disease, cystic fibrosis, or gastric or small-bowel resection). Low levels also may be linked to hepatic diseases that directly affect vitamin D metabolism. Elevated levels may indicate toxicity. Elevated levels associated with hypercalcemia may stem from hypersensitivity to vitamin D, as in sarcoidosis.
Sleep studies (polysomnography) • Aid differential diagnosis of breathing disorders in patients with a history of excessive snoring, narcolepsy, excessive daytime sleepiness, insomnia, cardiac rhythm disorders, and restless leg spasms	While sleeping overnight in a sleep laboratory, the patient is monitored for cardiac rate and rhythm, chest and abdominal wall movement, nasal and oral airflow, oxygen saturation, muscle activity, retinal function, and brain activity. Electrodes are placed on the patient's skin, and an EEG is recorded for a baseline reading before the patient falls asleep.	*Normal findings* A normal sleep study shows a respiratory disturbance index (apnea-hypopnea index) of fewer than 5 to 10 episodes per study period and normal electrocardiogram (cardiac rate and rhythm), impedance (chest and abdominal wall motion), airway (nasal and oral airflow), arterial oxygen saturation (oximetry), leg electromyogram (for muscle activity), electro-oculogram (for retinal function), and EEG (for brain activity). *Abnormal findings* Abnormal recordings indicate obstructive sleep apnea. Abnormal movement during sleep indicates a seizure or movement disorder.

Guide to uncommon diagnostic tests (continued)

Test and purpose	Description	Findings
Soluble amyloid beta protein precursor • Aids diagnosis of Alzheimer's disease	A cerebrospinal fluid (CSF) specimen is collected by lumbar puncture, and a small portion is tested using enzyme-linked immunosorbent assay (ELISA). Presence of the amyloid beta protein in senile plaques of the brain is a hallmark of Alzheimer's disease. CSF of some dementia patients contains smaller amyloid amounts than CSF of healthy people, making this test a useful diagnostic tool.	***Normal findings*** Normal amyloid beta protein levels in CSF exceed 450 U/L, based on age-matched controls using the ELISA test. ***Abnormal findings*** Below-normal CSF levels suggest a change in amyloid beta protein precursor processing and amyloid beta protein formation. Low levels of soluble amyloid beta protein precursor correlate with clinically diagnosed and autopsy-confirmed Alzheimer's disease.
Tensilon test • Aids diagnosis of myasthenia gravis • Helps differentiate between myasthenic and cholinergic crises • Helps monitor anticholinesterase therapy.	The patient is observed after I.V. administration of Tensilon (edrophonium chloride), a rapid, short-acting anticholinesterase that improves muscle strength by increasing muscle response to nerve impulses.	***Normal findings*** Fasciculations indicate absence of myasthenia gravis. ***Abnormal findings*** Improved muscle strength within 30 seconds of Tensilon administration indicates myasthenia gravis. (Results are inconsistent when myasthenia gravis affects only ocular muscles.)
Urine vanillylmandelic acid (VMA) • Helps detect pheochromocytoma, neuroblastoma, and ganglioneuroma • Evaluates adrenal medulla function	A 24-hour urine specimen is collected and measured for levels of VMA, a phenolic acid and the most prevalent urine catecholamine metabolite. VMA results from hepatic conversion of epinephrine and norepinephrine; urine VMA levels reflect endogenous production of these major catecholamines. The patient should restrict foods and beverages containing phenolic acid, such as coffee, tea, cola, bananas, citrus fruits, chocolate, and vanilla, for 3 days before the test. During the collection period, he must avoid stressful situations and strenuous physical activity.	***Normal findings*** Normal urine VMA values range from 0.7 to 6.8 mg/24 hours (SI, 3 to 34 μmol/day). ***Abnormal findings*** A catecholamine-secreting tumor can cause urine VMA levels to rise. A precise diagnosis requires further testing, such as urine HVA levels, to rule out pheochromocytoma.

Index

A

Abdominal ultrasonography, 300-302
Abetalipoproteinemia, 75
ABG analysis. *See* Arterial blood gas analysis.
ABO blood typing, 125-127
  antigens and, 126
  blood compatibility and, 126i
  blood types in, 126, 126i
  naturally occurring antibodies in, 127
Acetest, 203. *See also* Ketones, urine.
Acetylcholine receptor antibodies, 151-152
Acetylcholinesterase, 70
Acid phosphatase, 66-67
Activated clotting time, 18
Adrenocorticotropic hormone. *See* Corticotropin.
Advanced Breast Biopsy Instrument procedure, 258. *See also* Breast biopsy.
Ahaptoglobinemia, congenital, 40
Alanine aminotransferase, 63-64
Albumin values, 38
  implications of, 39i
Aldosterone
  serum, 106-107
  urine, 182-183
Alkaline phosphatase, 64-65
Alpha-fetoprotein, 171-172
ALT. *See* Alanine aminotransferase.
Ambulatory electrocardiogram, 385-386
Ammonia, plasma, 43-44
Amniocentesis, 223
Amniotic fluid analysis, 223-226
  implications of findings in, 224t

Amylase
  serum, 59-60
  urine, 181-182
Angiotensin-converting enzyme, 73
Anion gap, 34-35
  metabolic acidosis and, 34, 35
Antibody, ABO blood typing and, 127
Antibody identification test, 133
Antibody screening, 133-134
Antidiuretic hormone, serum, 403t
Anti-double-stranded deoxyribonucleic acid antibodies, 153
Antigen, ABO blood typing and, 126
Antigen assay, 136-137, 138. *See also* Lymphocyte transformation.
Anti-insulin antibodies, 152
Antinuclear antibodies, 145-147
  incidence in various disorders, 146t
Antithyroid antibodies, 147
Aplitest. *See* Tuberculin skin tests.
Arterial blood gas analysis, 24-26
  measurements included in, 24
  obtaining sample for, 25
Arthroscopy, 286-289
  obtaining different views in, 288i
  triangulation and, 286
Aspartate aminotransferase, 61-62
Australia antigen. *See* Hepatitis B surface antigen.
Autoantibodies, 145-153
Automated coagulation time, 18

B

Bacterial meningitis antigen, 165-166
Barium enema, 324-327
Barium swallow, 319-321
Basophils
  effect of disease on, 4t
  normal percentages of, 3

B cells. *See* B-lymphocyte assay.
Bence Jones protein, urine, 192-193
Bicarbonate, measuring, 24
Bilirubin
  serum, 81-82
  urine, 198-199
Biopsy, 253-272
Bleeding time, 14-15
Blood compatibility
  ABO typing and, 126i
  crossmatching and, 130-131
  Rh typing and, 128t
Blood culture, 248-249
Blood gases, 24-27
Blood urea nitrogen, 35-36
B-lymphocyte assay, 135-136
Bone marrow aspiration and biopsy, 263-267
  common sites for, 266i
  methods of obtaining specimen for, 265, 267
  normal values in, 265t
  preparing child for, 266
Bone scan, 366-368
  comparing findings in, 367i
Breast biopsy, 257-260
  improving accuracy of, 258
  methods of obtaining specimen for, 257, 259
Breast cancer, using ultrasound to detect, 336
Bronchoscope, features of, 285i. *See also* Bronchoscopy.
Bronchoscopy, 283-286
  complications of, 286
  as specimen collection method, 247
BUN. *See* Blood urea nitrogen.

C

Calcitonin, plasma, 103-104

i refers to an illustration; t refers to a table.

Calcium
serum, 31-33
albumin level, serum, and, 32
urine calcium and phosphate,
207-208
disorders that affect levels of, 208t
Carbohydrates, 50-59
Carbon dioxide, total, 26-27
Carcinoembryonic antigen, 169-171
cancer treatment monitoring
and, 170i
Cardiac catheterization, 386-388
cardiac pressures in, 387t
Cardiac enzymes, 44-47
Cardiac nuclear imaging, 364-366
Cardiac proteins, 47-49
Cardiac stress testing, 294
Cardiac troponin T, 47-48
Catecholamines
plasma, 110-112
urine, 184-186
Cerebral angiography, 307-310
comparing findings in, 308i
Cerebrospinal fluid analysis, 230-233
interpreting results of, 232t
Cervical punch biopsy, 262-263
recovering from, 263
Chest radiography, 313-315
implications of abnormalities
in, 314t
Chest X-ray. See Chest radiography.
Chloride
serum, 33-34
urine chloride and sodium, 204-205
Cholesterol, total, 75-77
Cholinesterase, 70-71
Chorionic villi sampling, 225i
Cirrhosis, immunoglobulin levels
in, 139t
Clean-catch specimen, collecting, 240
Clinistix, 201, 202. See also Glucose,
urine.
Clonidine suppression test, 111
Coagulation tests, 1-2, 14-21

Cold agglutinins, 149-150
Colonoscopy, 273-276
clear liquid diet for, 275
Colposcopy, 280-281
Complement assays, 142-143
Computed tomography, 339-340
of biliary tract and liver, 343
of bone, 346, 351
of intracranium, 341-342, 348-349i
of kidney, 352-353, 353i
of pancreas, 344, 345i
patient teaching for, 342
of spine, 345-346
of thorax, 351
Contraction stress test, 374-375
Cope's needle, obtaining biopsy
specimen with, 256i
Corticotropin, 86-87
Cortisol
plasma, 108-109
secretion cycle and, 109i
urine, free, 183-184
Cosyntropin test. See Rapid
corticotropin test.
Creatine kinase, 44-46
isoenzymes of, 44
implications of abnormal levels of, 45
Creatinine
serum, 36-37
urine, 193
Creatinine clearance, 194
Crossmatching, 130-131
Cultures, 239-251
Cytomegalovirus antibody screen,
163-164

D
Dexamethasone suppression test, 401t
Diabetes mellitus, 50, 52, 54, 56
Diastix, 201, 202. See also Glucose,
urine.
Direct antiglobulin, 131-133
Direct Coombs' test. See Direct
antiglobulin.

Doppler probe. See also Doppler ultrasonography.
detecting thrombi with, 299i
mechanics of, 297i
Doppler ultrasonography, 296-300
Ductal lavage, 337
Dynamic monitoring, 385-386

E
ECG. See Electrocardiography.
Echocardiography, 291-293, 295, 347i
comparing types of, 293i
Electrocardiography, 379-382
normal waveforms in, 380i
12-lead, 382i
Electroencephalography, 376-377
comparing tracings in, 377i
techniques used for, 378
Electromyography, 378-379
Electrophysiology studies, 391-393
Endoscopic retrograde cholangio-
pancreatography, 327-329
Endoscopic ultrasound, 277-280, 350i
esophageal approach for, 278-279
opposite-end approach for, 279
Endoscopy, 273-289
Eosinophils
drugs that affect count of, 5
effect of disease on, 4t
normal percentages of, 3
Epstein-Barr virus antibodies, 159
Erythrocyte count. See Red blood cell
count.
Erythrocyte indices, 9-10
Erythrocyte sedimentation rate, 10-11
Erythropoietin, 112-113
Esophagography, 319-321
Estradiol. See Estrogens.
Estriol. See Estrogens.
Estrogens
serum, 117-119
urine, total, 186-187
Estrone. See Estrogens.

Excision biopsy, 270, 271-272. *See also* Skin biopsy.
Excretory urography, 331-333
   abnormal findings in, 332i
Exercise electrocardigraphy, 382-384
   stopping, 384
Expectoration as specimen collection method, 246
External fetal monitoring, 369-371

F

Factor II, 16
Fecal lipids, 219-220
Fecal occult blood, 218-219
   collecting specimen for, 219
Ferritin, 13-14
Fetal-maternal erythrocyte distribution, 129-130
Fibrin degradation products, 20-21
Fibrinogen, plasma, 19-20
Fibrin split products, 20-21
Fight-or-flight reaction, 111i
Flat plate of abdomen, 329-331
Fluoroscopy, 315-316
Folic acid, 401t
Follicle-stimulating hormone, serum, 92-93
Fungal serology, 164-165

G

Gallium scanning, 401t
Gamma glutamyltransferase, 65-66
Gamma glutamyl transpeptidase, 65-66
Gastric acid stimulation, 214-215
Gastric culture, 402t
Gastrin, 115-117
Gastrin stimulation tests, 116
Gastrointestinal disorders, causative pathogens for, 242. *See also* Stool culture.
Gastrointestinal motility study, 320
German measles. *See* Rubella antibodies.

GI disorders. *See* Gastrointestinal disorders, causative pathogens for.
Globulin values, 38
   implications of, 39i
Glucagon, plasma, 115
Glucose
   fasting, blood, 50-52
   loading, 89-90
   tolerance, oral, 54-55
administering glucose solution for, 55
   2-hour postprandial, plasma, 52-54
   age as factor in, 53i
   urine, 201-203
Glucose-6-phosphate dehydrogenase, 71-72
Glycohemoglobin test, 56
Glycosylated hemoglobin, 56
G6PD. *See* Glucose-6-phosphate dehydrogenase.
Growth hormone, 88
   suppression of, 89-90
Guthrie test, 42-43

H

Haptoglobulin, 40-41
Hb S test. *See* Sickle cell test.
hCG. *See* Human chorionic gonadotropin.
HCT. *See* Hematocrit.
Helicobacter pylori antibodies, 167
Hematocrit, 7-8
Hemoccult test, 218-219
Hemoglobin
   serum, 6-7
   fasting, total, 56
   urine, 196-197
Hepatitis, immunoglobulin levels in, 139t
Hepatitis-associated antigen. *See* Hepatitis B surface antigen.
Hepatitis B surface antigen, 155, 158
Herpes simplex antibodies, 161-162
Heterophil antibodies, 158-159

hGH test. *See* Human growth hormone.
High anion gap acidosis, 34
High-density lipoproteins, 77-78
HLA. *See* Human leukocyte antigen.
Hodgkin's disease, immunoglobulin levels in, 139t
Holter monitoring, 385-386
Homocysteine, 82-83
Human chorionic gonadotropin
   serum, 121-122
   urine, 187-188
Human growth hormone, 88-89
Human immunodeficiency virus antibodies, 162-163
   guidelines for positive test results of, 163
Human leukocyte antigen, 144-145
   antibodies to. *See also* Leukoagglutinins.
17-hydroxycorticosteroids, urine, 188-189
Hypercalcemia, 32
Hyperchloremia, 33
Hypercholesterolemia, 76
Hyperglycemia, 50, 51, 52
Hyperkalemia, 28-29
Hyperlipoproteinemia, congenital, 74
Hyperlipoproteinemia, familial, and classifying, 79t
Hypermagnesemia, 30
Hypernatremia, 27-28
Hyperphosphatemia, 31
Hypocalcemia, 33
Hypochloremia, 33
Hypocholesterolemia, 76
Hypoglycemia, 50-51, 52-53
Hypokalemia, 29
Hypolipoproteinemia, 80
Hypomagnesemia, 30
Hyponatremia, 28
Hypophosphatemia, 31
Hypertriglyceridemia, familial, 74

IJ

Immune complex assays, 140-141
Immunoglobulin levels in certain diseases, 139t
Immunoglobulins A, G, and M, 138-140
Indirect antiglobulin test. *See* Antibody screening.
Indirect Coombs' test. *See* Antibody screening.
Infarct avid imaging, 363-364
INR. *See* International Normalized Ratio.
Insulin
    resistance, 152
    serum, 113-115
    tolerance, 90-92
Internal fetal monitoring, 371-374
    intrauterine pressure readings and, 372t
    mechanics of, 374i
International Normalized Ratio, 17
Interstitial-cell-stimulating hormone test. *See* Luteinizing hormone, plasma.
Iron
    deficiency, 13
    overload, 13
Iron assay, 13
Iron-binding capacity, total, 13

K

Keto-Diastix, 203-204. *See also* Ketones, urine.
17-ketogenic steroids, urine, 191-192
Ketones, urine, 203-204
17-ketosteroids, urine, 189-191
Ketostix, 203. *See also* Ketones, urine.
Kidney-ureter-bladder radiography, 329-331

L

Lactate dehydrogenase, 46-47
    isoenzymes of, 46, 47
Lactic acid, 57-59

Lactose tolerance test, oral, 56-57
Laparoscopy, 281-283
LD. *See* Lactate dehydrogenase.
Leukemia, immunoglobulin levels in, 139t
Leukoagglutinins, 134-135
    transfusion reaction precautions and, 135
Leukocyte count, 2-3
Leukocytosis, 2
Leukopenia, 2-3
Lipase, 60-61
Lipoprotein-cholesterol fractionation, 77-78
Lipoprotein electrophoresis, 78-81
    lipoproteins measured in, 78-80
Liver-spleen scanning, 402t
Long-acting thyroid stimulator, 98, 147-148
Low-density lipoproteins, 77
Lower gastrointestinal examination, 324-327
Lung biopsy, 253-255
    methods of obtaining specimen for, 253-254
Lung perfusion scan, 357-358
Lung ventilation scan, 358-360
    comparing findings in, 359i
Luteinizing hormone, plasma, 93-95
    secretion cycle, 94i
Lyme disease serology, 166-167
Lymph node biopsy, 269-270
    methods of obtaining specimen for, 270
Lymphocyte marker assays, 137t
Lymphocytes
    effect of disease on, 4t
    normal percentages of, 3
Lymphocyte transformation, 136-138

M

Magnesium
    serum, 29-30
    urine, 206-207

Magnetic resonance imaging, 340-341
    of bone and soft tissue, 353-354
    of cardiovascular system, 354-355
    metal and, 341
    of neurologic system, 355-356
Mammography, 335-337
    follow-up probe for, 337
    screening recommendations for, 337
Mantoux test. *See* Tuberculin skin tests.
Mean corpuscular hemoglobin, 9
    concentration, 9
    volume, 9
Menstrual cycle, 94i
Metabolic acidosis, anion gap and, 34, 35
Methemoglobin, 11
Mitogen assay, 136, 138. *See also* Lymphocyte transformation.
Mixed lymphocyte culture assay, 137, 138. *See also* Lymphocyte transformation.
Monocytes
    effect of disease on, 4t
    normal percentages of, 3
Monospot test, 160
Mono-Vacc test. *See* Tuberculin skin tests.
Myelography, 311-313
    removing contrast media after, 313
Myocardial imaging
    cold spot, 364-366
    hot spot, 363-364
Myocardial perfusion scan, 364-366
Myoglobin
    serum, 49
    urine, 197-198

N

Nasopharyngeal culture, 244-245
    obtaining specimen for, 245
Neonatal thyroid-stimulating hormone, 96-97

i refers to an illustration; t refers to a table.

Neonatal thyroid-stimulating hormone
(continued)
collecting specimen for, 97
Neonatal thyrotropin test. *See* Neonatal thyroid-stimulating hormone.
Nephrotic syndrome, immunoglobulin levels in, 139t
Neutrophils
effect of disease on, 4t
normal percentages of, 3
Normal anion gap acidosis, 34

O
OGTT. *See* Oral glucose tolerance test.
Oral glucose tolerance test, 54-55
administering glucose solution for, 55
Oxygen content, measuring, 24
Oxygen saturation, measuring, 24
Oxytocin challenge test, 374-375

PQ
Papanicolaou test, 226-228
Bethesda system for grading, 226
ThinPrep and, 227
Pap test. *See* Papanicolaou test.
Parathormone. *See* Parathyroid hormone.
Parathyroid hormone, 104-106
effect of disease on, 105t
Partial pressure of carbon dioxide, measuring, 24
Partial pressure of oxygen, measuring, 24
Partial thromboplastin time, 15-16
Percutaneous liver biopsy, 402t
Pericardial fluid analysis, 233-235
classifying effusions in, 234
Pericardiocentesis, 233, 235i. *See also* Pericardial fluid analysis.
Peritoneal fluid analysis, 215-218
normal profile in, 216t
pH, measuring, 24
Phenylalanine, 42-43

Phenylketonuria, 42
confirming, 43
Phosphates
serum, 30-31
urine phosphate and calcium, 207-208
disorders that affect levels of, 208t
Pigments, urine, 196-201
bedside testing for, 197
Pinworm infection, collection procedure for, 221. *See also* Stool examination, for ova and parasites.
PKU. *See* Phenylketonuria.
Platelet count, 8-9
Pleural biopsy, 255-257
obtaining specimen for, with Cope's needle, 256i
Pleural fluid analysis, 211-214. *See also* Thoracentesis.
classifying specimen in, 212t
Polysomnography, 404t
Potassium
serum, 28-29
urine, 205
Premature labor, predicting, 118
Progesterone, plasma, 119-120
Prolactin, serum, 403t
Prostate cancer, prostate-specific antigen test and, 68
Prostate gland biopsy, 260-261
approaches used for, 261
automated cone procedure for, 261
Prostate-specific antigen, 67-68
Protein electrophoresis, 38-40
fractions measured in, 38
implications of abnormal levels in, 39i
Protein values, total, 38
implications of, 39i
Prothrombin time, 16-17
Pro time, 16-17
PSA. *See* Prostate-specific antigen.
Pseudocholinesterase, 70-71
Prothrombin time, 16-17

Partial thromboplastin time, 15-16
Pulmonary angiography, 316-318
Pulmonary arteriography, 316-318
Pulmonary artery catheterization, 388-391
catheter insertion sites and waveforms for, 390i
types of catheter used in, 389
Pulmonary function tests, 393-397
interpreting results of, 395-396t
Pulmonary transudate and exudate, characteristics of, 212t
Pulse oximetry, 393
Punch biopsy, 270, 271. *See also* Skin biopsy.
Pyruvate kinase, 72-73
Pyruvic acid, 58-59

R
Radioactive iodine uptake test, 360-361
Radioallergosorbent test, 143-144
Radionuclide thyroid imaging, 361-363
patient teaching for, 362
Raji cell assay, 141
Rapid ACTH test. *See* Rapid corticotropin test.
Rapid corticotropin test, 87-88
Rapid human immunodeficiency virus test, 162
Rapid plasma reagin test, 168
RAST. *See* Radioallergosorbent test.
Red blood cell count, 5-6
Red cell indices, 9-10
Renin activity, plasma, 68-70
Renal angiography, 333-335
Renin-angiotensin-aldosterone cycle, 68
Renovascular hypertension, screening test for, 68, 69
Respiratory syncytial virus antibodies, 160-161
Rhesus system. *See* Rh typing.
Rheumatoid arthritis, immunoglobulin levels in, 139t

i refers to an illustration; t refers to a table.

Rheumatoid factor, 148-149
Rh isoimmunization, screening for, 129
Rh_0(D) immune globulin, indications
    for administration of, 128, 129
Rh typing, 127-128
   blood compatibility and, 128t
Rubella antibodies, 154-155
Rubella exposure, evaluating risk
    of, 154

S

SalEst, 118
Scout film of abdomen, 329-331
Semen analysis, 228-230
Semen specimen, collecting, from
    rape victim, 229
17-KGS. *See* 17-ketogenic steroids,
    urine.
17-KS. *See* 17-ketosteroids, urine.
17-OHCS. *See* 17-hydroxycorticos-
    teroids, urine.
Shave biopsy, 270, 271. *See also* Skin
    biopsy.
Sickle cell test, 12
Siderophilin, 41
Skin biopsy, 270-272
   methods of obtaining specimen for,
      270, 271-272
Skull radiography, 305-307
   positioning for, 306i
Sleep studies, 404t
Sodium
   serum, 27-28
   urine sodium and chloride, 204-205
Sodium-potassium pump, 28
Soluble amyloid beta protein precur-
    sor, 405t
Somatotropin, 88
Sputum culture, 245-247
   methods of collecting specimen for,
     245, 247i
Stool culture, 241-242
   implications of pathogens present
     in, 242

Stool examination
   for ova and parasites, 220-222
   for rotavirus antigen, 222
Stress test, 382-384
Swan-Ganz catheterization. *See* Pul-
    monary artery catheterization.
Sweat test, 236-237
Systemic lupus erythematosus,
    immunoglobulin levels in, 139t

T

T cells. *See* T-lymphocyte assay.
T_3. *See* Triiodothyronine.
T_3 uptake test, 102
T_4. *See* Thyroxine.
Technetium-99m pyrophosphate
    scanning, 363-364
Tensilon test, 405t
Tes-Tape, 201, 202-203. *See also*
    Glucose, urine.
Testosterone, 120-121
Thallium imaging, 364-366
   patient teaching for, 365
ThinPrep, 227. *See also* Papanicolaou
    test.
Thoracentesis. *See also* Pleural fluid
    analysis.
   complications of, 214
   positioning patient for, 213i
Throat culture, 243-244
Thrombin clotting time test, plasma,
    18-19
Thrombocytes, 8
Thrombocytopenia, 8
Thrombocytosis, 8
Thyrocalcitonin, 103
Thyroid biopsy, 267-269
Thyroid hormones, 98-104
Thyroid-stimulating hormone, 95-96
Thyroid-stimulating immunoglobulin,
    98, 147-148
Thyrotropin test, serum, 95-96
Thyroxine, 98-99
   free, 103

Thyroxine-binding globulin, 101-102
T-lymphocyte assay, 135-136
TORCH test, 172-173
Tracheal suctioning as specimen
    collection method, 246, 247i
Transcranial Doppler studies, 302-303
Transesophageal echocardiography,
    295-296
Transferrin, 41
Triglycerides, 74-75
Triiodothyronine, 99-101
   free, 103
   uptake of, 102
Troponin I, 47-48
TSH. *See* Thyroid-stimulating
    hormone.
Tuberculin skin tests, 173-176
   follow-up for, 174
   reading results of, 175
   technique for performing, 174

U

Ultrasonography, 291-303
Upper gastrointestinal and small-
    bowel series, 321-324
Uric acid
   serum, 37-38
   urine, 195-196
Urinalysis, 177-180
   drugs that influence results of, 180
   implications of abnormal findings
     in, 179
   normal findings in, 178t
Urine cultures, 239-241
   collecting clean-catch specimen
     for, 240
   quick centrifugation test and, 240
Urine specimen, timed, collecting, 182
Urobilinogen, urine, 199-201
   using random specimen to test
     for, 200t

V

Vanillylmandelic acid, urine, 405t

i refers to an illustration; t refers to a table.

VDRL test. *See* Venereal Disease
    Research Laboratory test.
Venereal Disease Research Laborato-
    ry test, 167-169
    implications of reactive results
        of, 169
Viral hepatitis test panel, 156-157i
Vitamin B_{12}, serum, 404t
Vitamin D_3, serum, 404t

W

WBC. *See* White blood cell count *and*
    White blood cell differential.
White blood cell count, 2-3
White blood cell differential, 3-5
    effect of disease on, 4t
White cell antibodies. *See* Leukoag-
    glutinins.
Wound culture, 249-251
    aerobic specimen collection for,
        250-251
    anaerobic specimen collection for,
        250i, 251

XYZ

Xeromammography, 335

i refers to an illustration; t refers to a table.

Notes